FROHLICK, TIMOTHY J. CAPT, U
553-84-7700 AFSC 9286
PHYSICIAN ASSISTANT, CERTIFI
MALCOLM GROW MEDICAL CENTER

MW00998502

Practical
Radiologic Diagnosis

Practical
Radiologic Diagnosis

Donald R. Germann, M.D.

James K. Fisher, M.D.

Reston Publishing Company, Inc.
A Prentice-Hall Company
Reston, Virginia

To my wife, Ruth,
and my daughters, Janice and Patricia

Donald R. Germann, M.D.

To my wife, Kathy,
and my children, Stephanie, Jim, and Christopher

James K. Fisher, M.D.

Library of Congress Cataloging in Publication Data

Germann, Donald R
    Practical radiologic diagnosis.

    Bibliography: p. 297
    Includes index.
    1. Diagnosis, Radioscopic.   I. Fisher, James K.,
joint author. II. Title.
RC78.G464   616.07'572   80-24703
ISBN 0-8359-5590-7

© 1981 by Reston Publishing Co., Inc.
A Prentice-Hall Company
Reston, Virginia 22090

All rights reserved. No part of this book
may be reproduced, in any way or by any means,
without permission in writing from the publisher.

10   9   8   7   6   5   4   3   2   1

Printed in the United States of America

Contents

Preface

This book is offered to an important segment of medical personnel who have had limited access to the techniques and skills of roentgen interpretation. This group includes physicians and non-physicians. In order for these persons to find explanations of even the most frequently performed roentgen examinations, it has been necessary to search subspecialty encyclopedia-type texts. It is our hope that we can present the entities most frequently seen in practice in a simple narrative style that will be readily available to the non-radiologist. As nurses increase their clinical responsibility and expand their teaching roles, it is important that they learn some of the practical means of demonstrating pathology in the living patient. Radiologic technologists are always interested in the results of the films they have produced. This text can supplement their knowledge and add depth to their course in medical and surgical diseases. Medical students on their first radiological rotation need help in correlating the radiographic changes with the clinical features of disease and the pathological processes that they have seen under the microscope.

Likewise, many physicians in the fields of family practice and emergency medicine, and house staff officers on non-radiological services are occasionally forced to interpret x-rays that are unfamiliar to them. These radiographic changes can be confusing, and this text should offer the reassurance that is badly needed even when evaluating the most frequently occurring clinical disorders.

The descriptive portions of the text are written in the same style that would be used if the student were sitting beside the radiologist and experiencing a personal give-and-take teaching and learning relationship. It is for this reason that the bibliography is short. The science of medicine and radiology is hopefully not ignored, but we wish it to be presented as a subtlety in this more narrative form of teaching. We feel that teaching is still as much art as science.

This text does not include sections on the important subjects of physics and radiation protection. Our decision to delete these subjects was based on the fact that radiologic technologists and radiology residents get extensive exposure to these areas from other sources. Nurses, even those in postgraduate courses, have little or no involvement in the actual filming process. The same can be said for emergency room physicians, house staff physicians on non-radiological services, and other paramedical groups. It is granted that family physicians and non-radiological specialists who have x-ray units gravely need this type of information, but it is available from multiple sources.

We frequently comment on how other imaging techniques can supplement standard roentgen studies, but we have resisted using nuclear images, ultrasound studies, computer assisted tomograms, and vascular studies in our examples. These are specialized exams that need to be studied separately.

Radiology is rapidly becoming more sophisticated. As indicated above, other energy sources can be used in medical imaging. Computer-assisted transmission and emission studies are not just dreams. They are here. No one can predict the magnitude of their role over the next twenty-five years. Despite their increasing usage, there seems little doubt that for the next decade the primary tool for extending the physician's senses in examining patients will be the standard radiograph. Maintaining and expanding its usefulness will continue to be an exciting challenge.

Acknowledgments

Many people made contributions to the preparation of this manuscript. We wish to express our appreciation to:

The Department of Radiology, St. Luke's Hospital of Kansas City, our partners, and especially Helen Loe and the typing pool.

Our radiology office staff, especially Cathy Runnels, Judy Marvel, Sharon Watters, Shelley Richards, and Pam Vaughn.

The Department of Radiology at the Children's Mercy Hospital of Kansas City.

The Department of Radiology at the University of Missouri at Columbia. Especially we wish to thank Dr. Harold R. Hinsdorf and Beverly Bittle for their help in reproduction of films.

Mr. Jack Doht of Eastman Kodak Company.

Ms. Betty Barnett of CGR X-ray Corporation.

Introduction

The major function of all scientific writing in diagnostic medicine is to offer a planned approach to a diagnosis. Certainly, textbooks in diagnostic radiology are based on the premise that a variation from the normal appearance of the film is the starting point for diagnosis. This variant is carefully analyzed, and the probabilities of its origin are carefully weighed. After arriving at a working diagnosis, we may offer suggestions as to how this diagnosis can be firmly established. This may be through additional radiographic views, or it may move into specialized radiographic studies, such as arteriograms or computerized tomograms. We rarely suggest nonradiological studies, such as those done in the chemical or even pathological laboratory, for the clinician usually has pursued these areas.

All of these diagnostic exercises imply that a lesion has been found. But what about another type of problem—errors of omission, the most serious of all? How does one keep from overlooking a lesion on a radiograph? If a lesion is seen, consultations and other investigations can usually evaluate its importance. However, if a lesion is not seen, the film is filed; the patient is dismissed; and the process, possibly a very serious one, is unknown to patient and clinician alike. Our comments here are directed to all health care providers who are called on to interpret radiographs. Consultation with colleagues is extremely important. And while it may not be needed as frequently by the radiology professor as by the medical student, it should be used by all analysts of roentgenograms.

We will offer tips on how to keep from missing pathology. The discipline of radiograph interpretation is a self-discipline that each individual must agonize through in his own way. There are standard protocols for performing a physical examination included in virtually all textbooks in diagnostic medicine. No such protocols exist for roentgen examinations. Yet, roentgen examinations are just as surely a form of patient examination as the physical. Therefore, some standard routine must be defined and followed religiously. We will report to you our routines. Each area examined has its own routine. The routines suggested are certainly not the only ones that can be devised, and possibly not the best, but they are routines that, when adhered to, can reduce errors of omission.

Here are some examples of routines that can be used to analyze different roentgen examinations. The first technique may be referred to as "eye patterns," "analysis disciplines," or even "systems of examination." For analysis of a chest film, the routine that will be used here starts with heart, hilar structures, and mediastinum; drops to the hemidiaphragms; goes through each lung individually; and finally ends with evaluating the bone structure and associated soft tissue. In the skull, we use an "inside-out" analysis program starting with sella, pineal body, basilar structures, cranial vault, and finally soft tissues of the face and sinuses. For virtually all extremities, start with bony architecture and joint detail, and end with soft-tissue changes. Similar programs are used for the spine. But spine areas become more complex, for there are several types of joints. And the soft-tissue study must include evaluation of the kidneys, the liver, and the gastrointestinal tract. We emphasize these patterns of study, but, of course, other features are important in helping avoid errors of omission.

Errors of omission are also reduced when films are subjected to double reading, a second technique. For those of us based in hospitals where there is a teaching program, this is easy to accomplish, for residents and staff double read virtually all films. Certainly at our institution double reading, as well as eye pattern discipline, is used extensively to reduce errors of omission.

A third technique, review of the film with the clinician, is also important. This is of special value to the radiologist attempting to interpret films without history, for subtle lesions may become apparent or take on a very different degree of importance when clinical information is correlated with radiographic findings.

This brings up the role of history. How much history should be provided the radiologist who interprets the films? Everyone has an individual preference in this regard. We like enough history so that we feel that we know why the film was requested and understand the answer that the clinician wishes. However, history can be misleading as well as helpful. Certainly if the persons interpreting the films are prejudiced by the clinical story, they may find entities that they wish to find even though the supporting evidence is minimal. At the same time, they may overlook incidental findings that are more important.

Six months or even one month after the clinician's physical examination, no one can validate the findings. The roentgen examination of patients is different. The roentgenographic film made today represents the conditions existing today. The stored film is forever available for review and criticism. To avoid embarrassment and to protect patients, errors in roentgenogram interpretation must approach zero. The overreading of films that requires additional studies for evaluation of unimportant findings increases the cost of medicine. But the underreading of films and the missing of lesions may be even more important. Therefore, we would remind all of you interpreting radiographs of the following. Yours is a keen responsibility. Learn your lessons well.

Chest

FUNDAMENTAL PROCESSES

The most frequent examination in x-ray departments is the chest film. Its interpretation can be difficult, or it can be relatively easy if you are familiar with the anatomy and pathology of the chest. There are many normal variations in the chest, and the appearance of the chest film varies with age as well as disease. It is impossible to present all of these variations in any book, and in fact there is no substitute for seeing thousands of chest films. In this way your mind, the greatest of all computers, will be programmed with these variations and you will respond properly. A discussion of the basic anatomy of the normal chest will follow in the presented cases.

Unfortunately, the chest film does not come from the processor with pathological diagnoses printed on it. It is only through study of the film and identification of altered patterns that abnormalities can be identified and diagnoses suggested. Since radiography is dealing with the shadows of anatomy and pathology, the changes that we see on the radiograph are either those resulting from low absorption of the photons (decreased density or increased radiolucency) or increased photon absorption (increased radiopacity or decreased radiolucency).

We usually think of pathology in the lung as those processes increasing lung density. This is not always true. At this point, let me review some of the fundamental pathological changes that occur in the chest and relate them to radiographic findings.

Atelectasis

Atelectasis is one of the most important observations in the chest and refers to a loss of lung volume. With the loss of volume comes absorption of air. Hence, an atelectatic segment of lung is one that shows increased density and reduced volume. The development of atelectasis, especially as it occurs with respect to foreign bodies, demonstrates an important physiological process. Assume that a small foreign body drops into a major bronchus. It will proceed down the course of the bronchus to that point where its size equals the size of the tapering bronchus. It is known that on inspiration the bronchi tend to dilate and on expiration they tend to reduce their diameter. Therefore, there comes a point in the obstructive process where air can go by the foreign body on inspiration but will be trapped behind it on expiration. This phenomenon is called obstructive emphysema, and the portion of the lung distal to the foreign body becomes temporarily more radiolucent (air is trapped here). This important radiographic sign of a foreign body will be present before atelectasis develops. As time progresses and edema develops around the foreign body, air flow will be stopped both on inspiration and expiration. As time continues, the air behind the foreign body will be absorbed; atelectasis in a conventional sense will develop.

With any loss of volume in a portion of the chest, certain compensatory changes develop in the remainder of the chest. Therefore, if the lost volume is of some magnitude, the diaphragm on the involved side will elevate. This is best observed with lower lobe atelectasis. The heart and mediastinum shift toward the side of lost volume. This occurs in upper lobe collapse, especially of the right upper lobe. The remaining lung on both sides will tend to hyperinflate to fill the space. Of course, with obstructive emphysema or airtrapping, these processes will be reversed.

The first form of atelectasis is, as we have described above, related to endobronchial obstruction. This obstruction occurs with foreign bodies of any type: animal, vegetable, or metallic. It is a relatively frequent observation to see mucus plugs produce atelectasis in the chests of postoperative patients. Atelectasis is also important in malignancy, for many malignant lesions arise within the bronchus and eventually produce bronchial obstruction and lobar collapse.

In addition to the classical lobar or segmental atelectasis described above, another form of atelectasis occurs secondary to the extrinsic compression of alveoli. We refer to this as linear, platelike, or discoid atelectasis since its appearance on the radiograph is that of a relatively sharp line. It does not indicate the important endobronchial lesions mentioned above but may identify areas of reduced air exchange that result for a number of reasons. Pain in the chest or upper abdomen, whatever its cause, will limit the patient's ability to make the usual or even adequate respiratory effort; and linear atelectasis may result. Furthermore, this form of atelectasis may precede other signs of disease, such as pneumonia, pleurisy, or pulmonary embolus. It may also be nothing more than the poor motion of a high hemidiaphragm in an obese patient. Linear atelectasis usually does not involve sufficient volume of lung to produce the important anatomical shifts seen in lobar collapse.

Emphysema

Emphysema represents, from a radiological standpoint, the reciprocal of atelectasis. Emphysema implies overaeration, stretching, or distention of alveoli; therefore, the percentage of air per unit tissue is increased. Emphysema may be localized as indicated above, in the early stages of air trapping, or a diffuse process as seen in degenerative lung disease. Generalized emphysema is a chronic disease and will be discussed subsequently. As the air volume in the lung increases, on either a local or generalized basis, again shifts will occur. The hemidiaphragms will be flattened, pushed downward. The anterior-posterior (AP) diameter of the chest will be increased. The anterior portion of the ribs will be lifted. The chest will take on a more cuboid configuration. Intercostal spaces will be expanded. Mediastinal structures will tend to be compressed and elongated; the heart will even appear small. Localized emphysema will produce local shifts exactly the opposite of those that would be seen in localized atelectasis.

The fundamental change, then, in an emphysematous process is one of increased radiolucency or decreased lung density, and shift of anatomical structures, in a manner reciprocal to that described in atelectasis.

Infiltration and Consolidation

The term *infiltration* obviously implies adding a process to the lung that does not belong there. Usually, this refers to an infectious process; and this means pneumonia. Infiltrations involve neoplastic processes as well as infection. Our discussion here will be based on infection. With the addition of more solid tissue to the aerating lung, increased density on a localized basis occurs in the lung. The infiltrative process may start along the course of the bronchi and extend into the alveoli. It is the involvement of the alveoli that results in loss of air from the lung and increased lung density. The margins of an infiltrative process are usually fuzzy and ill-defined.

Infiltration involves a number of things. For instance, since infiltration and consolidation are related to pneumonia, one implies that there are bacteria, usually *pneumococcus* (of course other organisms can produce pneumonia), growing freely in this portion of the lung. It would take literally billions of organisms to produce a tiny radiographic density; therefore, the extensive change seen on radiographs with pneumonia is due to the body's response to this invasion. Increased blood flow, congestion, and edema are part of the initial defense mechanism. This is followed by pus formation and consolidation. Therefore, the fuzzy nature of the margins of the infiltrative process is related to interstitial fluid, increased blood flow in the area, and pus accumulation,

and even some necrosis that may occur to the lung.

The radiographic appearance of infiltration, while always one of increased density, does vary with the anatomical area involved. The pattern of interstitial pneumonia appears quite different from the consolidated pattern of lobar pneumonia or the acinar pattern of bronchial pneumonia. These changes will be described in the section "Roentgenographic Patterns" and will be reemphasized in case presentations.

PLEURAL PROCESSES

The pleural space is a potential space. Normally, there is just enough fluid between the pleural surfaces to permit free and painless movement of the lung on the chest wall as the lung expands and contracts. This is an important function, for if the pleural space is obliterated by scarring the ventilatory movements are reduced, and lung function is less efficient.

Radiographically, there are two important processes that occur in the pleural space. One is a pneumothorax that occurs when air from the lung ruptures through the visceral pleura, and results in collapse of the underlying lung; or pneumothorax can occur when the chest wall is injured, letting air from the outside into the pleural space. The extent of the pneumothorax is important. A small pneumothorax may produce pain with little or no reduction of pulmonary function. On the other hand, a pneumothorax in which the pressure in the pleural space is elevated will result in total collapse of the lung and shifting of the mediastinum to the opposite side. A pneumothorax is recognized by seeing the sharply demarcated retracted visceral pleura against an air background. Examples will follow.

The second process that occurs in the pleural space is abnormal fluid accumulation. Fluid, as it increases in the pleural space, results in increased density. If the volume is significant, it will produce shifting of the mediastinum toward the opposite side and/or collapse the lung on the side that is involved. Since normally there is no air in the pleural space, as the amount of fluid increases, the increased density of the pleural contents is seen as a meniscus density. This is true since the thickest portion of the fluid is that at the edge of the radiograph. If there is air in the pleural space at the same time, then a sharp air/fluid level is seen.

Fluid accumulates in the pleural space for a reason. Two processes account for most cases of pleural effusion. One is congestive heart failure with interstitial and alveolar fluid in the lung, and the other is metastatic disease of the pleural surface. A not infallible rule of thumb is helpful here—a right-sided pleural effusion (especially if the heart is enlarged) is due to congestive failure. Conversely, a left-sided effusion, especially in older patients, is malignant until proven otherwise. A third, and somewhat less frequent, cause (in our experience) of fluid accumulation in the pleural space may be a very small amount of exudate, secondary to pneumonia or tuberculosis, or it may actually represent a pocket of pus, empyema, in the pleural space. Empyema, as does other fluid, increases the density in the involved area.

Pulmonary Fibrosis

Pulmonary fibrosis and scarring carry the same connotation in the lung as elsewhere. They represent healed stages of inflammatory disease that may be due to infection, trauma, or autoimmune disease. It is not uncommon to see stellate scars in the lung secondary to previous infection. Apical pleural thickening results from scarring secondary to infectious disease (often granulomatous infection). In addition to these changes, one may identify increased fibrous tissue along the interstitial portion of the lung. This, too, is scarring, but in some instances it is a proliferative process or an actual increase in interstitial fibrous tissue. This may be without known cause or may be an autoimmune process associated with collagen diseases as scleroderma, or rheumatoid arthritis. Fibrosis also occurs secondary to radiation and some consider it part of the normal aging process. When associated with chronic obstructive pulmonary disease, the lung volume will increase. In all instances, the local areas of fibrosis and scarring result in increased radiodensity.

Pulmonary Edema

Since the lung is the organ where oxygen and blood come in contact with each other, disease processes may occur on either side of the oxygen-blood barrier. Our previous discussions have dealt principally with processes involving air exchange. In contrast to this, pulmonary edema is, at least initially, on the vascular side of the organ system.

The usual cause of pulmonary edema is a failing left ventricle. Heart muscle tone decreases, the heart dilates, the ejection fraction drops, and the vessels in the upper portion of the lung bed tend to become distended and larger than usual resulting from a relative increase in blood flow in upper lung fields as the pressure in the basilar pulmonary veins increases. The next phase is the accumulation of a small amount of fluid in the interstitial portion of the lung. Fluid collecting along vessels make the vessels less distinct but large. This is followed by development of alveolar flooding and pleural accumulation of fluid. The process described here is one of increasing venous pressure in the lung vascular bed.

Other causes of edema include fluid overload or an abnormally high vascular volume or decreased osmotic pressure and irritations within the airway. The latter irritation is seen in patients exposed to noxious gases or other irritants, even water in the airway. Edema produced by such irritation tends to be somewhat more localized, but this depends entirely on the irritant and the method of exposure.

Bone Pathology

This is included as a matter of completeness. One sees a generous sampling of the skeletal system on the chest film. This includes the ribs, the shoulder girdles, and to a large extent, the dorsal spine. The same processes described in the bone section in reference to fracture, infection, and destructive disease are pertinent here. No chest radiographic evaluation is complete without careful scrutiny of the bony structure; however, the technique of chest filming is designed to maximize visualization of the heart and lungs. The techniques that more clearly visualize bone detail may compromise our lung evaluation.

ROENTGENOGRAPHIC PATTERNS

In the preceding paragraphs major area changes in the radiologic appearance of the lungs were discussed. At this point radiologic changes will be described as they relate to the minute anatomy of the lung. It is hoped that this can serve as a further guide in differential diagnoses.

In oversimplified terms, the lung consists of two basic areas. One is the airway side where air is moved into and out of the lung. The other is the vascular side where oxygen is absorbed from the air in the alveoli and carried to peripheral tissues; and carbon dioxide is returned from peripheral tissues to the lung. An airborne pathological process may cause alveolar contamination and initiate an inflammatory response, eventually filling the alveoli with exudate, mucus, pus, or other debris. This results in the so-called alveolar pattern of disease. Such a process usually starts as very small lesions with poor margins. These lesions tend to coalesce, increase in size, and have a segmental or lobar distribution. This is the classical evolution of pneumonia. It is usually associated with an air bronchogram as the consolidation increases in extent, for the major airways remain open. The air bronchogram is one of the most important signs in chest roentgram interpretation. The bronchi are air filled and stand out against the airless consolidated lung. In contrast to this finding in consolidation an airless lung due to endobronchial atelectasis will show no air-filled bronchi.

The second area that gives rise to a different form of radiologic manifestation of disease is in the interstitium—space that contains the vascular structures of the lung, the lymphatics, and the framework of supporting fibrous tissue. Lesions that are bloodborne tend to manifest themselves first in the interstitium. A classical example would be a metastatic lesion which starts its growth as a minute struc-

ture in end capillaries and gradually expands. Its margins tend to remain smooth
as it grows and displaces adjacent alveolar
and other structures away from its epicen-
ter. Other disease processes that involve
the interstitium are those that result in
fibrous proliferation. These processes include scleroderma, rheumatoid disease of
the lung, sarcoid and even early pulmonary edema and interstitial pneumonia.
Defining the interstitial pattern is difficult. Read multiple authors and find multiple descriptions, for the appearance of
lesions in this space varies. As long as the
disease process remains in the interstitial
space, its edges are well defined—whether
nodular, as a metastasis, or linear, as
fibrosis. Examples will be shown.

Some lesions do not remain purely alveolar or purely interstitial. For these
processes the term "mixed interstitial-al-
veolar patterns" or possibly the term
coined by Felson, "destructive lesions of
the lung," would be even more descriptive. This latter term is not always appropriate for pulmonary edema—first interstitial, then alveolar—is not really destructive.
The term does apply to malignant lesions.
Regardless of the original site of involvement, the process extends to adjacent
parts of the lung, and a mixed pattern
develops.

Other modifications of these basic lung
radiologic patterns involve nodular development in either the alveolar pattern or
the interstitial pattern. Interstitial nodules
occur in such diseases as sarcoid, metastatic disease, tuberculosis, and the pneu-
monoconioses. An alveolar nodular pattern is probably best demonstrated by
bronchial pneumonia and lipoid pneumonia.

Examples of these patterns help differential diagnosis, but certainly there are

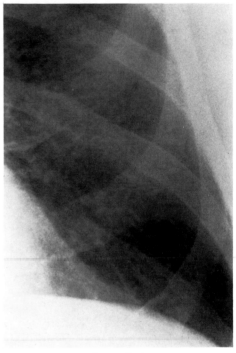

Example 1

times when the radiologic manifestations
seem to be far from typical. The underlying pathology in these roentgen maver-
icks then must be considered individually, but even here these may be clues as
to where in the lung the process started.

We have magnified local areas of chest
films for examples. Example 1 shows a
fine interstitial pattern. The linear markings of the lung are increased and more
irregular than normal. Example 2 also
shows interstitial disease that is more extensive and shows early nodular changes.
Note the horizontal lines near the lung
periphery. Example 3 is an area of consolidation—alveolar filling. It has a segmental distribution with a patchy appearance
at its proximal margin.

SOLITARY NODULES

Solitary nodules of the lung involve diagnostic fundamentals. Not all causes of solitary nodules can be presented in this type of text. Therefore, we hope to make a few pertinent comments and warn you of pitfalls. First, it is impossible to make a specific diagnosis from radiographic findings of most solitary nodules. We are doing a service if we can separate, by radiographic means, those patients that can with reasonable safety avoid surgery.

All types of disease processes can be responsible for the production of a solitary lung nodule. Only the more common causes will be listed for each major category.

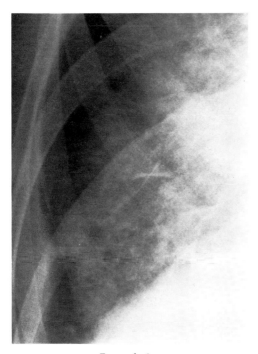

Example 2

I. Congenital anomolies:
   A. Bronchogenic cysts
   B. Pulmonary arteriovenous fistula
   C. Pulmonary sequestration
II. Infectious
   A. Tuberculosis
   B. Histoplasmosis
   C. Lung abscesses
   D. Aspergillus
III. Neoplastic
   A. Benign
      1. Bronchial adenoma
      2. Hamartoma
   B. Malignant
      1. Bronchogenic carcinoma
      2. Lung metastases
      3. Bronchial aveolar carcinoma
IV. Miscellaneous
   A. Rheumatoid necrobiotic nodule (rarely solitary)
   B. Lipoid pneumonia
   C. Organizing hematoma (trauma)

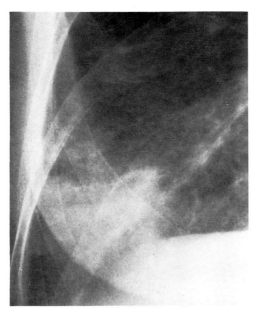

Example 3

The above list will provide the etiology for nearly 95% of lung nodules. If we were to list enough causes to account for the remaining 5%, the list would be infinitely

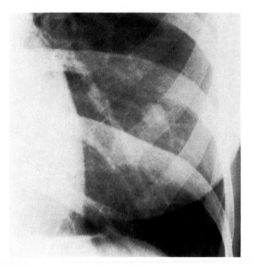

Case SN-1

ably most important, is the patient a smoker and what is his/her quantitative smoking history?

2. Request old x-rays: Regardless of the present appearance of the lesion on the radiograph, if a film can be found that is two or more years old showing no appreciable change in the lesion the chances of it being a surgical lesion are remote. It is granted that there have been some slow-growing primary tumors reported; but even though their growth is slow, there is growth. If one can be assured there has been no increase in size, neoplasia as a diagnosis is remote.

3. Laboratory findings: Is there laboratory evidence of an acute infectious process going on at the moment? Is there evidence of other systemic disease? This is additive to history.

4. Specialized x-ray examination: The use of tomography in solitary lung lesions is extremely important and should be done in adult indeterminant cases. There is no point in doing tomography in well-defined cases. Tomograms are done to evaluate the margins of the lesion in order to prove or disprove the presence of stellate lesions, the presence of associated adenopathy, and—probably even more important—the presence or absence of calcification within the lesion.

Angiography may be needed on rare occasions. It is used to prove the diagnosis of arteriovenous malformation and pulmonary sequestration. If the suspected arteriovenous malformation is relatively peripheral and over 2 cm in size, the study can be more safely carried out as an isotopic angiogram rather than with contrast material.

longer. Before trying to assign a category to the radiographic density being observed, our first responsibility is to be certain that the density seen is in the lung. Nipple shadows, skin papillomas, or hair braids may be very confusing and very embarrassing if not identified early as the cause of the radiographic density. Case SN-1 is classical nipple shadow—not all cases are this obvious.

Once we are assured that the lesion is not artifactual or readily explainable on bases other than pulmonary pathology, some form of logical approach will be needed to determine whether this is a surgical or nonsurgical lesion. The following general protocol is presented.

1. History: What are the patient's chest complaints? What is the patient's age and sex? Does he/she know of or is there some explanation for this radiographic finding? Has he/she been exposed to tuberculosis or other known infectious diseases? Prob-

Lesion	High Probability of Cancer	Low Probability of Cancer
Increasing in size	+	−
Shows calcification	−	+
Appearance of margins	Lobulated, indistinct, irregular	Smooth
Lung extension from edges of lesion	Fine fingerlike processes into the lung	None
Associated satellite lesions	−	+
Associated adenopathy	+	−
Patient smoking history	+	−
Patient history of CA elsewhere	+	−
Age over 50	Increased	Less likely

Computerized tomography of the lung should certainly be done prior to surgery if the more simple and inexpensive procedures have not explained or offered a sound diagnosis. CT scanning has improved our diagnosis of pulmonary metastasis, for many lesions thought to be solitary actually are found to be multiple when the patient is subjected to computerized tomography. Some clinics are using CT scanning instead of linear tomography for indeterminant solitary lesions. Its value is becoming apparent.

After collecting data decision making is in order. Either the patient has a benign disease that can be followed, or he/she still carries the risk of life threatening disease.

In the decision-making process, the table above may be of value in determining the need for surgical intervention.

Any one of these criteria can be wrong in a given instance; however, by taking advantage of multiple criteria, accuracy can be improved. Primary lung cancer has been shown to overgrow calcified granulomas; therefore, calcium in itself cannot be used as an all-or-none criterion, but calcification in a soft-tissue nodule of a nonsmoker is very likely benign. While satellite lesions, like calcifications, are not all granulomas, most of them are. It is also true that adenopathy can occur in infectious disease, but it is more frequently a finding of neoplastic extension. While it is also true that the fingerlike projections at the lesion margins may not be an infiltrating tumor but may represent contracting fibrosis about a granuloma decreasing in size, this is also an exception—not the rule.

The following film reproductions give some examples of the radiographic signs.

Case SN-2 is an example of satellite nodules. The major lesion has some very fine calcification indicated by the small arrow—the larger arrow is directed toward the satellite. This lesion proved to be histoplasmosis.

Case SN-3 is a lobulated nodule. There is no calcification. The margins vary in degree of sharpness. This was an adenocarcinoma. The patient, a smoker, was admitted with brain metastasis.

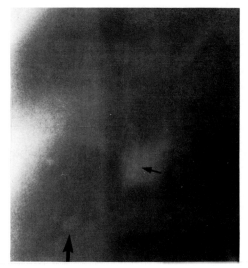

Case SN-2

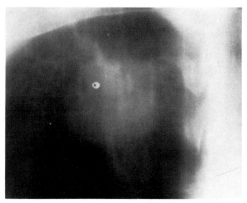

Case SN-4

Case SN-4 is tomograms of a large apical mass. There is no calcification. The edges are poorly defined and there are fingerlike projections from the mass out into lung. This was squamous-cell carcinoma.

Case SN-5 is a difficult lesion to categorize. In general, it is smooth but margins are very indistinct. No calcification is present—but there are varying densities due to small amounts of air in and through the lesion. This is alveolar carcinoma of lung, to be discussed later.

Case SN-3

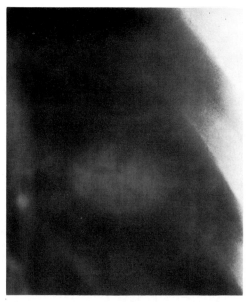

Case SN-5

CASE PRESENTATIONS

Cases C-1 and C-2

The first radiographs to be presented in this series are the posteroanterior (PA) and lateral chest studies of a 48-year-old woman. The films were made routinely prior to a surgical procedure. Except for special cases, all radiographs presented are standard chest technique—upright with target film distance of 72 inches.

Discipline on the part of the observer is important in interpreting all films. It is just as important to examine radiographs in a disciplined, orderly manner as it is to physically examine patients in a disciplined manner. There is no standard routine for examining radiographs, such as the system used in examining patients in physical diagnosis. Each observer tends to work out his/her own routine. Any routine is acceptable, but it must be a disciplined, orderly, never-abridged routine. The one used here has worked well for the author.

Start with evaluation of the heart. The heart, in this instance, is certainly normal in size. The heart has about a 95% chance of being normal in size if its transverse diameter is less than one half the inside diameter of the chest when this diameter is measured at the level of the highest point on the right diaphragm. The heart is basically a midline structure, although in most instances it does extend to the left. There are sharp cardiac margins all around, except at the diaphragm level where the heart comes in contact with the diaphragm. There is a very slight convexity to the left margin of the heart.

Move cephalad after the cardiac evaluation. At this point evaluate the hilar

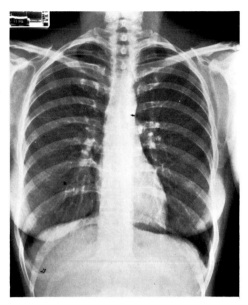

Case C-1

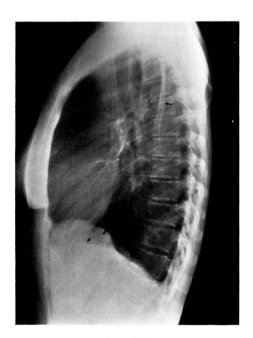

Case C-2

structures, the aortic arch, and the upper mediastinum. In this instance, there are several discrete calcifications in the left hilar area, the largest of which overlies the left pulmonary artery and is approximately a centimeter to the left of the aortic line. An arrow is used to point to the left lateral side of the descending aorta. This line can be followed inferiorly even to the level of the 11th rib. Here, the line is slightly medial to the vertebral body. A similar, less well-defined vertical line is noted on the right side of the vertebral bodies. This line is in a position quite comparable to that noted on the left, except that the upper portion of the aorta tends to place it farther to the left than is seen on the right side. This represents the medial pleural reflection, the margin of the mediastinum, or the so-called mediastinal stripe of the chest and is an important line in evaluating chest and mediastinal pathology.

Also of interest in the left hilar area is a small annular shadow. This shadow at the inferior margin of the posterior seventh rib is identified by a small black arrow. This shadow is frequently a source of confusion to students learning to interpret chest films. It does not represent cavitation but is evidence of a bronchus running parallel to the line of vision. We are, therefore, seeing the bronchial wall on end. Virtually all chest films, if they are examined carefully, will show one or more of these circular-type structures.

In the midline, there is a larger linear air-filled structure, the trachea; it is best seen in the upper mediastinum. As the mediastinal and chest contents become more opaque inferiorly, the airway becomes less apparent. There are techniques in doing chest radiography that will bring out the airway and still not interfere with visualization of the lung parenchyma.

These techniques involve high kilovolt exposures and use an air gap between the patient and the film. They are recommended in many instances, and, in fact, are routine in some institutions. However, since they do require specialized equipment, we elected not to use that type of film in this text.

The ringlike shadows seen in the midline over the upper three dorsal bodies are the spinous processes of the vertebral bodies extending posteriorly. The medial ends of the clavicle are also apparent as they approach the midline. An important criteria for determining rotation on a chest film is to note the medial ends of the clavicle. They should be symmetrically placed. Here the left medial clavicle is slightly closer to the midline than the right; however, this degree of rotation is acceptable.

Another source of confusion to the student involves the anterior medial portions of the first rib. There is frequent ossification of the cartilage at this site, and the ossification and the calcification may be quite bizarre in appearance. A great deal of variation occurs here. We will point them out as incidental findings on other chest films. At this point we have completed our visual examination of the midline structures.

Next, turn your attention to hemidiaphragms and costophrenic angles. This patient shows smooth hemidiaphragms on both sides. The superimposed breast shadow on the right does fall over the midportion of the hemidiaphragm, while the breast shadow on the left comes down to just the hemidiaphragm level. This points out the fact that the right hemidiaphragm is normally slightly higher than the left. It also emphasizes the slight change in the lung's appearance due to the attenuation of the x-ray beam produced by the patient's breasts. The radiograph is slightly more dense inferior and lateral to the breasts than that seen directly through the breasts. In this instance, the hemidiaphragm extends down to the eleventh rib. This is quite normal, but is somewhat lower than would be seen if the patient were stocky or obese.

An open arrow is placed on the right side of the lower chest or, in this instance, possibly the upper abdomen. The arrow reflects the posterior costophrenic angle, and shows the level of the aerating lung in the posterior chest. The midportion of the right hemidiaphragm that is seen as the dome is several centimeters higher than this point. In this patient the posterior reflection is much more evident on the right than on the left. This is generally true, for the underlying liver serves as a fine contrast agent to the air in the lungs. Pleural fluid will be seen first in the costophrenic angles. This is true because most chest films are made in the upright position. Actually, smaller amounts of fluid can be shown along the lateral portion of the chest if the radiograph is made with the patient in the decubitus position. The amount of fluid that can be detected radiographically depends largely on the size of the patient and the sharpness of the costophrenic angle. It is possible to see 200 to 300 cc. of fluid in a small patient with a very sharp angle, whereas several times that amount may be lost in a large patient with relatively flat hemidiaphragms.

The next phase of the chest film examination involves evluating the lung fields. Since we are just finishing with the hemidiaphragms this author's routine is to vertically examine each lung field moving the line of study from the hemidiaphragm level to the apex, crossing to the opposite side moving down, then reversing the

order. In this way, one examines the entire lung fields at least twice. Two small arrows are seen on the right. The tiny arrow in the third anterior intercostal space on the right simply points to the minor fissure that, in this case, is a delicate white line. If fluid were present, it would become more apparent. The heavier curved arrow is directed toward the anterior portion of the fifth rib. This actually is the end of the fifth rib, which, in this instance, points toward us more than is usually seen. It is one of the many normal variants noted in the rib cage, and should not be interpreted as lung pathology. Whenever a peculiar or unexplained shadow is noted, always evaluate it in relationship to bony structures. Note the fine lattice work of the lung fields, which represents a combination of blood vessels and bronchi.

It is impossible to be certain which are bronchi and which are vessels unless you can follow the tapering linear structure back to its origin. The pulmonary arteries are seen rather clearly as one approaches the hilar area. You will note that on the left the pulmonary artery comes out above the level of the upper lobe bronchus, but it comes out under the upper lobe bronchus on the right. This patient shows no evidence of lung infiltration. The apices are unusually clear. Only the sternocleidomastoid muscles are seen extending over the medial portion of the apices.

Up to this point we have said nothing about the lateral chest film. With practice you will learn to interpret the two films together and will be perfectly comfortable when evaluating the heart on both views. The same is true of the hemidiaphragms and the lung structures.

The lateral film is especially important when examining the bony structures and, with this routine of chest film evaluation, the spine and soft tissues of the chest wall become the final area of evaluation. The lateral film frequently gives an excellent view of the dorsal spine, as is the case here. There is some wedging of lower dorsal bodies and some minimal spurring. This is a reflection of the patient's age and is a degenerative process. Over the upper portion of the dorsal spine is a black arrow pointing towards a vertical density. This is the margin of the scapula when viewed in this projection. A similar but less sharp density paralleling it sits just anterior to the vertebral bodies. This is the scapula on the side away from the film. These paired bony densities are frequently a source of confusion to the novice. Another point to evaluate is the degree of diaphragm flattening. The largest black arrow pointing cephalad points to the inferior vena cava as it comes through the diaphragm. This is an important landmark since the left ventricle as it enlarges extends posterior to this dividing point. The smaller black arrow, which is directed inferior and anterior to the inferior vena cava, is directed to the point where the margin of the left diaphragm is lost. This is due to the silhouette effect of the heart as it comes in contact with the diaphragm. The silhouette sign in the chest radiography interpretation is extremely important. It has been popularized by Dr. Felson, and his text on the chest radiographic interpretation is a fine reference. We will discuss this more as we evaluate other chest films. At this point it is enough to say that when two structures with the same density contact each other, the result of that contact is the loss of the interface between the two.

Our evaluation of the bony structures is not complete until we have at least observed the sternum as well as the ribs.

With experience this can be done rapidly. To the beginner it may be a slow process. Each rib should be followed all the way from its posterior margin to its anterior end. Shoulder girdles are seen only in part on the chest film. It depends upon the patient's size. The humerus is always distorted due to the internal rotation and rolling forward of the scapula that is done routinely in taking films. Occasionally one can identify pathology in the scapula or distal clavicle. The shoulder joint itself is less reliably evaluated on chest studies.

We have already commented about breast shadows on the PA chest radiograph. Note them as well on the lateral view, and see that the inferior lateral portion of the breasts also extends over a portion of the anterior lung parenchyma. Another soft-tissue structure that is frequently visible and always worth looking for is the spleen. In this instance, it is not well outlined. On some PA chest radiographs, it is clearly seen and its size can be evaluated.

So ends our routine in evaluating the normal chest, with its innumerable variations. We are now ready to look at pathology.

Case C-3

The radiograph presented is the second of a series made on this patient who was admitted to the hospital with the clinical diagnosis of congestive heart failure. The initial study showed marked bilateral pleural effusion. The opacification of the lung bases was so great that the heart margins were not visible. Because of the patient's distress, bilateral thoracenteses were done, and the radiograph presented here was made following the bilateral pleural taps.

This study is presented to demonstrate

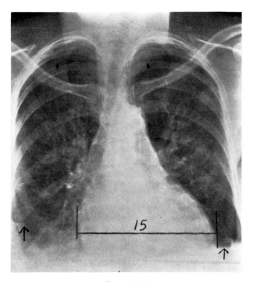

Case C-3

a number of fundamental observations. The heart is obviously enlarged. The measurements indicated on the radiograph are to demonstrate the simplest method of determining cardiac enlargement from the chest study. The greatest transverse dimension of the heart is measured at 15 cm. This is compared to the greatest internal transverse dimension of the chest, which in this instance is 26 cm. Other more complex methods of measuring the heart have been devised. However, in this author's experience, none has been any more reliable than this simple system.

In addition to the cardiac enlargement, there is engorgement of the pulmonary vessels in the infraclavicular area on both sides. This is additional evidence of the increased pulmonary venous pressure and altered pulmonary blood flow pattern consistent with congestive failure.

As a complication of the thoracentesis, the patient developed a pneumothorax on each side. The curved arrows on the upper chest on each side indicate the visceral pleural margin. The pleural margin on the left is sharper and easier to follow than that on the right. On the left the arrow is at the inferior margin of the posterior medial fifth rib. The pleural line can be followed downward toward the midline, and to a lesser degree, upward toward the first rib, and over the lateral chest. The arrow in the left costophrenic angle indicates a sharp fluid level. A sharp air/fluid level occurs only when there is an air/fluid interface. Even if the pneumothorax could not be identified in the left apex, the sharp line in the left costophrenic angle would be indicative of free air in the pleural space that also contains some fluid.

On the right, the pneumothorax is less obvious but the pleural line is noted directly beneath the arrow. The inferior portion of the right lung is not collapsed by the pneumothorax, and because of this we do not have a sharp air/fluid interface. The right side demonstrates the usual meniscus or cuplike density that occurs in the base of the upright chest film when the pleural space contains fluid. Even though the opacification of the pleural space is higher and more dense laterally, the fluid, of course, is at the same level all the way around the lung. This characteristic feature of fluid in the pleural space is explained by the relative thickness of the fluid at the edge of the pleural space compared to the relatively thin anterior and posterior thickness of the fluid.

Final diagnosis: Cardiomegaly with congestive failure and bilateral hydropneumothorax.

Cases C-4 through C-9

Cases C-4 through C-9 are presented together because they show a number of similarities. Their differences are primarily differences of location. All are either segmental or lobar in distribution. Pneumonia with a segmental distribution is now more frequent than total lobe involvement. This is probably due to early diagnosis and effective forms of therapy. In all cases, the area of pathology is reflected by increased radiodensity. Infiltration and consolidation simply replace the aerating lung tissue. The process of infiltration and consolidation was discussed under the fundamentals of the chest pathology. All of the cases show sharp demarcation by at least one pleural reflection. Straight dense arrows point to the significant pleural reflections in each instance. In general, the area of pathological involvement is of uniform density. There are some exceptions to this, as indicated by the curved arrows on Case C-7, AP projection, and Case C-5, lateral projection. Here curved arrows point to an air bronchogram, which is one of the classical radiographic signs of consolidation. Air in the bronchus surrounded by opaque lung implies that the bronchus is open, and that the pathology is alveolar or, less likely, interstitial. The cases presented here all show an alveolar-type consolidation. The air bronchogram sign is important in ruling out atelectasis.

Even though the process in all of these cases is one of consolidation, you will appreciate that the volume of the lung or segment involved is decreased. This is especially evident in Case C-4 and Case C-8, where the position of the fissure is displaced in such a way that the volume of the segment must be reduced. This universally occurs when a lobe shows total involvement, for with the loss of air from the parenchyma, even though fluid and inflammatory tissue tend to replace it, there is volume loss. The loss in volume

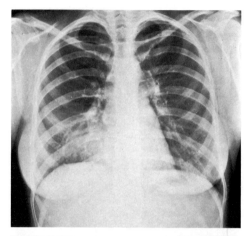

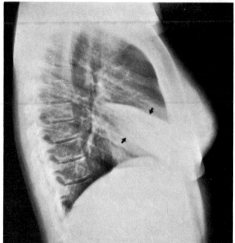

Case C-4

is generally less than that seen with atelectasis, but this feature tends to be a confusing point when learning to interpret radiographic findings. All cases presented here show other areas away from the primary pathology to be normal. There is little or no evidence of hilar adenopathy and no evidence of spillover into other lung areas, as might be expected with more chronic inflammatory processes.

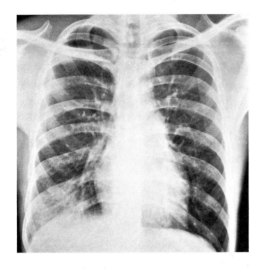

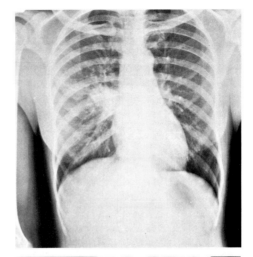

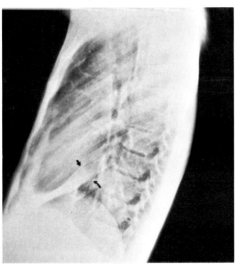

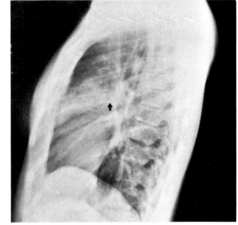

Case C-6

Case C-5

There is one well-known exception to the rule that pneumonic consolidation reduces lung volume, and that is consolidation due to Friedländer's bacillus. This consolidation characteristically expands the solid lobe or segment.

Case C-4: Classical right middle lobe pneumonia. Arrows indicate the major and the minor fissures, as seen in the lateral view. The loss of the right heart margin indicates a positive silhouette sign.

Case C-5: Infiltration in the lateral inferior segment of the right lower lobe. Infiltrate limited anteriorly by the major fissure. Air bronchogram is present. The sharpness of the right heart margin with normal aerating lung here indicates a lack of involvement of the middle lobe.

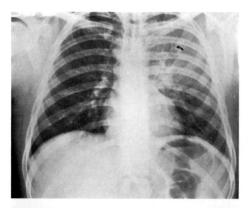

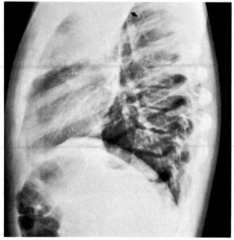

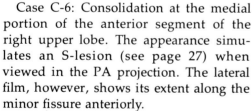

Case C-7

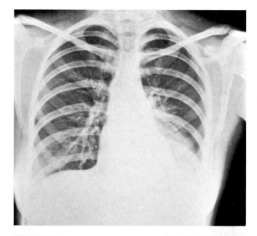

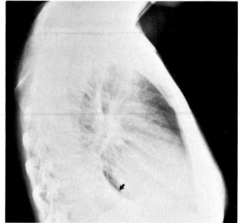

Case C-8

Case C-6: Consolidation at the medial portion of the anterior segment of the right upper lobe. The appearance simulates an S-lesion (see page 27) when viewed in the PA projection. The lateral film, however, shows its extent along the minor fissure anteriorly.

Case C-7: Left upper lobe involvement with the exception of the lingular segment (the lingular segment distribution on the left is the same as in the middle lobe on the right). The air bronchogram is indicated by a curved arrow; the major fissure is indicated by a heavy arrow posteriorly.

Case C-8: Left lower lobe pneumonia. There is posterior displacement of the major fissure. The left heart margin is well defined (negative silhouette sign), but the diaphragm is poorly outlined, as the consolidation silhouettes out the diaphragm.

Case C-9: When consolidation extends down to the minor fissure in the PA projection, this usually implies involvement of the anterior segment of the upper lobe. In this instance, an accessory fissure divides the apical segment of the lower lobe from the rest of the lower lobe (see the

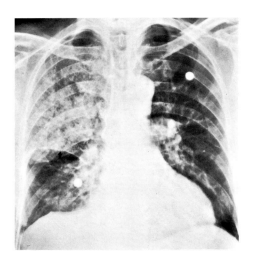

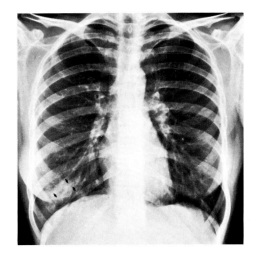

Case C-10

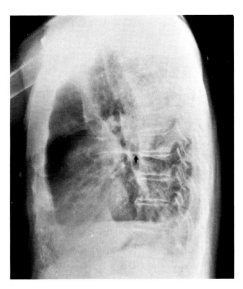

Case C-9

arrow on the lateral film), and the pneumonia seen here is actually in the apical segment of the lower lobe—a most unusual finding.

Case C-10

Case C-10 is a 35-year-old woman seen in the emergency room with a cough and fever. The PA radiograph of the chest demonstrates what is the most frequent radiographic presentation of pneumonia. In these days of readily available medical care and the prevalent antibiotics, we rarely see lobar consolidation. A small area of consolidation is noted just above the right hemidiaphragm. There are some radiolucent shadows that represent an air bronchogram. These are indicated by arrows. The infiltrate does extend into the costophrenic angle, but this is seen only as a very faint haziness, and is best demonstrated when compared to the opposite side. The area beneath the breast on the right is more opaque than the similar area on the left. The remaining lung fields are clear. The heart is normal in size and outline.

The localization of the infiltrate from a single PA radiograph is possible since the infiltrate goes into the costophrenic angle. This implies that it is in the lower lobe. This was confirmed by a lateral film, even though the lateral film is not presented here. Final diagnosis: Pneumonia, right lower lobe. The radiographic presentation seen here represents the usual manifestation of acute pneumonia, and certainly it is one of the most frequent radiographic diagnoses.

Cases C-11 through C-14

Cases C-11 through C-14 are all examples of metastatic disease. All have certain features in common, as well as certain dissimilarities. Metastatic disease may appear with a number of different faces. However, certain patterns dominate; and this, when associated with a history of a primary tumor, usually makes the diagnosis relatively easy. Of course there are those cases where no primary tumor is known, and metastases are the first finding. In those cases, the chest film helps establish the disease process and leads in the search for a primary tumor.

Case C-11 presents the usual textbook appearance of metastatic disease. There are multiple soft tissue densities scattered through both lung fields. The margins of the lesions are quite sharp and smooth.

Virtually no reactive change is seen in either the pleura or the lung parenchyma. The lesions tend to be peripheral, and tend to be more numerous in the lung bases. These latter features are reasonable since metastases are bloodborne, and approximately two thirds of the blood flow is to the lower half of the chest. (Not all metastases are bloodborne, as subsequent cases will show.) The peripheral location is also reasonable when one considers that these lesions are embolic, and that the initial tumor cluster is trapped in a peripheral capillary bed. Most metastatic lesions cause little in the way of host response, so no inflammatory changes are seen to complicate the picture. The varying sizes of the lesions seen in this case suggest that they are of differing ages.

In this case the primary source was the colon. It is always difficult to try to predict the primary source from the appearance of the metastatic pattern. Multiple large lesions are thought to be characteristically of sarcomatous origin, but certainly we see them from the kidney, testicle, and

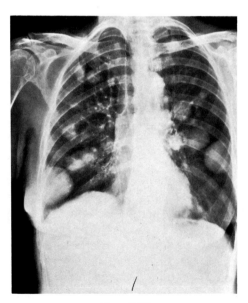

Case C-11

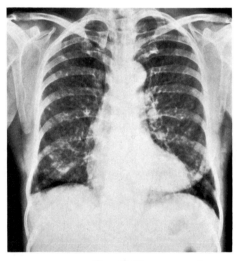

Case C-12

colon. No rules are hard and fast. Probably the most valuable rule in making the diagnosis of metastatic disease is that the lesion should be multiple, and yet we all know that solitary metastases do occur.

Case C-12 has many similarities with the first case. Multiple soft-tissue lesions are present. However, the obvious difference is that these lesions are much smaller, and they tend to be approximately the same size. This appearance suggests that the patient had a shower of tumor clumps into the blood stream at the same time, and multiple metastatic lesions resulted. These, we assume, are approximately the same age. This patient also had a colon neoplasm as the primary source of the metastatic disease. This pattern is less classical for colon metastasis than the previous case.

Case C-13 presents another type of metastatic pattern. With general inspection of the film, one is led to the diagnosis of metastatic disease. There is absence of the left breast and there are some small discrete nodules in the lungs, the most obvious of which is just above the left costophrenic angle.

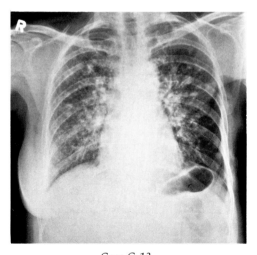

Case C-13

The pattern that is different is the linear and reticular nodular pattern that extends out from the hilar area on each side. This is the classical appearance of lymphatic spread of malignant disease. Tomograms through the hilar areas would show some adenopathy, although this is not an obvious part of the disease here. Masses of tumor cells actually are plugging the lymphatic pathways. There are times when lymphatic spread of a tumor looks very much like Kerley B-lines* with linear streaking best seen in the lung just above the costophrenic angle.

That is not the case here. The primary tumor is the breast. Such tumors frequently spread by the lymphatic route. Other tumors also spread by this route, most notably lymphomas and cancer of the stomach.

Case C-14 in our series of metastatic tumors is a different problem. This is a 76-year-old man, and there are obvious osteoblastic lesions noted throughout the skeletal structure. The right glenoid, the medial end of the right clavicle, and virtually all posterior and lateral ribs are involved. On first glance, one has the impression that there are also lung lesions present. However, this author cannot specifically identify a lung lesion that is separate from a bony area. The curved arrow on the right points to what appears to be a shadow separate from the posterior seventh rib, but the scapula is in the region, and the lesion is most likely in the bone substance of the scapula. The patient has cancer of the prostate—this is the most frequent cause of osteoblastic bone lesions in elderly men.

There are some rather coarse linear streaks extending into the lung bases. This pattern could represent lymphatic

*See description page 61, Case V-5 Cardiovascular Section.

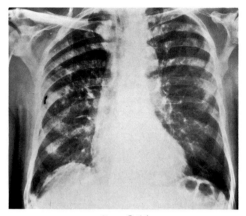

Case C-14

dissemination, but it is different from that of Case C-13, in that most of the streaking is extending into the bases, rather than the mid lung field and upper two thirds of the chest. Since this man was 76 years old, the changes here probably represent only a chronic basilar degenerative disease, which is principally fibrosis. It also helps to know that carcinoma of the prostate rarely metastasizes to the lung parenchyma. Therefore, our final impression on this case is multiple osteoblastic metastases with generalized degenerative disease.

Cases C-15 through C-17

Our next five cases will deal with the subject of primary lung cancer. We will make no attempt to present all of the ways this disease can present itself radiographically. We will show some rather classic examples.

Much has been stated about the increasing incidence of all forms of cancer in the American population. However, when one looks at the true statistics, the one cancer that has significantly increased in incidence has been lung cancer. The death rate from this disease has increased sevenfold over the past 30 years, and from the appearance of its mortality curve, there is no reason for optimism about the future. The changing disease patterns, as seen in the past 30 years, has altered our diagnostic approach to chest films. There was a time when tuberculosis was considered the great mimicker of other chest lesions, and with unusual types of infiltrate, tuberculosis was the prime suspect. Tuberculosis has decreased in incidence, and cancer of the lung has increased, so now the death rate from lung cancer is tenfold greater than tuberculosis.

If you are interested in preventive medicine or in disease epidemiology, and have looked at the literature that is so plentiful regarding cancer of the lung, you will be impressed at the overwhelming evidence that relates cigarette smoking to lung neoplasia. There is now a rapidly increasing incidence of lung cancer in women associated with their increased use of cigarettes.

Keep in mind the role of cigarette smoking in lung cancer; as you understand other problems associated with smoking, it will help in the differential diagnosis of pulmonary disease. Like lung cancer, pulmonary emphysema is virtually a smoker's disease, and in fact the two diseases frequently occur together. This, in itself, serves as a helpful diagnostic point. If we assume that tobacco smoke is the effective carcinogen, then the distribution of lung cancer should follow ventilation patterns more than perfusion patterns. This is precisely what happens. Cancer of the lung occurs in the upper half of the chest approximately two thirds to three fourths of the time while metastatic disease, which is usually bloodborne, tends to show a reverse pattern. This is logical when one recalls that blood flow is primarily in the basilar lung fields, and air flow is greatest in the upper lungs. Primary lung cancer is generally seen as a unilateral lesion, but primary lung tumors do metastasize to the opposite lung, and because of the expressed etiology of lung cancer lesions have been seen at different stages of development involving both lungs.

Case C-15 is that of a 68-year-old man with a relatively long history of chronic obstructive pulmonary disease and cough. Recently he developed hemoptysis, as well as accentuation of his shortness of breath. The overall appearance of the film is consistent with that of chronic obstructive pulmonary disease. The hemidiaphragms are flattened. The anterior-posterior dimension of the chest has increased with considerable radiolucency noted substernally (C-15b). There are coarse markings in the central lung fields and bases, with peripheral hyperaeration.

The striking feature of the film is the hilar enlargement seen on the left. There is some fine infiltrate in the left infraclavicular area. The lateral film shows the major fissure to be displaced posteriorly (this is pointed out by heavy dark arrows). A small dark arrow points to a soft-tissue shadow in the left apex. This may be only pleural thickening, but could also represent supraclavicular nodes.

The tomogram (C-15c) presented is extremely helpful (curved arrows point to a partially obstructed lower and upper lobe bronchus). The patchy infiltration distal to the upper lobe narrowing presumably represents infectious disease trapped behind the narrowed bronchus. The upper lobe is experiencing some obstructive emphysema, since we have already commented upon the displacement of the major fissure posteriorly and the moderate expansion of the upper lobe.

The lower lobe is certainly not hyperaerated; it shows reduced volume indicating that the narrowing of the lower lobe

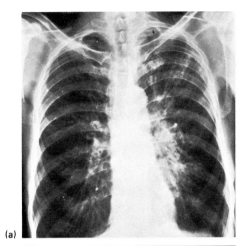

(a)

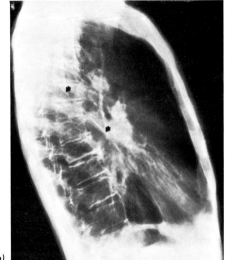

(b)

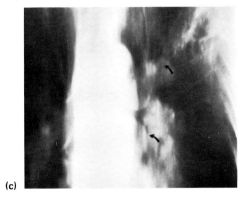

(c)

Case C-15

bronchus is more severe than that of the upper lobe. The tomogram also reveals lobulation of the hilar shadows, particularly in the area between the upper and lower lobe regions, and at a point medial to the narrowed upper lobe bronchus. These certainly represent lymph node extension of the primary tumor. At this point it is impossible to be certain whether the primary tumor originated in the lower or upper lobe. As we have indicated earlier, it is statistically more sound to suspect the upper lobe. This would imply that the lower lobe obstruction has occurred due to encroachment and lymph node spread.

It is always important to examine the bony structures of the chest in patients suspected of primary lung neoplasia. Bone destruction strongly supports the presence of malignant disease. None can be identified here.

Our final diagnosis is primary lung carcinoma with extension to the hilar nodes on the left. This was subsequently biopsied and shown to be a squamous cell tumor. The neoplastic process has developed in a patient with underlying chronic obstructive pulmonary disease (pulmonary emphysema).

The smoking history is extremely important in all patients with lung pathology. This patient had a long smoking history, which is strong supportive evidence of our initial diagnosis. The radiographic findings here are classical. Although findings like this occasionally occur in lymphoma, tuberculosis, and other granulomatous disease, given a long smoking history, the probability of any diagnosis other than primary cancer is unlikely.

Case C-16 is a 52-year-old woman. Like nearly all lung cancer patients, she had a long smoking history. Her complaints

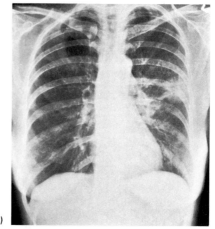

(a)

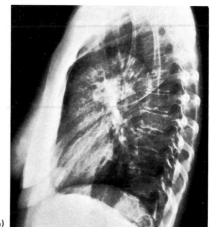

(b)

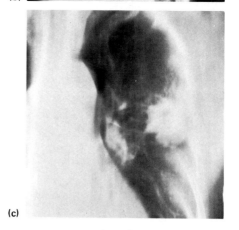

(c)

Case C-16

were those of tightness in the chest and a nagging cough.

This case presents no challenge in finding the pathology. A large soft-tissue mass is seen in the left midlung field. It is directly beneath the posterior axillary line. The lateral film (C-16b) indicates that it is approximately in the midchest. By studying both the plain film and the tomogram (C-16c), one can identify features that are highly suggestive of malignant disease. The tomogram particularly shows small fingerlike projections from the margin of the lesion. The margin is not smooth, but is quite serrated, and shows infiltrating strands. Heavy strands extend from the lesion toward the enlarged and lobulated left hilar area. This is characteristic of enlarged hilar nodes and mediastinal nodes. There is a poorly defined radiolucency in the central portion of the primary lung mass. This indicates central necrosis or cavitation within the tumor. Cavitation occurs most frequently in squamous cell tumors. However, in this instance, our patient's biopsy indicated an adenocarcinoma. Adenocarcinoma is more common in women than in men. As a general rule its margins are much smoother than are seen here, and it rarely cavitates. This case simply is an example of the fact that virtually all our rules for attempting to predict cell type have so many exceptions that they are of little value.

The lateral film (C-16c) shows a curved major fissure, as indicated by the arrows. Again, we are seeing the anterior portion of the major fissure elevated, but with enough fixation at the hilar region that the fissure does not move forward in a symmetrical manner.

An incidental finding on the PA chest film is a deformed second anterior rib on the right. It appears that this rib attempted to be a bifid structure, and the superior portion of the rib grew cephalad and now forms a false articulation with the first rib.

Our final interpretation is peripheral primary lung tumor, with extension to the hilar nodes. From its appearance we predicted a squamous cell lesion; however, this was an adenocarcinoma. The relationship of adenocarcinoma to smoking remains in question. As recently as 1978 some authors felt adenocarcinomas had no correlation to tobacco usage. Ernest Wynder, the epidemiologist who first showed the tobacco—cancer-of-the-lung connection feels that the correlation of smoking to adenocarcinoma, while less strong than with other primary neoplasms, is still a very real one.

Case C-17 is another in our series on primary cancer of the lung. The patient is a 50-year-old woman, who is asymptomatic so far as the chest is concerned. The study was made prior to an elective surgical procedure.

The initial PA chest radiograph (C-17a) shows normal findings except for a vague, poorly defined area of increased density between the second and third anterior ribs on the right. This is the type of shadow that might easily be considered an artifact, and certainly this radiograph offers evidence that whenever a poorly defined suspected artifactual lesion is seen, the film should be repeated. The tomogram (C-17b) shown with the film indicates that the lesion is not an artifact; in fact, the tomogram has quite a different appearance from the chest film. Note that while the lesion is reasonably dense, it is very poorly defined at its margins. It is located about the end of one of the branches of the upper lobe bronchus. There is no calcification in or about the lesion.

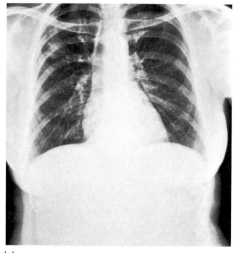

(a)

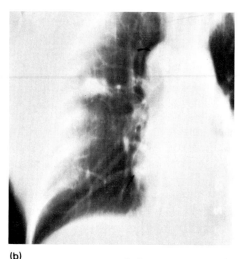

(b)

Case C-17

The curved arrow points to a soft-tissue ovoid structure in the right paratracheal area. This is considered to be a paratracheal node. This not only offers supportive evidence of the diagnosis of primary lung malignancy but also indicates that this lesion has a poor prognosis. The arrow at the inferior portion of the tomogram serves to point out a good demonstration of a pulmonary vein as it returns to the left atrium. Notice this branching structure as it enters the heart at a point well below the carina.

This case was proven to be an alveolar cell carcinoma of the lung (synonyms: bronchiolar carcinoma or bronchioalveolar carcinoma). This type of tumor is a fascinating variation from the usual lung tumor. It makes up approximately 10% of primary lung tumors, and tends to occur in two distinct types. One type is that demonstrated here in which the primary lesion appears to be localized but may actually be a slow growing tumor. If it can be identified prior to node metastasis, it carries a reasonably good prognosis. The other form of alveolar cell carcinoma is one that may be seen as acinar nodules through both lung fields. This has given rise to the speculation that it may be of multicentric origin. The diffuse type has a poor prognosis, and is associated in over half of the cases with excessive mucoid expectoration from the lungs. Because of its diffuse nature and high volume of sputum production, it was thought by some observers to have an inflammatory origin. This, however, has never been proven.

Both the localized and the multicentric types of this tumor are difficult diagnostic problems. Certainly if there had been no paratracheal node, here the diagnosis of malignancy would be less certain. Yet, if no node had been present surgical removal would carry as high as a 30% to 40% cure rate. Such a cure rate is unusual in primary cancer of the lung. Had this lesion fallen directly under the rib, rather than in the interspace, its identification would very certainly have been delayed. Note also the size of the paratracheal node and its failure to be demonstrated on the routine chest film.

Our final diagnosis here is that of a local type of alveolar cell carcinoma with extension to a paratracheal node.

Case C-18

The films presented are those of a 61-year-old man admitted with a history of shortness of breath and hemoptysis. He also admitted to a 40-pack-a-year smoking history. Even without his very suggestive history, this is one of the easiest diagnoses we will present. The PA radiograph presents a hilar mass on the right with some elevation of the minor fissure as indicated by the dotted lines. This indicates loss of aerating volume in the right upper lobe. The case is presented primarily to demonstrate the so-called "S" sign of the minor fissure. This sign as described by Ross Golden several decades ago was considered to be pathognomonic of primary carcinoma of the lung with mediastinal adenopathy. The sign is produced by loss of volume of the right upper lobe, thus elevating the lateral portion of the minor fissure; however, since the medial portion of the fissure is fixed by metastatic nodes or by a primary lung lesion, this portion of the fissure cannot rise freely with the lateral portion. This results in the curve or S configuration of the minor fissure. Of course, with more experience we know this sign occurs whenever hilar adenopathy produces fixation of the medial part of the minor fissure.

The tomographic insert (C-18c) is a nice demonstration of the "rattailed" narrowing of the upper lobe bronchus and the fixation or depression of the medial part of the minor fissure. The fine mottling and mixed aeration and consolidation seen in the upper lobe represents inflam-

(a)

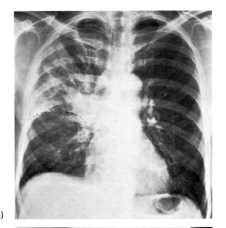

(b)

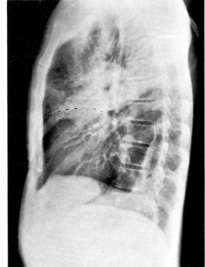

(c)

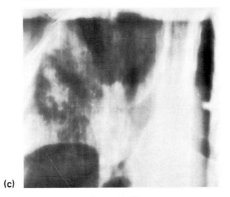

Case C-18

matory disease behind the poorly drain- ing upper lobe bronchus.

When biopsied this turned out to be an oat cell carcinoma of the lung. This was not predictable from this study. The find- ings here indicate hilar spread and me- diastinal fixation, therefore adding gravity to the prognosis.

Case C-19

The diagnosis of Pancoast's tumor is easy when the findings are as well defined as those demonstrated on this radiograph. Unfortunately this is not the usual case. Even after a relatively short experience in interpreting chest films, you will encoun- ter apical densities that may or may not be symmetrical. These are usually just pleural tags and indicate previous inflam- matory changes. You will recall from au- topsy experience that virtually all elderly corpses have apical adhesions at the time of the postmortem exam. These show up in varying degrees on chest radiographs.

In this case there is distinct asymmetry of the opacification of the apices. The

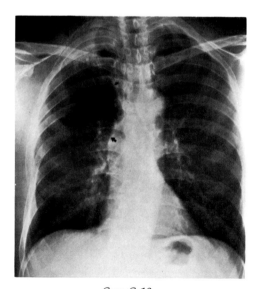

Case C-19

right side is opaque down to the level of the fourth posterior rib, while the left side remains well aerated clear to the ring of the first rib. In addition there is mottled bone destruction involving the right sec- ond rib directly beneath the dense arrow. If this bone destruction had not been present, a radiographic diagnosis of Pan- coast's tumor could be only suspected from the asymmetry of the apices. With the bone destruction, a diagnosis can be made with a high degree of confidence.

Pancoast's tumors are usually squamous cell carcinomas, as was true in this case. Pancoast's tumor derives its name from Dr. Pancoast, one of the early radiologists in this country, who described this entity in some detail. The clinical features of this tumor may include pain in the shoulder, and frequently there is involvement of the sympathetic nerve plexus giving the pa- tient a Horner's syndrome on the side involved.

The other two arrows on this film serve simply to point out features unrelated to the primary diagnosis. The arrow over the right sixth posterior rib is pointing to a line that is directed upward at approxi- mately a 15-degree angle from the vertical. This is an unimportant structure. It ac- tually represents the margin of the man- ubrium, which in this instance, is visible on the right because of the patient's slight scoliosis to the left. This can be a confus- ing shadow, and the finding here is ex- aggerated because of the scoliosis.

The third arrow, which is between the eighth and ninth ribs adjacent to the hil- um, is pointed toward the margin of the ascending aorta. This patient was 54 years old and is showing some of the signs of a tortuous aorta. Aortic tortuosity is a result of atherosclerotic changes. The as- cending aorta can be followed upward to the aortic arch, and a sharp descending line is seen on the left side of the mediastinum as the aorta descends.

Final diagnosis: Pancoast tumor in the right apex with bone destruction of the second rib. Moderate vascular degenerative disease. Slight scoliosis.

Case C-20

The radiograph here is of a 55-year-old obese diabetic man with fever and toxic disorientation. Even without this helpful history, the proper diagnosis should be included in the radiographic differential diagnosis. Previous films are always helpful, and in this instance a chest film made two months earlier showed moderate cardiac enlargement with clear lung fields.

The current radiograph shows cardiac enlargement, which is very little more than that seen on the earlier film, high hemidiaphragms related to the patient's stature, and, most important, extensive bilateral patchy-lung infiltration. We can evaluate this latter change even more extensively. The symmetrical nature of the pathology follows a "butterfly distribution," yet the process is more nodular than one associates with pulmonary edema. Pulmonary edema is the classical cause of butterfly or vascular distributed

density. In this instance, the nodularity is too indistinct to be considered metastatic disease (compare this film to the metastatic lesion shown on C-11). The distribution is not segmental or lobar. The distribution is that of pulmonary blood flow.

This is an example of pulmonary sepsis, in which the septic process is bloodborne. Some 90% of patients with this radiographic finding will have diabetes. Most of the remaining 10% are drug abusers or postoperative patients, usually with gram negative sepsis. The organism that produces the lung inflitrate is quite variable.

The differential diagnosis must include pulmonary edema, although study of the film reveals the indicated differences from pulmonary edema. Metastatic malignant disease must also be considered.

Some forms of anaplastic metastases may have indistinct margins, but this would be an unusual radiographic manifestation for such a process. History and clinical features will help make the differential diagnosis. Not all metastatic disease is cancer. Infectious processes may also be carried by the bloodstream to the lung with very serious implications. Prompt diagnosis may be lifesaving.

Cases C-21 and C-22

In the last quarter of the twentieth century, cases of miliary tuberculosis are quite uncommon. However, this is a most important radiographic diagnosis. This 50-year-old man had a chest film made ten days earlier, which showed the same very fine miliary pattern, except that it was less extensive than is seen here. The right diagnosis was made, and the patient, under aggressive therapy, recovered.

Close observation of the radiograph is worth a thousand descriptive words. In

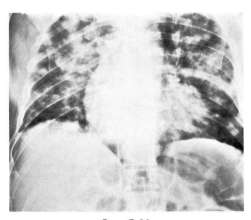

Case C-20

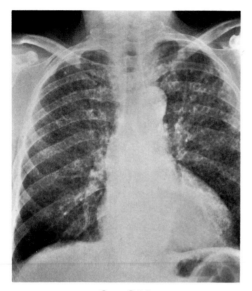

Case C-21

lobe infiltrate with tiny discrete nodules, and we must admit that there are many other things that can produce this type of radiographic change. Other processes that can produce this finding would include interstitial fibrosis, pneumonoconiosis, sarcoid, hemosiderosis, lymphoma, and even some metastatic processes. When this author is shown a film that has these characteristics, the first question is, "Is the patient in a toxic condition?" Most of the other entities that produce this radiographic picture do not result in fever, toxicity, and acute illness. When the patient is clinically ill, miliary tuberculosis is the first diagnosis. If the patient is relatively asymptomatic, the other entities mentioned above take precedence. It is also of interest that most of these patients have little in the way of physical findings in the chest. This is because an interstitial process is involved. Only after there has been reactive change in the lung for a period will physical findings result.

Our final diagnosis is miliary tuberculosis. It is an uncommon illness, but it occurs. Its diagnosis is extremely important, for prompt treatment is lifesaving.

Case C-22 is one of the few we will present of children. The patient is an eight-year-old girl known to have cystic fibrosis (mucoviscidosis) since shortly after birth. Cystic fibrosis of the pancreas involves many more tissues than the pancreas. In fact, the prognosis of the disease is more related to the lung changes than to the gastrointestinal findings. The pulmonary portion of the disease is one manifested principally by inability to liquefy and mobilize lung secretions. The patient therefore creates thousands of thick mucoid foreign bodies that result in air trapping, poor lung drainage, and repeated lung infections. Because of these infection

this particular case, we note some very fine nodular shadows in the right base, and some larger more confluent densities in the left upper lung field. The earlier one studies a patient with this disorder, the more normal the radiograph will look. As the cluster of tubercle bacilli stimulates host response, the nodular densities become larger and tend to become confluent. Most of the densities seen in the right base and the mid lung field are pinhead size or perhaps even smaller. On the left there are some densities at least 5 mm in diameter, and in addition there is pleural reaction in the infraclavicular area.

There are no cavities and really no evidence of a previous tuberculous process. A previous tuberculous process certainly does not give the patient immunity against a miliary spread, but patients with tuberculosis who are under treatment generally do not experience miliary spread.

There are no secrets in making the diagnosis of miliary tuberculosis. It is a five

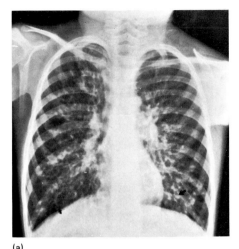

(a)

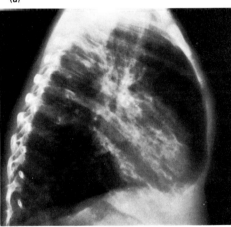

(b)   Case C-22

children do have problems with hypovolumnemia, due to salt loss through the skin.

This contracted blood volume does result in a small cardiac silhouette. Hilar structures are prominent. Most of this is due to reactive lymph adenopathy from the peripheral lung infections. In addition, there is fullness of pulmonary arteries due to increased vascular resistance in the lung bed.

One of the most striking features of this radiograph is the innumerable small cystic areas seen in the lung bases. The arrow on the left points to a structure approximately 4 × 8 mm in size. On the right the annular shadow identified by the arrow is approximately 3 mm in diameter. These are actually bronchiectatic cavities. Some of these bronchiectatic cavities contain pus, while others contain air. Those filled with air are more readily visible on the chest film. If you have an opportunity to see an autopsy on such a patient, it is a striking demonstration of the pulmonary problems these patients experience. The lungs do not collapse with opening of the chest. Cross sections show innumerable pus pockets and irregularly dilated bronchi. The "tram sign" has been used to diagnose bronchitis and bronchiectasis, particularly that which occurs in association with cystic fibrosis. The tram sign describes the abnormal appearance of the bronchi in which, running parallel to each other, they resemble a railroad track. The bronchi are dilated and do not taper as they should.

The lateral film C-22b adds to the diagnosis only by emphasizing the degree of obstructive disease in the chest, with the flattened diaphragm and the markedly increased anterior-posterior dimension of the chest.

and drainage problems, the patients develop pulmonary emphysema and bronchiectasis.

The film presented here shows the combination of emphysema, which we have discussed previously, and bronchiectasis, which is a disease that we are fourtunately seeing with less frequency now than in the previous 25-year period. The heart appears small. Part of this is an illusion due to the tamponade effect of the hyperaerated lungs, but at the same time these

Other incidental findings may be helpful in making the diagnosis if the chest
film is less than characteristic. These children also are greatly lacking in subcuta-
neous tissue. As you can observe in this
case, the skin virtually touches the rib
cage along the lateral chest wall. This is
part of their nutritional problem. Since
these children have problems with pancreatic secretions, they also have a great
deal of bowel distention. While very little
gastrointestinal tract is seen on this film,
it is not uncommon to see marked distention of the colon, and even some small
bowel distention on the chest film.

Cystic fibrosis is a familial disease, generally considered to be a genetic transmission of recessive order. It involves pre-
dominately whites. Mild forms of the
disease are known to occur, but as a
general rule the morbidity or mortality is
high, and the number of these children
that reach adulthood is small. It is a mul-
tisystem disease, but the chest findings
are probably the most important. It presents a rather classical radiographic appearance.

Case C-23

The thick heavy linear peribronchial
lung densities that extend into the lung
bases are the most striking feature. This
is seen on both the PA and lateral views.
The arrows on the left identify a Ghon
complex, the peripheral calcifications and
calcification in a lymph node directly beneath the left ninth posterior rib. The
upper lung fields do not participate in the
streaky appearing peribronchial densities
quite to the extent that we see it in the
bases. Yet even here, vascular markings
are prominent. The markings in general
remain linear, even though there may be
some that approach confluence in the lower left base.

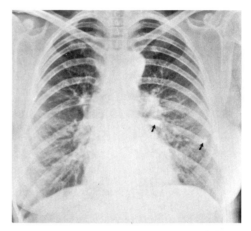
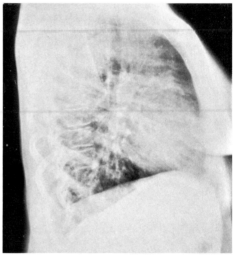

Case C-23

It also seems important that the hemidiaphragms are somewhat flattened. The
anterior-posterior diameter of the chest is
increased. While there are no specific
signs to indicate chronic obstructive pulmonary disease, the configuration of the
chest suggests that this may be a problem
in the future.

When one sees many chest films, the
findings we have pointed out here occur
frequently. Correlation with clinical findings is important. The changes may be
those of acute bronchitis, asthma, or per-

haps even early bronchopneumonia. In most cases none of these fits the clinical picture. A descriptive term that may be offensive to some has been used by a number of radiologists—"dirty lung." Possibly this is chronic bronchitis, and yet, chronic bronchitis should be a clinical diagnosis. Generally findings of this type imply chronic inflammatory disease. Usually the patients are heavy smokers, and the lung responds to this insult by excessive secretions and inflammatory changes.

Each radiologist tends to communicate this process to the clinician in his/her own way. Some use the term "diffuse increased lung markings." Others may use the term "dirty lung." This author prefers either of those terms to bronchitis, since by definition bronchitis implies a productive cough which cannot be determined from the radiographs. Environmental or industrial factors, or even allergies may contribute to this entity. This process probably has significant prognostic implication since it may precede chronic obstructive disease. Lung cleansing and strict preventive medicine techniques, especially stopping tobacco usage, should be applied.

Cases C-24 and C-25

Cases C-24 and C-25 are examples of lung abscess. By custom the term *lung abscess* refers to an acute pyogenic process. The organism is not defined. It may be either gram negative or positive, and again, usually by custom, the term excludes tuberculosis and fungus infestations. In general, the term lung abscess implies a solitary lesion. When the abscesses are multiple, the clinical problems are much the same, and perhaps worse, for their presence implies a bloodborne process. These are septic emboli. A solitary lung abscess is usually a complication of aspiration. Lung abscesses, therefore,

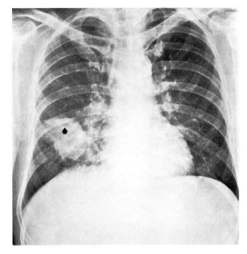

Case C-24

occur most frequently in patients that have neurological problems. This is especially true of stroke patients who cannot handle their own saliva effectively, or of patients in a coma. The most frequent coma-producing agent in lung abscess victims is alcohol. Unusual or extensive oral sepsis also predisposes to lung abscess, but even the normal flora of the mouth and pharynx, if aspirated, can produce a lung abscess. There are other predisposing conditions such as diabetes, immunosuppression, or immunodeficiencies that may result in greater susceptibility to forming a lung abscess.

The two cases of lung abscess presented here are reasonably representative of this disease. Case C-24 is a 24-year-old diabetic with an abscess in the lower lung field on the right. This was actually in the lateral segment of the middle lobe. The location is unusual, for abscesses usually occur in the posterior portion of the upper lobes, or in the apical segments of the lower lobes. Obviously, abscesses can occur in other locations depending upon the patient's position at the time of aspira-

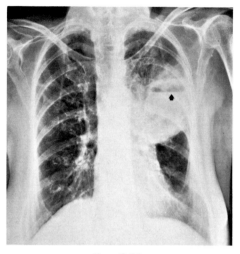

Case C-25

tion. This patient had been in a diabetic coma previously and apparently aspirated while lying prone and turned to the right.

Patient C-25 is a 70-year-old woman who had suffered a stroke, and the aspirant apparently went into the posterior portion of the left upper lobe.

Important radiographic characteristics can be demonstrated from these two radiographs. Both lesions tend to be rounded and solitary. Little or no reactive change is seen in other portions of the lung. Little or no marginal infiltration or fingerlike extensions are seen from the mass into the lung parenchyma. Both of these lesions show an air/fluid level; however, the air/fluid level can occur only when there is communication with the air-containing bronchus. Until such communication is established, the lung abscess exists only as a solid mass. Once cavitation occurs, it is noted that the wall of the cavity is thick (thick-walled cavities are generally considered having margins of greater than 2 mm). Even though this is a severe inflammatory process, hilar adenopathy is rarely a prominent feature

of the disease although it may be found to be present if searched for. For instance, case C-24 shows a more prominent hilar structure on the side of the lesion than is seen on the left. Even though abscesses may initially be of solid density, cavitation is the rule during the course of the illness. Not only is the diagnosis more firmly established with the presence of cavitation, but the drainage of the purulent material into the bronchus may be therapeutic. Since the abscess is generally well circumscribed and has relatively thick walls, pleural fluid when present is usually small in amount. Lung abscess and empyema do not usually occur in the same patient.

Heavy black arrows point to the air/fluid level in each case. A more delicate curved arrow in case C-25 is simply pointing to the vertical margin of the scapula. The film, in this instance, was made upright, as indicated by the air/fluid level, but the patient did not roll the shoulders forward in the usual manner to remove the scapula from the upper lung fields.

In summary, lung abscesses are usually solitary, thick-walled, cavitating lesions that produce minimal changes in the lung away from the area of consolidation.

Cases C-26 through C-28

Cases C-26 through C-28 represent sarcoid in varying degrees of involvement. Sarcoid is a chronic disease of unknown etiology. It involves organ systems other than the lung, but the radiographic manifestations of the disease are principally in the lung. This disease seems to vary in its frequency and, to some degree, its manifestations, according to geographical areas. Fraser and Paré in their classic text of the chest diseases describe four stages of sarcoid. They are as follows:

1. enlargement of hilar nodes only

2. pulmonary infiltration without adenopathy

3. peripheral lung infiltration with hilar nodes

4. fibrosis and scarring

This is a descriptive classification. Another concept might be that sarcoid presents a spectrum of pathology, varying from either minimal parenchymal infiltration or adenopathy all the way to severe fibrosis and scarring of the lung. Every case has the potential of going through the entire spectrum, with the patient becoming a pulmonary cripple, or it may end at any point along the course of the illness, with the patient losing little in the way of pulmonary function.

In any individual case the differential diagnosis of sarcoid may be a lengthy one. However, once the process can be established as a relatively chronic one, the differential diagnosis list can be shortened considerably. Invariably, the most important differential diagnosis involves sarcoid, tuberculosis, and lymphoma. Some general diagnostic points can be very helpful here. They are as follows:

1. Sarcoid rarely produces pleural effusion. If a pleural effusion is present, one must first consider that the diagnosis is either tuberculosis or lymphoma, or that there is a complicating factor in the disease, such as cardiac decompensation.

2. Despite high serum calcium levels in sarcoid, and the known metastatic calcification that occurs in multiple organs, calcifying lesions in pulmonary sarcoid are uncommon. Of course, sarcoid can develop in a patient who has calcifications prior to involvement with sarcoid; this may be confusing, but calcifications are uncommon in sarcoid.

3. Parenchymal infiltration may occur in lymphomas but is much less common in lymphomas than in either tuberculosis or sarcoid. Parenchymal infiltration among the lymphomas usually indicates Hodgkin's disease.

4. The adenopathy of sarcoid involves principally the bronchopulmonary nodes (hilar nodes) and mediastinal nodes with bilateral involvement. Lymphomas and tuberculosis tend to be predominantly unilateral. There are exceptions to this rule, especially in children and young adults.

5. Radiographic findings in sarcoid are usually more striking than the clinical features. There are obvious exceptions to this, especially when the process is very advanced.

6. When there is pathological examination of the parenchymal infiltrates, pathologists note that there is little or no reaction of the lung to the lesion. This is manifested radiographically by poorly defined reticulo-nodular type infiltrates. Lesions tend to be soft and poorly demarcated, in some instances even mimicking the septic metastases described previously.

The three cases presented here are rather typical samples of the spectrum of disease described above. All of our cases are women (the incidence is three times higher in women than in men). The ages of our patients varies from 24 to 38 (the age predilection for this disease is between 20 and 40). All of the cases presented here are black women. The incidence of the disease is at least ten times greater in blacks than in whites.

Case C-26 demonstrates rather classical hilar adenopathy, as viewed in both the AP and lateral projections. There is no silhouetting out of the heart, and there is a relatively clear space between the ad-

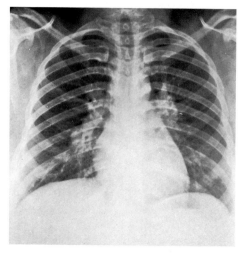
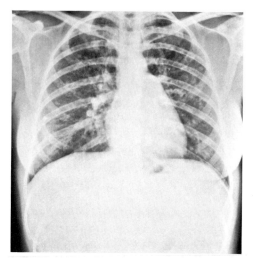
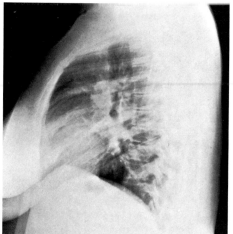
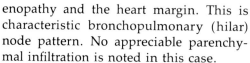

Case C-26

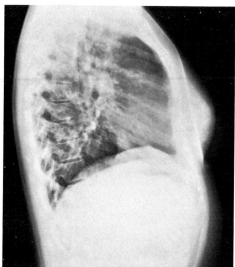

Case C-27

enopathy and the heart margin. This is characteristic bronchopulmonary (hilar) node pattern. No appreciable parenchymal infiltration is noted in this case.

Case C-27 is principally a reticulo-nodular parenchymal infiltrate, but the lateral film does show some hilar adenopathy. There is apparently some calcification in the adenopathy, indicating that the patient probably had histoplasmosis or

possibly tuberculosis at some previous time. The soft ill-defined peripheral lung lesions are quite classical. They tend to be predominantly in the upper lung field, but the bases are also involved. This patient has moderate splenomegaly that was evident on the original films, but has not been included on the print.

Case C-28 is a 38-year-old patient who

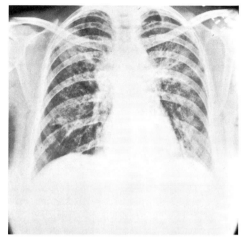

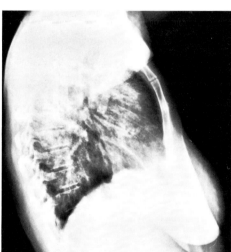

Case C-28

develop. At that point the identification of the initial process as sarcoid is impossible unless there are films that show the course of the illness. End stage lung disease can develop from many etiologies all manifesting a common end.

Sarcoid is an important disease in the differential diagnosis of chest pathology. Tissue for the pathology laboratory clinches the diagnosis, but the radiographic findings and the course of the disease are very important and are, in themselves, quite diagnostic.

Cases C-29 through C-31

As recently as 1900, tuberculosis was the leading cause of death in the United States. Since that time, the mortality rate from tuberculosis has steadily decreased. Now, approximately 80 years later, tuberculosis is no longer among the leading 20 causes of death in this country. This dramatic improvement has been brought about by improved living standards and public health measures. Antibiotic therapy has also helped reduce the mortality from tuberculosis over the last 20 years, but the death rate from this disease was already on the decline before drug therapy became available. During this period the incidence of tuberculosis has decreased, and the incidence of lung cancer has increased. This changing pattern of chest disease has dramatically influenced the thinking of those of us who interpret chest roentgenograms. In this section we will present three cases of the reinfection type of tuberculosis. In each case the differential diagnosis must include primary lung neoplasm.

has obviously had the disease for a number of years. The hilar adenopathy has become prominent. Scarring has retracted the nodes cephalad. There is still little, if any, calcification. A great deal of interstitial fibrosis and scarring is noted. This case does not necessarily represent the end point of the pulmonary changes in this disease. Actually, the process can progress to the point where severe emphysema and extensive fibrotic changes

The radiographic diagnosis of tuberculosis can best be made by studying the disease process over a period of time. This is not always practical. We need to review some of the radiographic characteristics of this disease as manifested by the reinfection process. There should be signs of a previous granulomatous lesion. A Ghon complex may be identified, possibly even in the opposite lung of the current involvement. Almost without exception there are areas of calcification in the lung, and these may or may not be in the area that is currently infected. Pleural effusion and hilar and mediastinal adenopathy are more frequent products of primary tuberculosis than of the reinfection type, but there are certainly exceptions.

It has been a long-standing radiographic axiom that reinfection tuberculosis involves the upper lungs. There are some numbers available to emphasize the importance of this axiom. One study reports that 85% of tuberculous lesions involve the apical and posterior segments of the upper lobes. An additional 10% involve the superior segment of either lower lobe. This implies that 95% of tuberculosis involves the upper lung fields. However, it is equally important to note the predominance of apical and posterior segment involvement. It has been stated that if only the anterior segment of the upper lobe is involved, the diagnosis should be either histoplasmosis or neoplasia. The 5% of tuberculosis that occurs in the mid- and lower-lung fields are rarely diagnosed radiographically.

Cavitation is another hallmark of the active exudative type of reinfection tuberculosis. Needless to say, this occurs only after the process has been active for some time. The tuberculous cavity is usually thick walled, of varying size, frequently associated with calcification; and it may rarely show a fluid level. Another form of cavitation, which is more properly considered a bleb or pneumatocele, is seen in the burned-out or inactive form of tuberculosis. These are thin walled and rarely contain fluid. Other areas of scarring and calcification generally occur in the same region.

Books have been devoted to the radiographic manifestations of tuberculosis. It is not our intent to be that thorough in our coverage here. We will present only the more frequent patterns of the disease, and hope that this, with your basic understanding of the disease process, will make it possible for you to diagnose tuberculosis, or at least be suspicious of this disease pattern whenever it is encountered.

Film C-29a and its associated tomogram C-29b were taken on a 49-year-old man as a routine film. His heart, hemidiaphragms, mediastinum, and left upper lung appear normal. However, the heavy arrow is placed in the right infraclavicular area to direct your attention to a linear area of infiltration. This area becomes much more apparent with tomography. The area involved is reasonably well demarcated on its inferior margin; but the superior portion of the infiltrate lacks definition, and shows some fingerlike projections extending into lung parenchyma. A second curved arrow on the tomogram points to an area of calcification extending around an upper lobe bronchus. The apical portion of the right lung shows considerable cystic change, as well as some fibrosis and scarring. The long, slender straight arrow pointing toward a soft-tissue density adjacent to the wall of the trachea on the right is pointing out the azygos vein. This should not be misinterpreted as a node. Nodes may occur here, but they must be identified in addition to this standard anatomical landmark. There is no evidence of cavitation nor adeno-

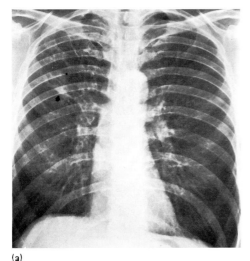

(a)

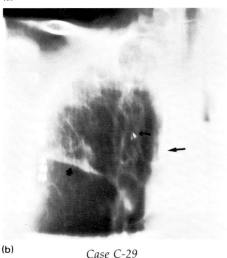

(b)   *Case C-29*

calcification in the right upper lung would make you feel that, hopefully, this might be a granulomatous process, and if the patient were a nonsmoker, this would offer additional weight to the diagnosis of tuberculous reinfection. The scarring and honeycombing in the right apex also indicate that the disease process may be a long standing one, and in this way favor the diagnosis of tuberculosis. Subsequently, acid-fast bacilli were found in this patient's sputum.

It is customary to classify tuberculosis as minimal, moderately advanced, or far advanced. The definition of these terms is dependent upon the volume of lung involved. The determination of active tuberculosis can rarely be made from a single film of the chest unless there is clear-cut cavitation. Active tuberculosis is suggested when the inflammatory process is seen to be either progressing or decreasing radiographically.

Our findings here indicate a minimal tuberculous lesion; since acid-fast bacilli were found, it is determined to be active from the clinical standpoint. Subsequent films will be necessary to confirm this radiographically. The cystic changes in the upper lung field imply that this is probably a secondary or even tertiary infection and that the scarring seen here is the residue of previous disease.

Case C-30 shows a more advanced stage of the disease than that seen in the previous case. A tomogram (C-30b) is also included here. Tomography is a vital part of the evaluation of chest lesions, particularly when the diagnosis of tuberculosis is suspected. Here, the infiltrate again involves the right upper lung, which is the most common site. There is some involvement of the anterior segment as evidenced by the continuation of the in-

pathy, and the calcification is indeed minimal.

This film demonstrates some of the real problems in the diagnosis of tuberculosis. Twenty years ago this would be called tuberculosis until proven otherwise. With disease patterns of the 1980s, one would consider this chest film highly suggestive of a neoplastic process with tuberculosis being in the differential diagnosis. The

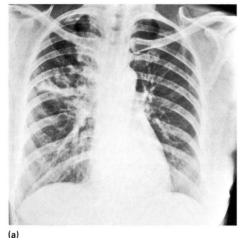

(a)

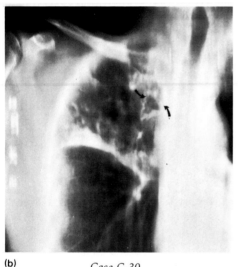

(b)   *Case C-30*

The two curved arrows indicate the medial and lateral wall of the unsuspected cavity. No adenopathy is identified, but the fixation of the medial portion of the minor fissure suggests that there is adenopathy present. Here again, we are producing the so-called "S sign" that we discussed with lung cancer. Again, the diagnosis of cancer of the lung must be in the differential. The points that swing our diagnosis away from neoplasia is the rather discrete cavity as well as the infiltrative lesion. It is surprising that calcification is a minimal factor here. Since the anterior segment is involved, it is a reasonable assumption that the patient is having primary tuberculous infection (there is no way that this can be proven; the assumption is made because of the absence of calcifications in the chest). There is no evidence of pleural fluid, and the left lung remains entirely clear. It is a diagnostic axiom that in active exudative tuberculosis there are contralateral heavy peribronchial-type densities in the opposite lung base. In this instance one would expect heavy markings in the left base, and these are not evident.

This patient was a 55-year-old woman. She was febrile and coughing. The history was of relatively short duration. Only location of the infiltrate and the cavity led to the proper diagnosis. Acid-fast bacilli were prevalent in the sputum.

Case C-30 represents an active exudative-type of tuberculosis. It probably represents the patient's primary exposure.

Case C-31 is that of a 65-year-old woman admitted with chronic pulmonary complaints and some weight loss. The routine film of the chest shows a small vertical heart, rather strikingly elevated hilar shadows, bilateral blebs in the apices, with scarring and some calcification, flat-

filtrate to the minor fissure. The infiltrative process is quite confluent. There is an alveolar exudate, and therefore the term *exudative* or active process is a logical one here. This is true despite the fact that we have a single film. The tomogram confirms the fact that this is an active process since an unsuspected cavity is seen in the medial portion of the right upper lung as indicated by the arrow.

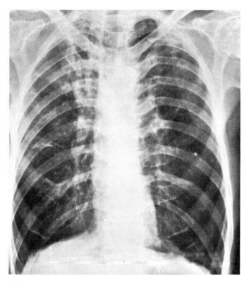

(a)

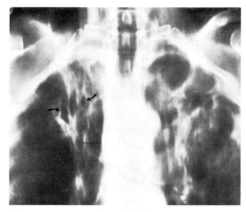

(b)   *Case C-31*

chiectatic cavities. The most common cause of upper lobe bronchiectasis is tuberculosis. Scarring is present; there is also some calcification in the left hilar area and in the right apex. No clear-cut cavities are identified except for the bronchiectatic changes mentioned above. The large pulmonary outflow tract on the left, as seen in the tomogram, would raise the question of either adenopathy or a primary neoplasm; however, this is most likely explained by retractions and scarring of the hilum due to the changes in the upper lung field.

The changes here would appear to be chronic and consist principally of scarring. The radiologist's report should indicate upper lung granulomatous disease principally scarring, but an active process cannot be ruled out. This latter statement is important because of the bronchiectasis; tubercle bacilli could be surviving in this region. This patient did not have tubercle bacilli in the sputum, so the findings here are principally those that represent the residue and scarring of such an infection.

The small vertical heart also deserved some comment. We frequently associate this finding with Addison's disease, which is frequently associated with tuberculosis. Clinically, this patient did not have Addison's disease; however, this radiographic picture is consistent with that diagnosis, and such a comment should be made by the radiologist to warn the clinican of that entity. The small vertical heart of Addison's disease is produced in part by the hyperaeration of the lung fields and also by the loss of blood volume secondary to sodium depletion.

Three cases of tuberculosis in varying stages have been presented. It is not implied that this represents the entire spec-

tening of the hemi-diaphragms, and a Ghon-type complex in the mid-lung field on the left.

The tomograms (C-31b) presented here reemphasize this technique's value. The pneumatoceles and blebs in each upper lung are striking, but also there are some rather thick-walled ovoid cavities in the right upper lung, indicated by curved arrows. These probably represent bron-

trum of tuberculosis. Tuberculosis can
mimick almost any disease in the chest.
One of the toughest radiographic differ-
entials that exists is that between primary
cancer of the lung and tuberculosis. Obviously, both have typical characteristics,
and if these are present, the differential
can be made with relative logic. Too many
times, as in the first two cases presented
here, there are overlapping signs and
symptoms. Sputum studies and/or bron-
choscopy is necessary to establish a diagnosis. Follow-up films of any suspect
lesion are important. Previous films are
frequently invaluable. Certainly the course
of the illness is extremely valuable in
making a differential diagnosis not only
in the chest, but in all areas of medicine.
Tuberculosis may be a very subtle or a
very fulminant disease. Fortunately it is
becoming less frequent in its occurrence,
and as a cause of death it is becoming
relatively unimportant. Even so, it still
occurs with enough frequency that any-
one seeing chest radiographs must be familiar with its many faces.

Case C-32

Case C-32 is a 57-year-old man admitted to the hospital for reconstructive joint
surgery. The patient had severe rheumatoid arthritis.

The chest film shows a very fine reticular pattern throughout the lung fields.
The tiny linear densities are interstitial
changes. Only a few tiny nodules, probably less than pinhead size, are noted in
the left lung base. The bases tend to be
more involved than the upper lungs, and
in fact the right infraclavicular area is
more radiolucent than the left. The appearance of the heart and aorta is not
unusual. The patient does show some

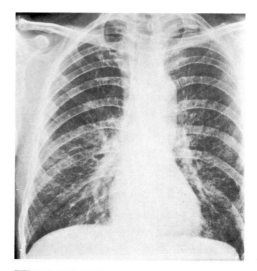

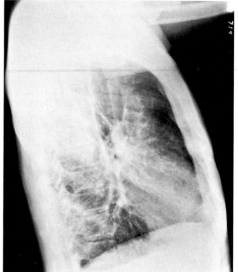

Case C-32

apical pleural thickening, especially on
the left.

Rheumatoid arthritis, as other collagen
diseases, produces a spectrum of changes
in the lung. The process is one of pulmonary fibrosis. The radiographic manifestations of pulmonary fibrosis may vary

all the way from a very faint ground-glass appearance through the reticular pattern seen here, and on to more nodular and cystic changes. It is easy to understand how progression of this interstitial fibrotic process would entrap small alveolar or lobular air spaces and produce cystic areas. As this entrapment progresses, pulmonary function decreases.

The films shown here are an excellent example of interstitial disease demonstrating principally a fine reticular pattern with minimal nodularity, and some air trapping in the right infraclavicular area.

Final diagnosis: Rheumatoid lung (pulmonary fibrosis secondary to a diffuse collagen disease).

2

The Mediastinum

No discussion of chest radiography would be complete without discussing the mediastinum and its contents. The mediastinum is a place or an area where important structures exist. Anatomists are inclined to divide the mediastinum into a superior and inferior portion, with the inferior portion of the mediastinum being subdivided into anterior, middle, and posterior sections. The superior mediastinum is defined as extending from the thoracic inlet down to the sternal manubrium junction and posterior to the D4-D5 joint space. This area contains a number of vital structures, but most of these are only as important as their inferior sites of origin. For this reason, radiologists tend to ignore the superior mediastinum and divide the entire mediastinum into anterior, middle, and posterior segments. There are more elaborate definitions but the practical boundaries described by Ben Felson are used by most radiologists. A line from the posterior edge of the heart upward above the margin of the anterior trachea separates the anterior from the mid-mediastinum.

The anterior mediastinal compartment is bounded anteriorly by the sternum, and posteriorly by the posterior pericardium and the trachea. The line separating the mid-mediastinum from the posterior mediastinum is a vertical line 1 cm posterior to the anterior edge of the dorsal bodies. The radiographic importance of the anterior mediastinum is related to pathological processes that occur here. In this relatively small space nearly 90% of the mass lesions will belong to one of the "three T" lesions. The three Ts referred to are thymus, thyroid, and teratoma. Thymic masses or thymomas obviously would occur in this area because of the presence of the thymus at this site during early life. The thyroid referred to implies a substernal extension of the thyroid, and at least 95% of substernal thyroids extend anteriorly into the anterior mediastinum. We have no good explanation as to why teratomas occur in the anterior mediastinum, but it is an observed clinical fact that they do.

There are some anterior mediastinal lymph nodes. Normally, these are not seen since most lymph nodes occur in the mid mediastinum. There is one striking exception to the latter statement—this is in the young adult with Hodgkin's disease or, less frequently, other forms of lymphoma. In these diseases the anterior mediastinum may be filled with involved nodes.

Of course, the internal mammary artery is in this space, but aneurysms of this vessel are quite rare. Aneurysms of the ascending aorta extend into this space. By our definition the heart with all its variable appearance is in the anterior mediastinum.

The middle mediastinal compartment contains the transverse portion of the aorta, the entire trachea, and major bronchi; pulmonary arteries and veins; and a relatively large collection of mediastinal lymph nodes.

Traditionally, mid-mediastinal masses are lymph node masses until proven otherwise. Obviously, there are other structures that can produce mass lesions here, for example, the esophagus, the trachea, and their variations. Neurogenic tumors of the vagus or phrenic nerves would occupy this space, as well as aneurysms of the vessels indicated.

The posterior mediastinal compartment contains the descending thoracic aorta, the hemiazygos system, and the sympathetic nerve chain, as well as a few posterior mediastinal lymph nodes. Classically, masses occurring in the posterior mediastinum are of nervous-tissue origin until proven otherwise. This accounts for at least 90% of the masses in the posterior mediastinum, and most of the exceptions that occur are in children where congenital lesions of the spine (anterior meningoceles) occur in this anatomical space.

The lateral margins of the mediastinum are defined by the medial pleural reflections and are distorted by the aorta and the heart-containing pericardium. Because of this distortion, the mediastinal reflections, as viewed in the PA projection, are usually best seen at the upper and inferior parts of the chest film. The presence of this mediastinal stripe emphasizes the fact that the mediastinum is more of a potential space than a real one. That is, it exists as a space only when anatomical structures or pathological processes separate the medial pleural reflections.

CASE PRESENTATIONS

Case M-1

The first case to be presented in our series of mediastinal masses is that of a 62-year-old white man. This patient had a chest x-ray study at his hometown hospital as part of a routine physical. A mass lesion was reported in the chest, and the patient was referred for additional workup.

In the PA projection (M-1a), the mass is seen to the right of the midline. It is identified by a dark curved arrow. In the lateral view (M-1b), two curved arrows point to the mass. which is low in density and superimposed on the vertebral bodies. The margins of the mass are very smooth. No variations in density are seen within the mass itself.

M-1a demonstrates the so-called "hilum overlay" sign, in which the hilar structures are seen clearly superimposed on the mass lesion. One could predict that the mass was either far anterior or far posterior, since hilar structures are not silhouetted out. No associated bone erosion is demonstrated, although a film to bring out the bone detail of the spine would be necessary to prove this point. There is some scoliosis of the spine to the right. This is presumably an incidental feature.

Another heavy arrow is directed to the anterior portion of the first rib on the left. This is simply to identify the chondral calcification that frequently occurs at the end of the first rib. A similar type of patchy density is seen on the right.

Overall evaluation of the radiograph shows some hyperaeration. This probably represents a mild degree of chronic obstructive pulmonary disease, although as people approach the age of 70 a certain

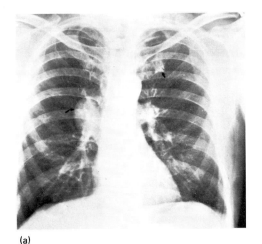

(a)

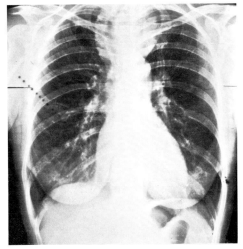

Case M-2

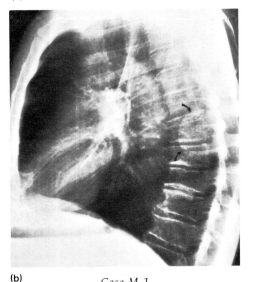

(b)   Case M-1

amount of hyperaeration results from degenerative changes in the lung but does not carry the disability associated with chronic obstructive lung disease.

Our final diagnosis was that of a neurogenic tumor in the posterior mediastinum. This was subsequently proven to be a neurofibroma. It follows the rule that we have previously listed in that neurogenic tumors are the most frequent mass lesions

in the posterior mediastinum. Generalized degenerative changes are also noted in the spine, lungs, and, to a lesser extent, vascular structures.

Case M-2

The next case in our series of mediastinal masses is the one that is probably the most frequently seen of all mediastinal bulky tumors. It has quite characteristic findings. The mass is in the superior portion of the mediastinum, and it displaces the trachea rather strikingly to the right (the trachea may be displaced in either direction). The displacement of the trachea implies that the lesion is relatively high in the anterior mediastinum, and the soft tissue margins of the mass extend above the clavicles indicating that there is a cervical component. Since these tumors are high they are difficult or impossible to visualize in the lateral view. We are not presenting a lateral film here since it did not add to our findings. The displacement of the trachea and the opacity extending above the clavicles localized the mass lesion quite adequately. Calcification may be seen in substernal lesions. Here, just above the clavicle, fine densities may represent calcifications. However, you will note that there are some small calcific densities in the first anterior interspace, just lateral to the lesion. Therefore, the patient presumably has some apical calcification separate from the mediastinal mass.

Substernal thyroids generally are extensions of the lower pole of one or the other thyroid lobes. These then extend inferiorly under the sternum and anterior to the trachea. A relatively small percentage of substernal thyroids will extend posterior to the trachea, and into the middle mediastinum. When this occurs it is invariably on the right, and the trachea is displaced to the left and slightly forward.

Our final diagnosis here is substernal thyroid. Its classical presentation is that of an anterior mediastinal mass with tracheal displacement.

Case M-3

Our next case in the mediastinal series is that of a 75-year-old woman who had myasthenia gravis. This is important clinical information since approximately 15% of the patients with myasthenia gravis have thymic tumors. Another statistic indicates that approximately 50% of patients with thymic tumors have myasthenia gravis.

Evaluation of the chest study (M-3a and M-3b) presented shows that there is a lobulated mass adjacent to the heart on the right side. M-3b shows that it is substernal, and definitely in the anterior mediastinum. A small arrow in the lateral film points to some very fine punctate calcification that is present within the mass. Calcifications in thymic tumors are usually peripheral and, as in this case,

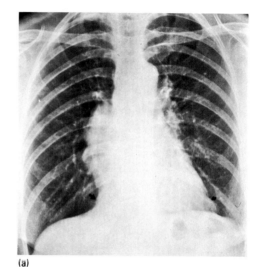
(a)

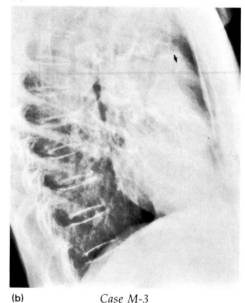
(b)   Case M-3

very fine and difficult to see. Some will only be demonstrated with tomography.

The short, heavy, dark arrow in the right cardiophrenic angle is directed toward a sharp line extending from the diaphragm up to the cardiac silhouette. This is a structure frequently visible on chest films, especially in slender, asthenic-type patients. This represents the venous trunk extending from the abdomen to the heart. It may be either the hepatic veins or the inferior vena cava. In the left cardiophrenic angle, a dark curved arrow is directed toward a soft-tissue density that is separate from the heart. This is a pericardial fat pad. These fat pads may be seen on either side and may become quite large. They are difficult to distinguish from pericardial cysts. The differential between these two entities is relatively unimportant since both are quite benign.

Our film (M-3a) also shows some asymmetry of the apical pleura with the right side being somewhat thicker and more dense than the left. This is always a point of concern, but it presumably is the residue of a chronic inflammatory process. Since our primary diagnosis here is that of thymoma, we will not pursue other differential diagnostic possibilities.

Thymic tumors may be either benign or malignant. The present case is a classical example. They tend to have smooth but lobulated margins. In general they are smaller than teratomas, and may even be so small that special studies such as tomography or air insufflation of the mediastinum or CT scanning may be needed to visualize the mass. They may occur on either side of the mediastinum, and as would be expected they are usually lower than substernal thyroids.

Our final diagnosis is lobulated thymoma in the right anterior mediastinum.

Case M-4

Our next case is a six-month-old infant. The chest film was made because the patient was having noisy respiration that was quite persistent. The infant had also had several respiratory infections.

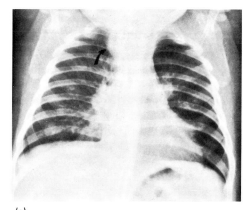

(a)

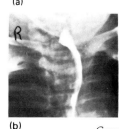 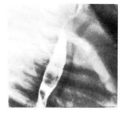

(b)   *Case M-4*

We have not discussed the infant chest, and only a few pediatric cases will be presented. The curved arrow on the PA projection (M-4a) shows a fullness in the upper mediastinum. The spot films (M-4b) made during a barium swallow shows that the esophagus and the trachea are displaced to the left, and the trachea is slightly displaced forward. Since the mass is behind the trachea, it must be classed as a middle mediastinal mass. Since approximately 5% of substernal thyroids do extend posterior to the trachea, this entity cannot be ruled out. It is to be recalled that when the thyroid does extend into the mid mediastinum, it is invariably on the right. However, a thyroid scan failed to show pickup in this area and showed the thyroid to be in a normal position. In a child the scan is at least 95% reliable in ruling out substernal extension.

Neurogenic tumors, including neuro-blastoma, arise in the posterior mediastin-um. This helps rule out the common child-hood tumor. Reduplication cysts of the tracheobronchial tree or esophagus tend to be in the middle mediastinum. As a general rule, they occur in or about the carina but can occur at any level within the mediastinum.

It is known that neurogenic tumors tend to accumulate technetium pyrophospate (the agent used frequently for bone scan-ning); and a bone scan therefore might be helpful in the differential diagnosis be-tween a neurogenic tumor and a redupli-cation cyst. In this case that study was not done. The patient was operated on.

The final diagnosis was that of a bron-chogenic cyst. The findings are rather typ-ical for that diagnosis, but the differential listed must be considered.

Case M-5

Case M-5 is a 12-year-old boy who was admitted to our hospital for the evaluation of a known chest mass. The child was currently asymptomatic. A previous chest film had been taken because of a respira-tory infection.

The chest film in each projection (M-5a and M-5b) is quite normal in appearance except for the large anterior mediastinal mass. Note that its margins are smooth, and in this instance there are no variations of density within the mass itself. The lesion is basically a hemisphere with the base of the mass sitting substernally and the dome of the mass extending toward the hilum.

The lesion is too low for a diagnosis of substernal thyroid, and there is no evi-dence of cervical extension and/or tracheal displacement. As a general rule, the lesion is larger than the usual thymoma, al-

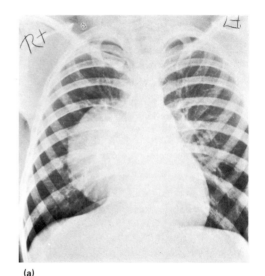

(a)

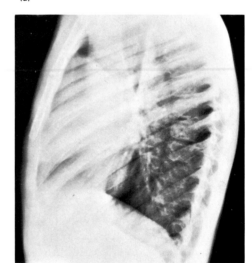

(b)   Case M-5

though size alone should not be consid-ered a major differential diagnostic point. It would be helpful if there were areas of decreased density (fat) within the mass or areas of increased density (bone or carti-lage) within the mass. These density var-iations may be demonstrated with CT scanning. The mass is too smooth to be considered lymph nodes of the type seen in lymphomas.

The final diagnosis and logical radiographic diagnosis is that of an anterior mediastinal teratoma.

Case M-6

Case M-6 is a newborn infant with respiratory distress. The PA radiograph (M-6a) of the chest shows a convex radiolucent line in the mid-chest as indicated by the curved black arrow directed toward the margin of the radiolucency. A sharp margin is not visible on the left. The lateral (M-6b) film shows increased radiolucency beneath the sternum. Other than this, the lung fields appear clear. The total lung volume may be somewhat reduced. The width of the superior mediastinum, separate from the radiolucency, is related to the thymus. Other findings are considered normal.

This is an example of pneumomediastinum in the newborn. This is the age group that has the highest incidence of this disorder. It may occur spontaneously, or it may represent a complication of respiratory distress syndrome. Certainly the incidence of pneumomediastinum rises in high-risk nurseries. Institutions that see many high-risk infants see a great deal of this entity. No one knows the incidence of pneumomediastinum but it may occur in as many as 1% of newborns.

Air can get into the mediastinum by rupture of an alveolus adjacent to a blood vessel, and the air dissects the tissue medially along the course of the vessel. The dissection can also occur peripherally, and a pneumothorax and pneumomediastinum result in the same patient.

In infants, unlike adults, the air in the mediastinum rarely dissects into the neck. The air may spread the lobes of the thy-

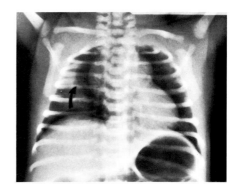

(a)

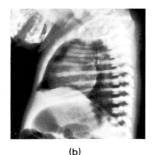

(b)

Case M-6

mus apart, and elevate them. The entity rarely needs treatment as it is a self-limiting process, but if the pressure is high and respiratory distress evident, the pressure can be easily relieved with a mediastinal tap.

Case M-7

Our next case, Case M-7 is that of a 21-year-old man who reported to the emergency room with chest pain. His history includes chest pain and coughing that developed while he was eating potato chips.

The chest study shows clearly the signs of air in the mediastinum. The PA projection shows vertical reflections of the medial pleura on each side, as evidenced by

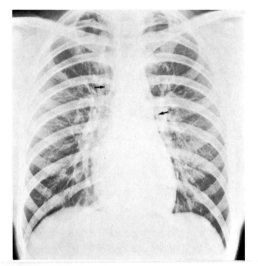

(a)

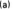

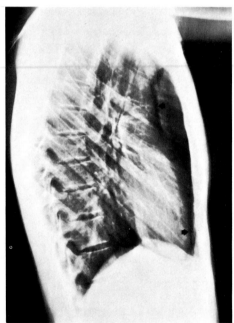

(b)   Case M-7

the arrows. Air is seen in the mediastinum up to the level of the clavicles and all the way down to the apex of the heart on the left. Air in the lateral film is identified by the heavy dark arrow in the anterior mediastinum. Air is also seen extending into the substernal area between the heart and the chest wall. It is identified by the heavy arrow pointing toward the xiphoid.

Assuming the history was important, we made an attempt to identify a tear in the esophagus. Our esophageal study was unsuccessful in finding extravasation.

Trauma is one of the causes of pneumomediastinum in adults. Usually this is closed chest trauma, but certainly laceration of the esophagus, whether it be from vomiting or from foreign-body ingestion can produce the same findings. Tracheostomy may permit leakage of air into the mediastinum, and probably this is the most common cause of this entity.

Just as pneumothorax can occur on a spontaneous basis, so can pneumomediastinum. Symptoms are much the same.

Air has also been reported in the mediastinum secondary to pneumoperitoneum. This is quite uncommon, but it is a reasonable explanation when air is known to exist in the peritoneum.

As in infants, pneumomediastinum in adults rarely requires treatment. If it is secondary to laceration of the esophagus, the question of infection and chemical mediastinitis must be considered. Air will dissect into the soft tissues of the neck in adults, but rarely is the pressure in the mediastinum high enough to warrant tapping.

Case M-8

Case M-8 is a routine chest film made on a 77-year-old woman.

This film is presented to demonstrate a

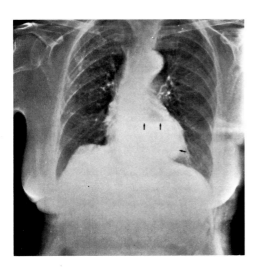

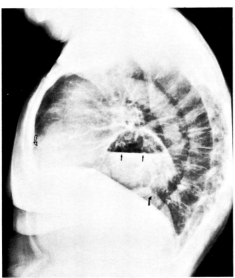

Case M-8

frequent and sometimes confusing radiographic finding. On the PA radiograph there is a midline air/fluid level. It is even more evident on the lateral since it is behind the heart. Two vertical arrows indicate the fluid level here. A third similar solid arrow points to the left lateral margin of the mass where it superimposes on the heart silhouette.

The solid curved arrow on the lateral film points to a section of diaphragm that has not contracted or descended in a uniform way with the rest of the diaphragm. Since this is below the level of the dome of the diaphragm, it is not visible in the PA view. It is of no clinical significance.

An open curved arrow at the anterior portion of the lateral view is directed toward a calcified coronary artery. Other than moderate kyphosis and some generalized degenerative disease, there are no other pertinent findings on the film. Final diagnosis: The lesion behind the heart is not an abscess or other mediastinal tumor of significance; it represents instead a large hiatal hernia. This is a frequent finding in the chest of elderly patients. The air/fluid level makes the diagnosis easy. If there is no air in the stomach, it appears as a solid mass; however, a swallow of barium or simply the realization that not all gastric structures above the diaphragm have air will lead to a diagnosis of a persistent hiatal hernia. Final diagnosis: Hiatal hernia, generalized degenerative change.

3

The Cardiovascular System

To this point most of our discussion involving the chest has centered about lung pathology. Obviously there is another major component to the chest that is very much involved in the health and disease of patients. This is the heart and vascular system as visualized on the chest radiograph. Volumes have been written on the radiographic evaluation of the cardiovascular system. Our discussion will deal with fundamental changes seen on the chest radiograph and will not include special procedures. However, if you can accurately evaluate the processes described here, virtually all of the possible nonangiographic diagnosis can be made.

The following is a relatively simple approach to the plain chest film diagnosis of cardiovascular disease:

1. Is the heart enlarged? We have previously indicated that the maximum permissible heart-size measurement is equivalent to one half the maximum inside diameter of the chest. This is a determination that can be made very simply by the use of a ruler. This author prefers the cardiothoracic ratio in estimating overall cardiac enlargement, but this ratio has its critics. Certainly if you insist that general rules cover all circumstances, this rule will occasionally fail. Its failures can be covered if you use judgment and accept that rules can be broken. Certainly if hemidia-

phragms are markedly elevated as in late pregnancy or ascites, the ratio will be distorted. At the other end of the spectrum of hemidiaphragm levels, in severe chronic obstructive pulmonary disease with low diaphragms, a vertically positioned heart distorts the rule. In such a circumstance, serial films showing changes in heart measurement are much more important. Another very important part of this determination is to find out which, if any, of the chambers are enlarged. It is possible for the overall heart size to be normal, but for one chamber to be disproportionately enlarged. This is obviously significant. Therefore, it is important not only to know the heart size from an overall standpoint, but also the size of the chambers. The left ventricle is rarely enlarged without the overall size of the heart being increased. However, subtle left ventricular enlargement can be identified as the heart mass extends posteriorly to the inferior vena cava, as we reported on page 14 in the Chest Section. Right ventricular enlargement is much more difficult to evaluate, for it is defined only as the filling of the substernal space. Here the contour of the chest is important, as well as the size of the cardiac mass. Left atrial enlargement will be identified on the lateral film as the portion of the heart extending posteriorly at the level of, or slightly below the level of the carina. This is usually seen in mitral valve disease. Right atrial enlargement is an infrequent, isolated finding. It can be identified as a disproportionate fullness of the right heart margin as seen in the PA projection without apparent enlargement on the lateral film.

2. Is the pulmonary vascular bed normal? The size of the pulmonary bed reflects the volume of blood in the lung fields. It may also reflect pulmonary vascular pressure, and it is certainly representative of the output of the right ventricle. The pulmonary vascular bed includes everything distal to the pulmonary valve. In the presence of pulmonary valvular stenosis with post-stenotic dilatation, the pulmonary outflow tract will be disproportionately large compared with the remaining pulmonary bed. This may also be true with increased peripheral lung resistance, where the proximal pulmonary vessels may be dilated. Asymmetry of the blood flow in the lungs may represent a pulmonary embolus or unilateral lung anomalies. Pulmonary edema and changes in lung vascular patterns are important in establishing the diagnosis of congestive failure. It is granted with right heart failure that the chest film may be normal, but this, in itself, would be an important finding. The presence of Kerley B-lines, while not 100% specific for increased pulmonary venous pressure, certainly are very important diagnostic findings in mitral valve disease or in any process that elevates the pulmonary venous pressure.

3. Is the aorta normal in size and appearance? Just as the pulmonary vessels are the reflection of the right heart output, the aorta is the reflection of the left heart output to the systemic circulation. All diseases that reduce the filling of the left ventricle are associated with a relatively small aorta. Those diseases that shunt blood from the left ventricle to the right are also known to demonstrate a small diameter aorta. Examples would include a defect in the atrial septum and mitral insufficiency. On the other hand, lesions that increase aortic volume increase its size. An example would be tetralogy of Fallot where the right heart outflow is reduced by pulmonary stenosis and the overriding aorta receives blood from both ventricles.

Rarely will the area of coarctation be demonstrated when this entity is present. However, a prominent ascending aorta and rib notching provide strong evidence of this disease entity. Dissecting aortic aneurysm is a much more difficult diagnosis, but when the aorta is increasing in size or changing its contour, this diagnosis should be suspected.

4. Are there vascular calcifications present? Most elderly patients show calcification in the aortic arch. Certainly if calcification occurs here, it can be anticipated in other vascular structures. This offers supportive evidence for the diagnosis of arteriosclerotic heart disease. Other calcifications (including calcification of heart valves) may be of diagnostic help in establishing a cardiovascular diagnosis. Valvular calcification is best seen with fluoroscopy, but frequently the heavy calcification that occurs in the annulus of the valve is evident in radiographs. Calcification of the pericardium is uniformly indicative of constrictive pericarditis. Calcifications in the coronary vessels may be identified; however, while this does not necessarily mean obliteration of the lumen of the vessel, it is a significant observation.

On every chest radiograph one should mentally process the questions raised in the preceding section. If the findings are such that the questions can be answered with a high degree of confidence, there is no doubt that most cardiovascular conditions amenable to plain film diagnosis can be made. On the other hand, some subtle changes may be very difficult to evaluate. When this occurs, other more specialized forms of examination, such as angiography or nuclear imaging, may be required.

CASE PRESENTATIONS

Case V-1

Case V-1 is a 33-year-old man admitted for a routine chest study (V-1a and V-1b). The heart is normal in size and outline. Lung fields are clear throughout; however, the case is presented because of what might be interpreted as a mass beneath the medial end of the right clavicle. It is also noted that there is a vertical stripe along the right vertebral margin, as indicated by the lower arrow on the PA projection. Note also that there is no aortic arch seen on the left, and no descending aortic stripe on the left.

The lateral film is also very important in the diagnosis here since it shows the trachea to be displaced slightly forward at the level of the aortic arch. This is marked by the black arrow.

This is a classical demonstration of a right-sided aortic arch. The findings may vary in degree. Certainly a tortuous aortic arch will be more striking in the PA projection, and it will also produce more displacement of the trachea. This must not be confused with a mediastinal mass, and the plain chest film appearance is so classical that further studies need not be done. The most important criteria for the

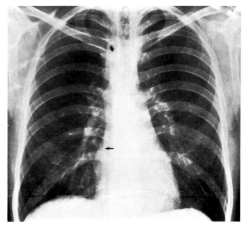

(a)

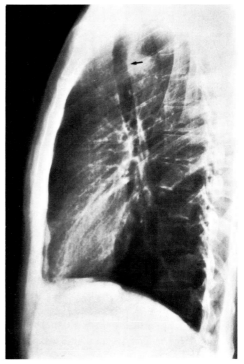

(b)

Case V-1

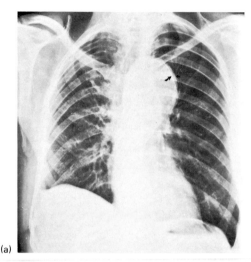

(a)

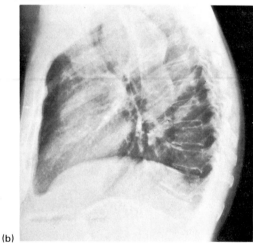

(b)

Case V-2

diagnosis are absence of the left aortic arch and forward displacement of the trachea as seen laterally.

A right-sided aorta may be part of more complex cardiovascular congenital anomalies, such as tetralogy of Fallot; but in this case it is an unimportant, isolated anomaly.

Our final diagnosis is right-sided aortic arch.

Case V-2

This patient was admitted for a follow-up study for a known diagnosis of aortic arch aneurysm. The aneurysm had been discovered approximately a year earlier, and it was elected to follow the patient rather than to intervene surgically. Our current films (V-2a and V-2b) showed no significant change from that seen a year before.

The heart is normal in size and outline. The absence of left ventricular prominence seems to rule out any aortic valve involvement. The dilated aorta, as visualized in the PA projection, clearly shows the calcification in the aortic arch. This is indicated by the dark arrow directed laterally. A small arrow directed medially points to the outline of the soft tissues over the calcification. The soft-tissue thickness or the distance between the points of the two arrows has been used as a guide for a dissecting aneurysm. However, this can only be used with confidence if there is a distinct change between two films. One would expect that if this soft-tissue thickness were quite marked a dissection would be present. Despite the logic of this assumption, we know that slight differences in projection may exaggerate the thickness of this soft-tissue plane. Therefore, it cannot be used as an index for dissection unless a previous film is available for comparison. In the lateral view, the aneurysm appears to be sharply demarcated on both its superior and inferior margins. Therefore, this is a saccular aneurysm. The anterior edge of the aneurysm starts at the level of the posterior trachea and results in slight forward angulation of the trachea. It is generally considered that the cervical cephalic vessels arise anterior to this point. However, an aortogram would be necessary to be certain that the left subclavian was not involved in the aneurysm.

Other observations should be made on this film. There is blunting of the right costophrenic angle. When an aortic aneurysm dissects, fluid may leak into the pleural space and produce blunting of the costophrenic angle. However, this is rarely seen on the right. This dissection and subsequent pleural fluid, almost without exception, occurs on the left. Again, comparison with an old film would be helpful in ruling out an acute process. This patient also has a moderate degree of scoliosis of the dorsal spine to the right, which is unrelated to the vascular pathology. Final diagnosis: Saccular aneurysm of the aortic arch, presumably degenerative in origin. Scoliosis of the spine with old pleural reaction on the right.

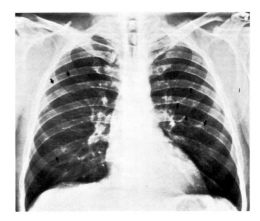

Case V-3

Case V-3

The patient is a 50-year-old man with hypertension.

The heart is normal in its overall size, with no special chamber enlargement noted. The open arrow to the right of midline identifies the ascending aorta. The pulmonary vascularity and lung fields are not remarkable in their appearance.

The case is presented principally to show the classical rib notching that is associated with coarctation of the aorta. In patients with coarctation of the aorta, rib notching occurs due to erosion from the pulsating, dilated intercostal arteries that are part of the collateral flow. Rib notching rarely occurs above the level of the third rib or below the level of the ninth rib. Notching due to coarctation always involves the inferior margin of the rib. There are a few other conditions that result in rib notching, namely neurofibromas along intercostal nerves, or other vas-

cular malformations. Rib notching has also been reported on the superior portion of the rib, but this is usually not related to coarctation, but is secondary to pressure from some other source. One explanation has been that rib notching is due to pressure from the scapula, described in patients with paralysis secondary to poliomyelitis.

The rib notches seen here show considerable variation in their prominence. On the right the two heavy arrows show very small rib notches, which if seen alone might be considered less than diagnostic. On the other hand, the inferior margin of the eighth rib on the left reveals a deep deformity.

The prominence of the ascending aorta would be anticipated secondary to the large volume of blood in the ascending aorta compared with the volume in the descending aorta. Rarely can the coarcted segment be seen on plain radiographs. Certainly the narrow segment is not seen here.

Final diagnosis: Coarctation of the aorta with classical rib notching.

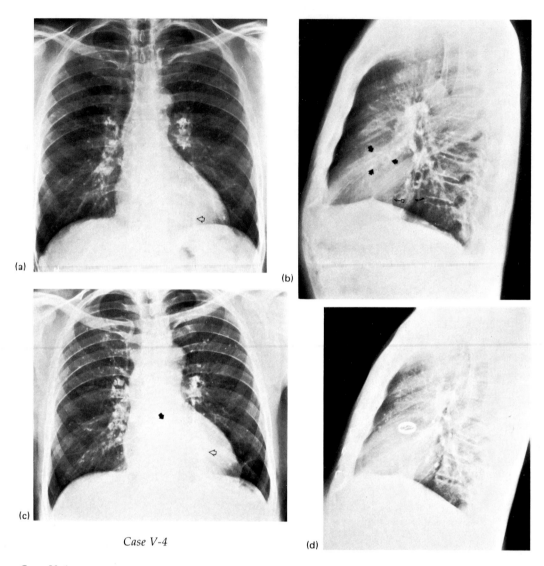

(a)

(b)

(c)

(d)

Case V-4

Case V-4

Case V-4 is a 49-year-old white man admitted to the cardiovascular service with a working diagnosis of aortic stenosis. The patient was being considered for aortic valve replacement.

The cardiothoracic ratio is just within the normal limits. The apex of the heart is somewhat prominent, and the axis of the heart as viewed in the PA projection (V-4a) tends to tilt downward toward the left. The ascending aorta and the arch are prominent. The descending aorta is quite well visualized along the paraspinous area on the left.

In the lateral projection (V-4b) the left ventricle projects posteriorly as indicated by the curved solid arrow. It is posterior to the inferior vena cava, indicated by the open arrow. This implies left ventricular enlargement. This rule, like the cardiothoracic ratio, requires reasonable judgment; either a depressed sternum or kyphosis will negate the rule. It is also reasonable to expect at least 1.5 cm of heart behind the inferior vena cava before it is significant. The three solid arrows outline some scattered, illusive, calcific densities. These calcifications could easily be overlooked because of the extensive calcification seen in the hilar areas and in the lung parenchyma. However, this is the characteristic appearance of calcification in the aortic valve when viewed in the lateral projection. Fluoroscopy is helpful, for with it one can identify the pulsations and movements of the calcifications that are characteristic of valvular densities. Aortic calcifications can be seen only on the lateral and left anterior oblige projections; they are obscured by the heart and spine in the PA projection.

The calcifications seen scattered throughout the lung fields are not an unusual finding in persons living in the midwestern United States. In fact, most chest films show some degree of calcification. However, it is not usually this extensive. These calcifications were biopsied at the time of valve replacement and found to be histoplasmosis, which is no surprise in this locality.

The open-faced arrow in the PA projection points to a vertical line behind the heart. This is a very small area of linear atelectasis. It is only pointed out so that you can compare this with the following films.

Films V-4c and V-4d are postoperative radiographs. They are shown to demonstrate the position of the aortic valve prosthesis. A heavy arrow is directed toward the valve prosthesis in the PA projection. It overlies the heart and spine, and even on review of the initial PA radiograph it would be difficult to identify the fine calcifications of the aortic valve because of the overlying spine and the heart density.

The open arrow on the PA projection shows heavy vertical streaking at the same location where an arrow of the same type showed a very fine vertical streak. This is linear atelectasis in this postoperative patient. The patient is now approximately eight days postoperative. The linear atelectasis is a frequent finding in patients having had cardiac surgery. It is seen so frequently that it is considered part of the postoperative recovery process and of very little clinical significance. Final diagnosis: The study shown here is a demonstration of the changes that occur with aortic stenosis. There is left ventricular prominence with some dilatation of the ascending aorta (post-stenotic dilatation), and valvular calcification, which is seen in at least 30% of patients with this disease. Incidental findings include calcific histoplasmosis and the usual postoperative linear atelectasis and demonstration of the position of the aortic valve by the presence of the valve prosthesis.

Case V-5

Our next case is that of a 34-year-old man who had been the victim of blunt abdominal trauma. He had internal bleeding and was initially in shock. Later in the course of his illness, he developed a pseudocyst of the pancreas. However, this is unimportant to us in evaluating his chest radiograph.

The chest radiograph (V-5) was made nearly two weeks after admission. The patient had a constant problem maintaining fluid and electrolyte balance.

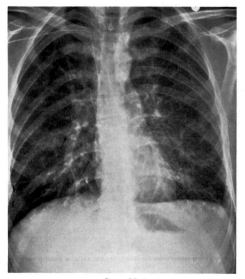

Case V-5

The heart is small (this is important) and in the midline. There is a central venous catheter entering from the right subclavian area with the tip directed into the superior vena cava. An oxygen tube is also seen running diagonally across the upper chest.

The most striking feature of the chest film is the demonstration of interstitial fluid. The small arrow, one pointing vertically and one inferiorly in the right lateral base, are directed toward classical Kerley B-lines. This is one of the most important observations to note in evaluating the vascular status of the lung bed in any patient where this may be a problem. It was initially thought to represent only distended lymphatics, but now we feel it represents increased fluid or tissue in the interstitial space of the lungs, not all of which need be in the lymphatics. These lines are characteristically less than 2 cm in length, and less than 1 mm in diameter. They are seen in fluid overload

as is the[1] case here or in patients with increased pulmonary pressure, such as congestive failure and mitral stenosis. These entities are the most common process that produces these lines.

The long slender arrows directed at an angle, but basically cephalad in the midportion of the right lower lung field, are pointing toward lines that are over 2 cm in length and approximately 1 mm in diameter. These longer lines in the midportion of the chest exist approximately halfway between the pleura and the hilum. They do not follow the arteries or veins precisely. These are Kerley A-lines. Kerley A-lines follow the distribution of lymphatics, but are much heavier and larger than a lymphatic. Their visibility probably depends on edema fluid along paralymphatic connective tissues, again an interstitial process.

Kerley also described C lines; however, some authors feel that they represent only Kerley B-lines projected "en face." Clinically, they are considered unimportant. Actually, even the Kerley A-lines are of little importance, other than to demonstrate the observer's diagnostic sophistication. Kerley B-lines are practical.

The vascular structures seen here are also somewhat distended, and there is blunting of the left costrophrenic angle indicating a small amount of pleural fluid. It is important to recognize that this edema is not cardiac in origin. The fluid volume is generally increased with all vessels dilated but no reversal of lung distribution pattern and no heart enlargement. Lung edema of cardiac origin may occur prior to detectable heart enlargement—the classical example is acute myocardial infarction. However, even in such a case, the upper lung vessels show disproportionately high flow.

The final diagnosis here is that of fluid overload, with a good demonstration of the radiographic findings associated with this entity.

There are entities other than pulmonary edema and increased pulmonary pressure that produce prominent Kerley B-lines on films. Extensive lymphatic infiltration with tumor will produce interstitial lines. This has been reported from cancer of the stomach or breast, as well as from lymphomas. Coarse interstitial lines are prominent in cases of pulmonary fibrosis, where the interlobular portion of the lung becomes thickened and scarred.

Case V-6

Case V-6 is a 50-year-old white man who was admitted to the hospital with a history of decreasing ability to perform physical activity over the past two months. His history was important in that he had a myocardial infarction 18 months earlier, and the infarction was in the distribution of the left anterior descending coronary artery with an anterior lateral wall infarction.

The heart is enlarged. Changes in the heart contour are indicated by the solid black arrows. In the PA (V-6a) projection, the arrow points to a bulge along the superior margin of the heart at a point approximately halfway between the apex and hilum. The lateral view (V-6b) shows the bulging segment to be anterior, again consistent with the anterior wall of the left ventricle. The lateral film also shows some fullness of the left ventricle posteriorly. These changes are considered those of a ventricular aneurysm.

The rest of the chest findings are unremarkable. There is no evidence of congestive failure. The costophrenic angles are sharp, indicating no significant fluid.

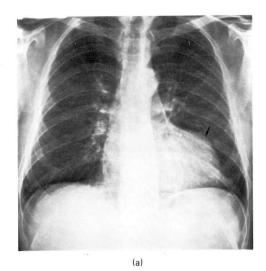

(a)

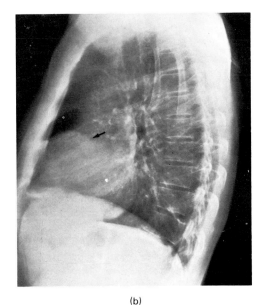

(b)

Case V-6

There are some coarse vertical lines noted through the heart silhouette, again consistent with some minor linear atelectasis.

It is now possible by using radioactive materials to determine the ejection fraction in a noninvasive way. This patient's ejection fraction was 35%, which represents a significant decrease from the normal (normal is usually considered 50% or higher). In addition to this calculation, it is possible to observe the wall motion, and get an idea as to how extensive and how detrimental the aneurysmal segment is to the left ventricular ejection fraction. If it can be shown that the rest of the ventricle is contracting very well, but that efficiency of the ventricle is lost due to the localized aneurysm, it can be predicted that surgery will be helpful. This same type of data is useful in identifying the inoperable patient.

Final diagnosis: Left ventricular aneurysm. This patient was operated on, and the diagnosis confirmed; his functional status improved.

Case V-7

The patient is a 54-year-old white woman admitted to the hospital because of peripheral edema. She had been known to have a heart murmur for a number of years.

Inspection of the PA chest radiograph (V-7a) shows that there is, without a doubt, overall cardiac enlargement. Identification of the chamber that is enlarged is more difficult. The lateral film (V-7b) shows the inferior vena cava (indicated by the curved dark arrow) to be in the midchest and very little heart silhouette is seen extending posterior to this line. There is prominent fullness in the anterior superior portion of the heart, as indicated by the inferiorly directed dark arrow over the heart margin. At this point we are inclined to believe that the cardiac enlargement is principally on the right. The differentiation between enlargement of the right ventricle and the right atrium may be difficult. Usually, right ventricular

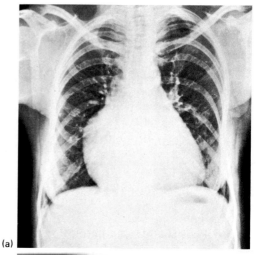

(a)

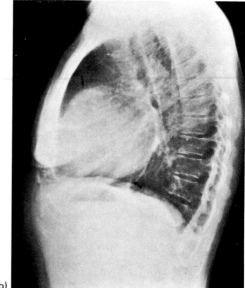

(b)

Case V-7

enlargement produces more intimate association of the heart silhouette and the inferior margin of the sternum than we see here. Another maneuver that this author uses that is sometimes helpful, but not always diagnostic, is to take a piece of paper and cover the right half of the chest. When this is done it is amazing how normal the left heart appears when viewed in the PA projection. This maneuver, plus the appearance of the heart in the lateral projection, indicated that the enlargement here is principally right atrial.

Clinical correlation is always valuable. Here the clinical findings of evident transmitted pulsation from the heart to the jugular veins and the liver is indicative of tricuspid valve insufficiency.

Final diagnosis here is tricuspid valve disease, most likely insufficiency. This was confirmed, and the patient improved with tricuspid valve replacement.

Tricuspid lesions are infrequent in our experience, but we felt that they deserved mention, if for no other reason than to offer some comments in regard to the identification of right atrial enlargement.

Case V-8

Case V-8 is that of a 58-year-old woman admitted to the hospital with moderate shortness of breath and considerable peripheral edema.

The heart is only slightly enlarged (V-8a and 8b). By actual measurement the heart size is equal to one half the inside dimension of the chest. The open arrow to the right of the midline points to a superimposed curved type of density seen through the heart shadow. This is the classical radiograph appearance of the so-called double density of left atrial enlargement. A second open arrow is directed just to the left of the midline, and points to an area where the left mainstem bronchus is slightly elevated. This, too, is a characteristic feature of left atrial enlargement. The third open arrow, which is slightly curved, points to a very faint bulge in the straightened left heart mar-

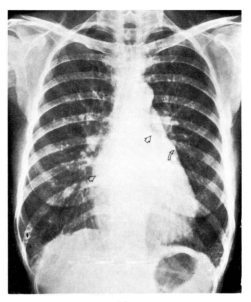

(a)

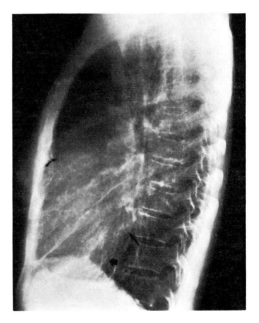

(b)

Case V-8

gin. This slight prominence is considered secondary to the left atrial appendage, as it rises slightly over the margin of the heart. In general, left atrial enlargement results in straightening of the left heart margin, but if the atrial appendage appears above the usual heart margin there is a convexity away from the heart at the level just below the hilum. In the lateral projection a heavy solid arrow identifies the inferior vena cava as it enters the right atrium. Little or no cardiac silhouette is seen extending posterior to this point, indicating that enlargement of the left ventricle is not a feature in this patient's cardiac problem.

The curved arrow seen beneath the lower portion of the sternum simply points to the filling in of the substernal space. The patient does show slight depression of the xiphoid and the distal part of the sternum. The long solid arrow in the lateral projection, which is above the short heavy arrow, and just anterior to the tenth dorsal vertebral body indicates the level of the lower margin of the left atrium. It is always surprising to show that the left atrium is relatively high when viewed in the lateral projection. Significant displacement of the esophagus will be demonstrated between the level of the pulmonary artery and the inferior margin at D10, as indicated here.

The aortic arch, as viewed in the PA projection, is certainly not large, but relatively small considering the overall cardiac size.

Short dark arrows are seen in the right costophrenic angle. These identify Kerley B-lines, which represent increased pulmonary venous pressure. The vessels in the upper lung fields are prominent, but show no evidence of edema. The minor fissure between the middle and upper lobe is visible in the PA view, indicating a very small amount of fluid in the fissure. In the right lateral view the major fissure is visible inferiorly.

In summary, in our radiographic findings, we are demonstrating modest overall cardiac enlargement—specifically, chamber enlargement involving the left atrium. There is also right ventricular enlargement. The left ventricle is considered normal, and the aorta, that is the outflow tract of the left ventricle is also normal or small. Pulmonary vessels in the upper lungs are heavy, and Kerley B-lines are present. All of these findings indicate that there is pathology in the mitral valve, with transmitted increased pressure behind it. Since the left ventricle is not enlarged, and the right ventricle is prominent, our findings indicate mitral stenosis. With mitral stenosis there is reversal of the pulmonary blood flow patterns, with increasing blood flow in the upper lung fields, and the presence of Kerley B-lines, which reflect the increased pressure in the pulmonary venous bed.

Final diagnosis: Mitral stenosis.

Case V-9

Case V-9 is a 47-year-old woman admitted to the hospital with intermittent shortness of breath and nocturnal dyspnea.

The chest radiographs (V-9a and V-9b) are quite striking in their appearance. The heart is markedly enlarged, and the enlargement appears generalized. However, open-faced arrows in the right chest outline the double density so characteristic of enlargement of the left atrium. In this instance the left atrium extends even more laterally than the right atrium. The superior arrow in the right chest identifies the left atrium, which is now outside the margin, as indicated by the curved open arrow. This, again, is considered to be the left atrial appendage. The aorta actually appears small when compared to a heart of this magnitude.

The lateral view also shows the marked cardiac enlargement. However, the curved arrow anteriorly indicates that there is no remarkable substernal filling by the cardiac silhouette. The heavy inferior arrow points to the inferior vena cava, and there is evidence of the heart extending posterior to this landmark. The upper diagonal arrow on the lateral chest radiograph indicates the rather evident displacement of the left mainstem bronchus posteriorly by the enlarged cardiac mass. A barium swallow in this instance would show marked displacement of the esophagus posteriorly from the level of the hilum, probably all the way to the hemidiaphragm.

The lung fields are quite clear. Pulmonary vessels in the hilar area are somewhat prominent. There are no Kerley B-lines. The black branching type of density seen overlying the upper dorsal spine and the left infraclavicular area (indicated by the short solid arrow) are static electricity artifacts—of no significance. They do detract from the quality of the film, but once recognized they do not handicap the evaluation.

To summarize the radiographic findings, there is evidence of heart enlargement. The enlargement is principally in the left atrium and left ventricle. Despite the enlarged left ventricle, the aorta is small; and the pulmonary vasculature shows only a modest increase with no evidence of heart failure. The presence of left atrial enlargement implies mitral valve disease.

The fact that the left ventricle is more strikingly enlarged than the right would

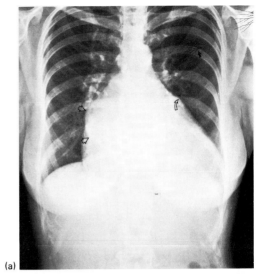

(a)

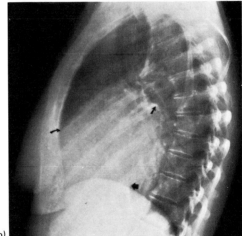

(b)

Case V-9

indicate that the patient has mitral insufficiency, but, in this instance we cannot rule out an associated aortic stenosis. The aorta is also small, reflecting low forward stroke volume of the ventricle. Final diagnosis: Mitral valve disease, considered to be mitral insufficiency. This radiographic study cannot rule out associated aortic stenosis.

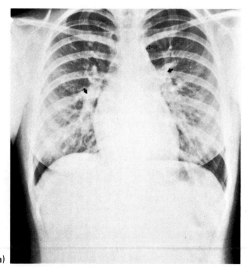

(a)

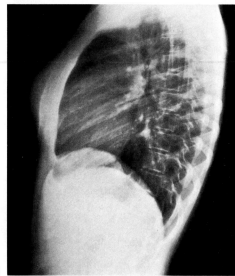

(b)

Case V-10

Case V-10

Case V-10 is a 13-year-old girl admitted to the hospital because of purpura. In the course of her workup, it was noted that she had a significant systolic heart murmur. Her past cardiovascular history was negative, although the family did admit

that they had been told that the child had a murmur several years before.

The overall size of the heart falls well within normal limits (V-10a and V-10b). The lateral radiograph shows no cardiac mass extending posterior to the inferior vena cava. There is moderate substernal fullness.

The most striking features on this film relate to the outflow tracts of the two chambers. Pulmonary vessels indicated by the heavy dark arrows are large and extend as relatively large trunks to the peripheral lung. On the other hand the aorta is so small that it is barely visible. It is indicated by the open arrow just beneath the left medial clavicle.

Since the aorta reflects the output of the left ventricle, and the pulmonary vessels reflect the output to the right ventricle, we must assume that the pulmonary circulation is carrying an additional load. This is further supported by the indication of right heart enlargement on the lateral film. These findings are very characteristic of an intracardiac left-to-right shunt. This shunt could be found at either the ventricular or atrial level. Some patients with an intracardiac left-to-right shunt have some enlargement of the left atrium. This generally occurs with a ventricular septal defect. This is due to the increased pulmonary venous return to this chamber. When this occurs, it usually indicates a larger or more significant defect. The case here does not show significant left atrial enlargement.

The pattern differs from what we see with a patent ductus. With a patent ductus, the shunt is outside the heart. In this case it is the left ventricle that must pump, not only the systemic blood, but also the blood that is shunted through the third circuit, namely, that recirculating through the ductus. It is also true, with a patent ductus, that the left ventricular outflow tract is increased because the proximal aorta must carry not only the systemic blood, but that blood shunted back to the pulmonary circuit.

Our final diagnosis here is intracardiac left-to-right shunt, in this case an atrial septal defect.

Case V-11

Case V-11 is a 49-year-old man admitted to the hospital because of a stroke. His past medical history indicated that he had known of a septal defect in his heart since the age of five. He had dyspnea on exertion, and four days prior to admission had the sudden onset of symptoms indicating an embolus to the brain.

We are presenting only a PA view of the chest for it shows the pertinent points in this case. The heart is at the upper limits of normal in size. The pulmonary outflow tracts are grossly enlarged. An arrow on the right side is directed toward a level of the large right pulmonary artery where the diameter sharply decreases. All peripheral vessels beyond this point appear to be relatively small. Similar findings are noted on the left, but the heart itself obscures most of the large pulmonary trunks. The aorta is so small that it is not definitely visible on the film.

The history and radiographic findings certainly indicate that the patient has an intracardiac left-to-right shunt. However, the chopping off of the large vessels in the mid lung field indicates that the patient has had the lesion for such a long time that pulmonary hypertension has developed. In this instance the patient's pulmonary pressure approached that of his systemic pressure. It was shown that the patient had venous thrombosis in the

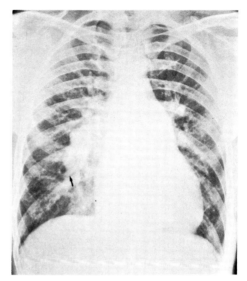

Case V-11

legs, which resulted in the embolus going to the heart, but instead of infarcting the lungs as would be expected, the embolus was shunted through the defect into the left heart. Patients with this much pulmonary hypertension usually have cyanosis. However, this may be an intermittent phenomenen.

Final diagnosis: Atrial septal defect with complicating pulmonary hypertension and reversal of the usual left-to-right shunt to intermittent right-to-left shunting.

Case V-12

Case V-12 is a 16-year-old boy admitted to the hospital because of a known heart murmur, with the development of dyspnea and reduced ability to perform physically.

The overall size of the heart is within the upper limits of normal. The lateral film shows no cardiac mass extending behind the inferior vena cava, but there

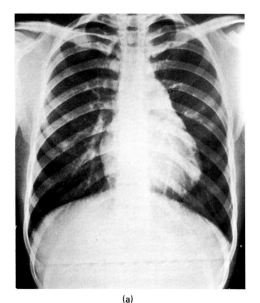

(a)

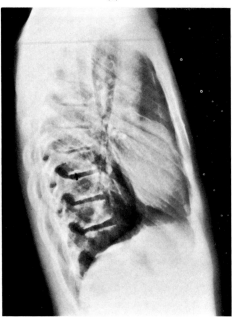

(b)

Case V-12

is apparently fullness in the region of the right ventricle since there is a heart density extending into the substernal space to a relatively high level. A curved open arrow points to a prominent pulmonary outflow tract, the pulmonary conus. The vessels distal to this fall off sharply in diameter, and practically no vessels are visible in the peripheral half of the lung fields. The aorta is barely visible. The arch, apparently on the left, is so small that it is difficult to differentiate it from the shadows of the manubrium and transverse processes of the spine.

One incidental variant is noted in the bony structure. There is a smooth indentation in the inferior margin of the ninth dorsal body. This is indicated by a heavy dark arrow on the lateral film. This is an incidental finding, a Schmorl's nodule, a pressure defect from the nucleus pulposus against the vertebral body, which is usually seen in young adults and considered of no clinical importance.

Our final diagnosis is that of valvular pulmonary stenosis. This diagnosis is made on the basis of reduced pulmonary blood volume and a dilated pulmonary conus. This dilatation is poststenotic and does not reflect a high blood volume going into the lung fields. The Schmorl's nodule is an incidental finding.

Case V-13

Case V-13 is a 5-year-old boy admitted to the hospital for cyanosis.

The heart size is at the upper limits of normal. The lateral film does show some cardiac density behind the inferior vena cava, but there is proportionately more filling of the substernal space than there is evidence of left ventricular prominence. The pulmonary outflow tract is poorly outlined. Hilar vessels are relatively small, and the peripheral vascular markings are virtually absent. In this instance, the aortic arch is to the right side of the trachea, as evidenced by the indentation of the trachea, and a curved arrow points to the tracheal margin where the aorta indents it. The size of the aorta is difficult to evaluate due to overlying structures, but one gets the impression that it is prominent.

This radiograph represents a rather typical appearance of tetralogy of Fallot, but there are some unusual features. In a simple tetralogy there is rarely cardiac enlargement. Usually cardiac enlargement occurs only after a ductus has been created surgically for the patient. In tetralogy of Fallot, neither ventricle works against a high pressure. Even though there is pulmonary stenosis, the pressure is relieved by the dextroposition of the aorta. Typically, this means that the aorta carries the left ventricular output, as well as some of the right, and that therefore, it is larger than the pulmonary vessels. There is no poststenotic dilatation of the pulmonary artery in tetralogy of Fallot—which comprises: (1) pulmonary stenosis, (2) right heart enlargement, (3) septal defect, and (4) dextroposition of the aorta.

Dextroposition of the aorta, in the usual case, does not necessarily imply a right-sided aortic arch. However, in this case there is a right-sided aortic arch and descending aorta. The septal defect is high and related to the aorta overriding the septum, which as indicated above, relieves the pressure that might otherwise develop behind the stenotic pulmonary valve. Final diagnosis: Tetralogy of Fallot.

Case V-14

Case V-14 is a 31-year-old moderately obese woman admitted to the emergency

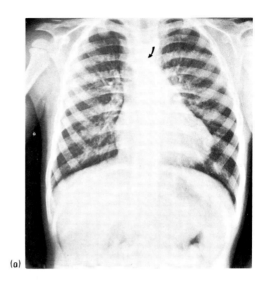

(a)

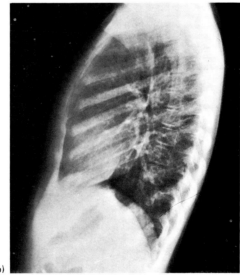

(b)

Case V-13

room with dyspnea, cyanosis, and hypotension. Except for the findings associated with her acute distress, the physical examination was not remarkable. The only pertinent information in her history was that of an inguinal hernia repair ten days earlier. She had been home from the hospital five days.

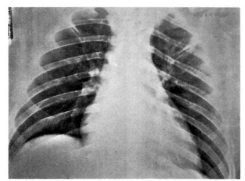

Case V-14

The chest radiograph shows findings pertinent for the diagnosis. The heart is mildly enlarged. Since this was a portable supine film, a lateral view is not available. There is some elevation of the right hemidiaphragm, although this is only slightly more than is usually seen. The most important feature here is the asymmetry of the vascular trunks. The right lung is very "anemic." The upper lung field on the left shows relatively normal vascular trunks. Peripherally in the left base, the vessels are poorly delineated, but one gets the impression that the vessels through the cardiac silhouette are essentially normal in size.

When the radiographic changes are correlated with the history, the diagnosis of high probability is a massive pulmonary embolus. The embolus is assumed to be blocking the right pulmonary artery. This explains the reduction in vascular shadows on this side. Elevation of the hemidiaphragm has been described on the side involved with the pulmonary embolus. It may be related to pain. The patient is not taking a full breath, or it may represent some segmental atelectasis with volume loss on this side.

The patient presented here did not survive, and the autopsy confirmed the suspected diagnosis of massive acute pulmonary embolus.

Case V-15

Case V-15 is a 35-year-old woman who had complained of shortness of breath, at times quite severe, over the past four to five years. In general, her problems had become progressively severe.

Evaluation of the chest shows the heart to be definitely enlarged, with the enlargement in the right ventricle. The lateral film shows fullness substernally (note the heavy solid arrow beneath the sternum). The inferior vena cava, as evidenced by the heavy arrow at the level of the diaphragm on the lateral film, is clearly posterior to any portion of the heart silhouette. The PA chest radiograph shows remarkably clear lung fields with a change in the caliber of pulmonary vessels at the level of the hilum. The open arrow on the right is directed toward a relatively small descending pulmonary artery, while the artery proximal to this point is normal or even somewhat enlarged.

The patient's symptoms were such that a cardiac catheterization was done. This resulted in a diagnosis of pulmonary hypertension without evidence of a left-to-right intracardiac shunt.

The differential diagnosis at this point (even without the cardiac catheterization data) is that of pulmonary hypertension.

There are three classical etiologies of pulmonary hypertension not associated with chronic obstructive pulmonary disease:

1. Long-standing intracardiac left-to-right shunt.

2. Multiple small pulmonary emboli.

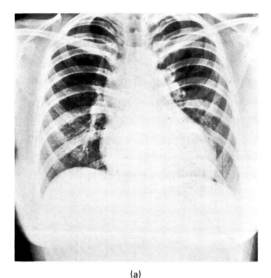

(a)

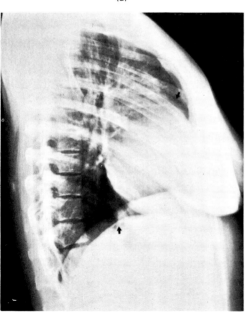

(b)

Case V-15

3. Idiopathic or totally unexplainable pulmonary hypertension.

In this instance, the catheterization data had ruled out the intracardiac shunt. Differentiation between pulmonary emboli and idiopathic pulmonary hypertension is much more difficult. Isotopic lung scanning and angiography are best used to make this differential, but even these tools may not solve the differential diagnosis.

This patient died of her illness. Autopsy showed multiple small pulmonary emboli of varying ages. The final diagnosis is, therefore, multiple pulmonary emboli (Castlemann-Bland syndrome).

We have presented two manifestations of the pulmonary embolus; however, we have not presented the most frequent manifestation of this disease which is that of acute symptoms with a normal chest film. The diagnosis is based on clinical suspicion, isotopic lung scanning, and possibly angiography. In the usual pulmonary embolus, the chest film may be totally normal or may show such minor, nonspecific findings as slight elevation of a hemidiaphragm on the side involved, linear atelectasis of varying degrees on the side involved, or a small amount of pleural fluid.

SUMMARY

The cases presented in the cardiovascular section were presented because they offered examples of basic radiographic determinations. Certainly tetralogy of Fallot and isolated pulmonary stenosis are not frequent radiographic diagnoses, but these entities offer the opportunity to demonstrate pulmonary perfusion and its variations, as well as to observe the size of the aorta in persons without degenerative disease. We did not present an example of pure hypertension, which is one of the most frequently occurring cardiovascular diseases. However, in light of what was presented, it seems that the reader should have no difficulty in determining what the appearance of the chest should be in hypertension. If you can identify the chamber that is enlarged, identify alterations in the blood volume being pumped by the two chambers, most of the cardiac lesions that are diagnosable by plain films can be identified. It was not our purpose to offer great detail in cardiovascular radiology of the chest, yet certain changes are so fundamental that knowledge of them should be a part of every physician's armamentarium.

4

Gastrointestinal Tract

The abdomen contains a multitude of organs and structures. Many of these are interrelated, such as the gastrointestinal and genitourinary tracts. Other structures such as the bones, vessels, muscles, and spleen are also present. A fundamental knowledge of this anatomy of the abdomen is needed for constant reference, so that a differentiation between normal and pathological entities can be distinguished.

The radiographic examination of the abdomen is difficult, and at times confusing, but can be made easier by using a systematic approach. There are three types of images on the abdominal radiograph. The opaque or white structures represent dense matter of the body, i.e., calcifications and skeletal structures. The least dense structures of the abdomen, the black or lucent images, represent gas shadows. Between these two extremes of density are the remaining structures of the abdomen. These gray images are the soft tissues that consist of all of the organs of the abdomen including muscles, blood vessels, and various fluids. Growths or masses in the abdomen will also show this soft-tissue-type density. The only way that structures of similar density can be separated radiographically is when they are outlined with fat, which has a slightly lower density than soft tissues, or by outlining either their inner or outer aspect with air, gas, or contrast (barium or io-

dinated substances) whose density is different than the adjacent soft tissues.

Normal ossified structures in the abdomen include the spine, the pelvis, the hips, and the ribs. Detailed examination of these structures may show not only focal disease processes, such as bony destruction or fracture, but may also delineate systemic problems such as may occur in metabolic and metastatic disorders. There are other normal, but infrequent, calcifications that may be confusing. Calcification of the costal cartilages in the upper abdomen may cause difficulty in excluding renal stones. These are curvilinear calcifications extending from the bony aspect of the anterior ribs as they course toward the sternum.

Small, round calcific densities measuring less than a centimeter in size, usually with lucent centers, are found in the pelvis of virtually all adults. These phleboliths, calcifications associated with pelvic veins, frequently are placed over the bladder or distal ureteral areas, making it difficult to distinguish them from urinary calculi. Our rules of thumb for distinguishing phleboliths from lower ureteral calculi involve both the appearance and the location of the calcification, and are as follows:

1. If there is a radiolucent center, it is most certainly a *phlebolith.*

2. If it is conical, or pyramid-shaped, it is most likely a *ureteral calculus,* since it developed its shape in a renal calix.

3. If the calcification in question lies outside a line drawn 2 cm. from the margin of the bony pelvis, it is most likely a *phlebolith.* As a general rule the ureter enters the bladder more medially than this 2 cm. margin.

Other smaller calcifications can be commonly seen in the left upper quadrant usually in the spleen representing an old healed granulomatous inflammation, most likely tuberculosis or histoplasmosis. Nodes in the abdomen can also calcify following inflammation or necrosis. These will be seen as irregular calcifications, usually measuring less than two cm in size and located in the lower abdomen and pelvis. Calcified nodes are most likely mesenteric and can be identified by their changing positions and locations. A lateral radiograph may also be of value. Retroperitoneal nodes rarely calcify, but such calcification when present occupies a periaortic position.

The gas shadows of the abdomen are easily recognized, being darker than the surrounding structures. However, differentiation between stomach, small bowel, and colonic gas may be difficult. Remember that the gas lies within the lumen of the gastrointestinal tract and will be located where these structures are located. For instance, gas in the stomach will be in the left upper quadrant and will outline the folds or rugae of the stomach. Colonic air will be located in the periphery of the abdomen, filling in various portions of the ascending and descending colon, which occupy the flanks. The transverse colon is across the upper abdomen below the gastric shadow, and the rectosigmoid colon is in the pelvis. Haustrations (the contractive folds of the colon) are usually seen mainly in the right colon and are easily identified, signifying that this is colonic gas.

Gas mixed with waste material or food can be identified in these respective organs of the abdomen as a granular substance. While gas is commonly seen in the stomach and colon, it is infrequently seen in the small bowel of normal adults, or at least in only very short nondilated segments. Conversely, a large quantity of small-bowel gas is normal in children. When small-bowel gas is present, it is usually centrally located and may contain transverse striations representing folds of the small bowel (valvulae conniventes). Normal small-bowel gas segments are short (less than 6 cm in length) and serpiginous and may be intermingled or scattered throughout the abdomen.

The soft tissues of the abdomen are more difficult to visualize. There are several specific structures that can be visualized because of adjacent fat outlining the organ. Each kidney is usually well seen on either side of the lumbar spine, and is bean-shaped and slightly diagonally oriented. Closely associated with the kidneys are linear structures in the paraspinal area, extending diagonally down toward the hips. These represent the psoas muscle shadows and are also outlined with fat. The superior aspect of the bladder may also be visualized in the pelvis by noting its surrounding perivesicular fat. The liver is a triangular homogeneous structure lying in the right upper quadrant. No gas shadows are usually seen in this area. The posterior, inferior aspect of the liver is usually well identified near the inferior aspect of the costal margin because of surrounding fat density. The spleen is a smaller homogeneous structure lying beneath the left diaphragm in the left upper quadrant, rarely extending below the costal margin unless enlarged. A spleen of normal size may be seen on a chest radiograph, as well or even better than on a film of the abdomen. Visualization of the remaining structures of the abdomen must be outlined internally by contrast material.

FUNDAMENTAL ABDOMINAL PROCESSES

There are several fundamental processes occurring in the abdomen that can be identified by the radiographic examination of the abdomen. There changes are secondary to basic pathology. Each will have a distinct radiographic appearance.

Ileus

Ileus is the obstruction of the bowel. There are two varieties. The first is an adynamic or paralytic ileus, in which there are no physical abnormalities which obstruct the bowel. Many pathological states act on the intestine in such a way as to inhibit its peristalsis and motility. Nonobstructing ileus can be a response to severe pain. Metastatic disease involving the mesentery can inhibit the bowel's motility, as can certain medications, trauma, electrolyte disturbances, and metabolic disorders. Frequently, inflammatory conditions of the abdomen such as peritonitis (which can result from many causes) or postoperative conditions will show a presentation like this. Radiographically, the abdomen will show gas throughout the gastrointestinal tract, but with more small bowel gas than normal and considerably elongated small bowel loops, which

retain their serpiginous character with or without distention of their lumen. This may be a diffuse condition within the abdomen, or a localized form of adynamic ileus can exist. Usually this is associated with a focal area of inflammation or trauma to a specific organ, and the overlying small bowel loops become paralyzed. It is frequently seen in cholecystitis, appendicitis, pancreatitis, and duodenal hematoma. For example, a focal area of small bowel loops will be seen in the right upper quadrant in cholecystitis. Similarly, small bowel loops can be seen in the left upper quadrant in pancreatitis. Small bowel loops located in the right lower quadrant would imply appendicitis.

The second form of ileus is a dynamic obstruction of the bowel. There is actually a physical obstruction narrowing the lumen of the bowel either partially or totally, causing distention of the bowel loops more proximal to the stenotic area. There are several varieties of this type of obstruction. Gastric outlet obstruction is a condition that prevents food and fluid from leaving the stomach and entering the duodenum in a normal fashion. Obstruction of the pyloric channel or duodenum will lead to a distended, dilated, food-and-fluid-filled stomach easily recognized on a radiograph of the abdomen. If the obstruction is further down as in the small bowel, there will be dilated small bowel loops proximal to the stenotic area. These small bowel loops lose their serpiginous character and become elongated, sometimes lying in a stepladder configuration across the abdomen. It must be remembered that, not only will gas be entrapped in the bowel, but also fluid. Therefore, fluid-filled bowel loops with minimal gas can also be identified, indicating small bowel obstruction. These appear as homogeneous shadows in the lower abdomen, often resembling a mass with small air bubbles in a string-of-beads configuration. If the obstruction is complete or total, there will be no gas in the small bowel or colon distal to the obstructive point. However, if the obstruction is only partial, the distal bowel beyond the obstructive site will contain gas, but without distention (disproportionate dilatation). The greatest dilatation of the bowel occurs immediately proximal to the obstructed point. Upright radiographs of the abdomen will show air/fluid levels in both obstructive and paralytic ileus. Frequently, but not always, air/fluid levels within a given loop will be at different heights in obstruction, while those in nonobstructive ileus will be at the same height.

Colonic obstruction is as easily identified as other obstructive problems. As you would expect, there is dilatation of the colon proximal to the obstructive point with little colonic gas beyond that area. If the ileocecal valve is competent, the cecum will distend and enlarge until it ruptures, unless surgery is performed to alleviate the obstruction. When the cecum becomes dilated more than 9 to 12 cm in diameter in either kind of ileus, surgical decompression is usually performed. Decompression of small bowel obstructive lesions can be obtained by passing orally a long intestinal drainage tube (Cantor or Miller-Abbott) into the bowel, advancing the perforated tip of the tube into the dilated fluid-filled bowel loops. While this does not usually cure the obstructive problem, it will decompress the bowel so that the surgeon will have an easier time in correcting the bowel obstruction. Decompression of a gastric outlet obstruction can be done simply with a nasogastric tube.

Intra-Abdominal Fluid or Air

Normally, the abdomen contains only a small amount of free intra-abdominal or peritoneal fluid without any free intra-abdominal gas. There are many processes that cause an accumulation of fluid in the abdomen. This fluid may be purulent as is seen in peritonitis. Or it may be a transudate as seen in the ascites of cirrhotic patients. Neoplastic cells can stud the abdominal cavity producing an accumulation of fluid within the abdominal cavity. Blood may also accumulate, as is commonly seen in lacerations of the spleen and liver following trauma.

All of these conditions will exhibit a similar radiographic appearance. The abdomen may be diffusely hazy with bowel loops separated by fluid between them. The more fluid that accumulates, the more the tendency for the gas-filled bowel to accumulate at the highest point of the abdomen when the patient is lying supine. This means that the bowel loops collect in the paraumbilical area, with the free fluid found more laterally in the flanks and along the lateral abdominal walls. Since fluid tends to collect in the most dependent portions of the abdomen, it therefore will not only be located in the gutters, but also can be seen in the pelvis as a soft tissue mass or dog-ear effect above the bladder.

Perforation of the intestine, whether due to a perforating gastric or duodenal ulcer or a ruptured colon from a neoplastic or inflammatory process, will allow gas to escape from the bowel lumen into the peritoneal cavity. Small amounts of air are difficult to demonstrate radiographically and are best seen by either (1) an upright chest radiograph looking for air to accumulate under the diaphragm leaves or (2) a left lateral decubitus radiograph of the abdomen looking for air beneath the right lateral chest and abdominal wall. The patients must be placed in these positions for at least ten minutes before the radiograph is made, to maximize the chance of air accumulating in these areas. The more gas that accumulates in the peritoneal space, the higher is the incidence of other signs of pneumoperitoneum. Normally, only the inside of the bowel wall or lumen is identified on a film of the abdomen. When the outer bowel wall is easily seen, this is an indication of free intra-abdominal air. Occasionally the falciform ligament coming from the liver to the umbilicus is easily demonstrated as a linear opaque density never otherwise seen on plain films of the abdomen.

Organomegaly and Masses

Unless organs of the abdomen contain gas, these structures will appear as a homogeneous density in the abdomen. For example, the liver, lying in the right upper quadrant, appears as a triangular density extending just below the costal margin. Enlargement of this organ will rarely be identified unless it extends to the iliac crest, displacing adjacent bowel loops to the left and inferiorly. It will retain its homogeneous character. Similarly, the spleen, kidney, bladder, and other organs of the abdomen and pelvis may displace adjacent gas-filled structures and appear as a homogeneous density in a certain location in the abdomen. Masses or tumors, whether solid or fluid-filled cysts, also present as soft-tissue shadows in the abdomen. Diagnosis as to the type of mass present will usually be based upon its location in the abdomen or its shape or the manner in which it displaces other structures. For example, pelvic masses will displace gas shadows up out of the pelvis.

Abdominal Calcifications

Certain disease processes will allow the deposition of calcium in structures that can be visualized on the radiograph. Usually, a small nidus or central core is formed, around which calcium and other debris may be deposited due to inflammatory processes or saturation with metabolites. The most common calcifications occurring in the abdomen are stones that develop in the gallbladder and urinary tract. Less frequently, stones can develop in the pancreas and appendix.

Gallstones can develop in the gallbladder, either due to inflammation or because of high concentrations of substances such as cholesterol or bilirubin. However, only 20% to 30% of these stones are calcified, and the rest are of soft tissue density. Therefore, most gallstones are seen only after contrast material has filled the lumen of the gallbladder during an oral cholecystogram. The contrast will be denser than the less opaque stones, allowing the stones to appear as lucent intraluminal densities. These can vary as to size, shape, and number, and will usually gravitate to the most dependent portion of the gallbladder in the upright position. Occasionally, the stones are of a specific gravity that differs enough from the contrast that they float in a straight line in the upright position. Calcified gallstones also appear as round, triangular, or multiple-faceted thin-rimmed calcific objects in the right upper quadrant. They can be of various sizes, ranging from one to hundreds in number.

Urinary tract stones, on the other hand, calcify more commonly than gallstones. Renal stones are calcified 80% of the time, the other 20% of the stones being non-opaque on the radiograph. These stones can be of various sizes and shapes, usually located in the fornices of the calices, in the calices themselves, or in the renal pelvis. When stones are being passed, they will gravitate into the ureter and can be seen to hang up at three common areas. The most common area is that of the ureterovesical junction, as the stone approaches the bladder. The other areas of momentary hangup are at the ureteropelvic junction and at the pelvic brim. Bladder stones typically are homogeneous or laminated in appearance when they are calcified. Stones of the urinary tract that are not calcified will appear as radiolucent or negative defects in a contrast-filled organ during excretory urography. They may also present with a hydronephrotic collecting system proximal to the point of obstruction.

Pancreatic stones usually form secondary to recurrent pancreatitis. Multiple small sandlike calcifications can be seen draped diagonally across the upper abdomen at the L1 (first lumbar vertebra) level in the area of the pancreas. Appendicoliths are calcified structures of various sizes and shapes occuring in the right lower quadrant. A patient with right lower quadrant pain and an appendicolith has appendicitis until proven otherwise. Occasionally, patients with appendicoliths will undergo elective surgery for removal of the appendix, not because there is a higher incidence of appendicitis, but because there is a greater risk of perforation when the patient does develop appendicitis.

KUB

The radiograph of the abdomen is called a flatplate or KUB. KUB stands for kidney, ureter, and bladder, which are at the extremes of the abdomen and, therefore, a radiograph that includes these structures

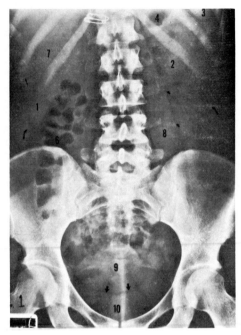

Figure 4-1

will cover most of the organs and structures within the abdominal cavity. The observer of the radiograph should examine the abdomen in a systematic fashion so that no information is deleted. He/she will usually do this in a sequence, that is comfortable for him/her and used over and over. Most commonly, the items of interest are skeletal ossifications and calcifications, masses, and abnormal gas shadows.

The accompanying radiograph (Fig. 4-1) shows five lumbar vertebral bodies and the lower half of the twelfth dorsal body, identified because of its paired ribs. The alignment of the spine and sacrum is usually straight, with the sacral wings or alae joining the pelvic bones at the sacroiliac joints. The pelvic bones are made up of three bony structures (ilium, pubis, and ischium) joining at the acetabulum forming a cup for the head of the femur, making the hip joint. Small calcifications are seen in the pelvis of this adult female (open arrow) which are phleboliths. Curvilinear calcifications, usually confluent with the bony ribs, are seen in the upper abdomen, and represent calcifications of the cartilage portions of the ribs as they extend toward the sternum (small straight arrow). These calcifications can, at times, be confusing when trying to exclude urinary or gallbladder calculi. No other significant calcifications or ossifications are seen in the abdomen.

As previously explained, the organs of the abdomen are not well defined unless they are surrounded by fat or contain contrast material. This individual's abdomen contains just the right amount of adipose tissue to distinctly outline various structures of the abdomen. Both kidneys are identified (2,7), as well as the tip of the spleen (3). The posterior aspect of the liver edge (1) is identified, and can be traced along the right lateral abdominal wall, toward the midline. The curved solid arrows demonstrate the edges of muscle bundles, commonly seen in the abdomen. The larger curved arrow represents the abdominal wall muscles, and the peritoneum seen in profile. The smaller curved arrows represent the edge of the iliopsoas muscle (8), attached to the lower dorsal, lumbar bodies, and running towards the hip. In the pelvis the bladder (10) is visualized as a semilunar structure lying on its convex side in the lowest aspect of the pelvis. Large solid arrows point to the perivesicular fat needed to visualize that structure. Directly above the bladder sits the uterus (9) in this female-type pelvis.

Few gas shadows are observed in this abdomen. The stomach is usually the highest organ in the left upper quadrant containing gas (4), but the gastric rugal folds are not well defined in this patient.

No definite small-bowel gas is seen, which is normal for the adult abdomen. Colonic gas (6) is identified in the ascending colon and hepatic flexure area and is characteristic because of its haustral folds. Other smaller gas-containing structures are seen, and probably represent cecal, transverse, and sigmoid colon gas. Incidentally noted are two safety pins overlying the lower dorsal spine, which apparently were holding the patient's bra straps together.

NORMAL GASTROINTESTINAL CONTRAST STUDIES

Before being able to identify pathological anatomy, you must be familiar with the contrast-filled appearance of the normal gastrointestinal tract. Barium swallowed by the patient is necessary to examine the upper gastrointestinal tract, and that radiographic examination is called an upper GI. If only the esophagus is needed, the radiologist will limit the study to the esophagus, the so-called barium swallow examination or esophagram. The accompanying radiographs will demonstrate the structures of the upper gastrointestinal tract. It must be remembered that the contrast material is within the lumen of the organs, not surrounding it.

The esophagus is a tubular structure beginning in the lower cervical spine area, and extending to just below the diaphragm. It passes through the mediastinum from the pharynx, entering the abdomen through the esophageal hiatus, an opening in the diaphragm. Normally, the esophagus is closed at each end and contains no structures. However, with swallowing, the upper esophageal sphincter will open; peristalsis will move the bolus

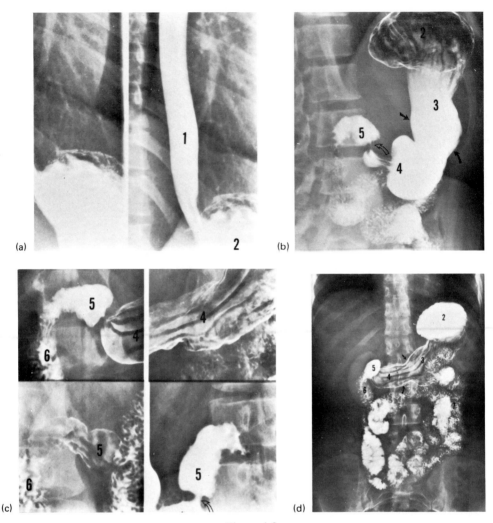

Figure 4-2

into the abdomen with the lower esophageal sphincter opening as the food approaches and closing after it enters the stomach. Normally, the gastric contents will not enter the esophagus in a retrograde fashion. Figure 4-2a demonstrates the distal esophagus (1) relationship to the stomach (2).

Barium and air will enter the stomach during the upper gastrointestinal exam.

Each coats and outlines different parts of the stomach and duodenum, depending upon the position of the patient when the radiograph was obtained. Gas will seek the nondependent portion of the organ, and barium will seek the most dependent portion. It must be remembered that barium will be the opaque or white density on the radiograph.

The stomach (Figs. 4-2b to d) is a backwards C-shaped structure in the left upper quadrant crossing the midline in the epigastric area. The medial margin is the lesser curvature (solid straight arrow), and the lateral margin is the greater curvature (curved solid arrow). The stomach contains several regions: the fundus (2), the body (3), and the antrum (4). Peristalsis in the distal half of the stomach will change the stomach's configuration, as noted on the radiographs. The contents of the stomach will empty through the pyloric channel (curved open arrow) as it intermittently opens.

The duodenum (Figs. 4-2b to d) is the next structure to be filled with contrast material. The first part of the duodenum is a spadelike structure, the duodenal bulb (5). This then leads to the vertical second portion of the duodenum, the descending duodenum (6). The duodenum, a C-shaped structure approximately 30 cm. long, then turns to the left directed toward the left upper quadrant before it meets the jejunum near the spleen at the ligament of Treitz behind the stomach. A proximal small bowel pattern can be observed incompletely on an upper gastrointestinal study. However, the more conventional approach in examining the small bowel in an antegrade fashion, is by giving the patient larger quantities of barium and observing the small bowel by fluoroscopy and radiographs obtained at one half hour intervals until the entire small bowel is seen. Figure 4-3 demonstrates such an examination. The jejunum (7) and ileum (8) contribute the majority of bowel loops to the small intestine. The duodenum is the first 30 cm. of small bowel with the jejunum and ileum contributing the remaining 500 cm. The jejunum lies in the left upper quadrant and left midabdomen with the ileum occupying the midabdo-

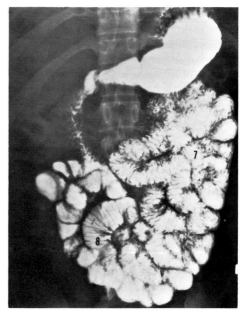

Figure 4-3

men and right lower quadrant. The small intestine is approximately 2 to 3 cm in diameter and constantly changes contour because of peristalsis. The distal aspect of the small bowel is the terminal ileum. This is the short section that enters the colon at the ileocecal valve.

The stomach and small bowel contain folds so that a greater absorptive area can be achieved. The stomach folds, seen as lucent or black stripes running lengthwise, are the rugae, which measure less than 1/2 cm in width. The duodenum and jejunum contain folds across the lumen of the intestine called valvulae conniventes, which are delicate and feathery in appearance. As the ileum is approached, the folds, which are less than 2 mm in width, become better defined and less frequent. Examples of the folds of the intestinal tract are demonstrated in Figure 4-2d and 4-3 using the small solid arrows.

There are other specialized techniques used today in examining the upper gastrointestinal tract and small bowel. These procedures are routine in some practices, but each has specific indications, advantages, and disadvantages. This book will use the more conventional studies as these are believed more likely to be familiar to the reader. By coating the stomach and duodenum with viscous high-density barium, and then distending the lumen with carbon dioxide produced by an effervescent agent, an air contrast effect can be achieved. This type of exam is best suited to demonstrate erosive changes of the mucosae (ulcers) and early carcinoma. Intramural or wall abnormalities are less well defined. While this method is excellent for examination of the stomach's surface, it can be enhanced by using an agent to reduce or abolish peristalsis. Glucagon is such an agent, which must be given IV or IM. It acts rapidly and lasts for various lengths of time depending upon the amount and route of injection. An air contrast exam of the esophagus can also be done as part of the foregoing exam or as a separate technique.

The mucosal coating and gaseous distention of the duodenal loop alone can be studied in a similar fashion. Glucagon is used to stop active duodenal peristalsis, and an intestinal tube or effervescent agent is used to distend the lumen and achieve the double-contrast effect (air and barium). This is called hypotonic duodenography. It was developed to find erosive changes and the alterations produced by carcinoma of the pancreas. The remainder of the small bowel can be examined in an antegrade fashion by using the same type of intestinal tube. Its tip is placed at the ligament of Treitz or proximal jejunum, and a barium solution is infused through the tubing using gravity. This achieves maximum distention of the bowel lumen needed to demonstrate areas of stenosis or partial small bowel obstruction. This small bowel enema or infusion technique is also indicated in gastrointestinal bleeding and suspected mucosal abnormalities. The distal small bowel can be similarly examined by refluxing barium into the small bowel across a patent ileocecal valve after filling the colon during a barium enema. To prevent superimposition of the ileum on the sigmoid colon, water is used instead of barium to fill the last aspect of the colon. This exam is best used for quick detection of distal small bowel obstruction and is called a retrograde small bowel exam.

Examination of the colon requires a different approach. The colon must be prepared to eliminate waste particles from the bowel as these will often be mistaken for small polyps. A small plastic tip is placed into the rectum. Attached to the tip is plastic tubing, which leads to a bag of barium hanging approximately 90 cm above the fluoroscopy table. Using gravity, barium is allowed to flow into the colon. The amount of barium needed to fill the colon will vary according to the size of the patient. When filling the colon, the terminal ileum will intentionally be filled, if possible, and the appendix may also be visualized.

Figure 4-4 demonstrates the 1½ m long colon, which is larger in diameter than the small bowel, and placed in the abdomen about the periphery. The terminal ileum (8) can be seen entering the colon at the ileocecal valve (large solid arrow). The cecum is the most proximal portion of the colon, and is a saclike structure (1) containing the appendix on its medial border (open arrow). The cecum usually

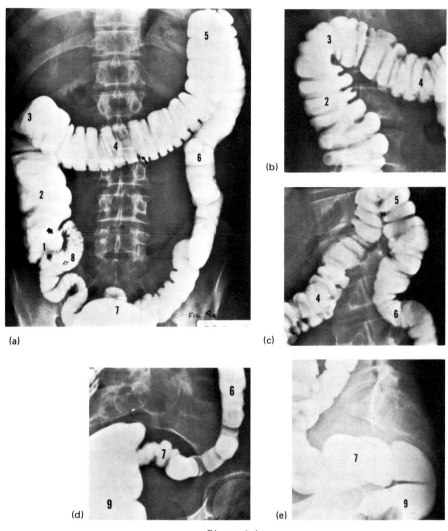

(a)

(b)

(c)

(d)

(e)

Figure 4-4

lies in the right lower quadrant, and leads to the ascending colon (2) along the right lateral abdominal gutter. The ascending colon then extends to the hepatic flexure (3) located in the right upper quadrant. As the hepatic flexure turns toward the left it comes forward forming the transverse colon (4), which lies anteriorly across the upper abdomen. The transverse colon then gives rise to the splenic flexure (5), which lies in the left upper quadrant, and leads to the descending colon (6) in the left lateral abdominal gutter. The descending colon then joins the sigmoid colon (7), which will eventually end in the rectum (9). Because of redundancy, the

flexures and sigmoid colon are best visualized on oblique films (Figs. 4-4b to e).
The outline of the colon is pleated due to
three longitudinal muscle bands, causing
haustral folds (Fig. 4-4a, curved solid arrow).

Visualization of the biliary system, including the gallbladder, is done by several
techniques. Most commonly, oral contrast
material is given the night before the
exam. This allows the medication that
contains iodine to dissolve and be absorbed by the gastrointestinal tract. The
material will flow into the intestinal blood
stream (portal system) to the liver where
it is extracted and excreted in the bile and
its duct system. Oddi's sphincter is at the
end of the bile duct system and only
intermittently opens. Therefore, fluid will
accumulate in the bile ducts and gallbladder. The contrast material, which is mixed
with the bile, must be concentrated by
the gallbladder and the excess water removed, so that the contrast material will
be opaque on the radiograph. Normally,
several radiographs are obtained in the
recumbent and upright positions. Figure
4-5 demonstrates the normal size and configuration of the gallbladder.

Another, less frequently used, method
of visualizing the biliary system is by
injecting aqueous iodinated contrast material, which goes to the liver and is secreted unchanged into the biliary ductal
system within one hour in normal patients. This technique does not need the
gallbladder to concentrate the material,
and therefore, is best used to demonstrate
the biliary system when the gallbladder
has been removed. Because the duct system is very delicate and thin, body section
radiographs or tomography is useful in
demonstrating the anatomy. Figure 4-6
shows the intrahepatic duct system (open

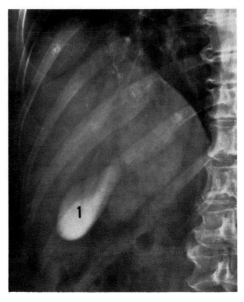

Figure 4-5

arrow) and the extrahepatic biliary ducts
(2). Occasionally, contrast material will
reflux into the pancreatic duct (solid arrow). The common biliary duct generally
measures less than 10 mm in diameter;
and the most distal aspect of this duct is,
at times, not well defined because of intermittent opening and closing of Oddi's
sphincter located in the duodenal wall.

There have been other sophisticated
techniques developed in the last few years
to define abnormalities of the biliary system. Ultrasound, which utilizes no radiation, can define the gallbladder and bile
ducts whether or not the gallbladder is
visualized with contrast material or the
patient is jaundiced. When the serum bilirubin is above 2 to 3 mg%, the chance of
seeing the gallbladder or ducts during oral
cholecystography or intravenous cholan-
giography is small. An even more refined
technique to see the same areas in the
jaundiced patient is computerized tomography (CT). It radiographically slices

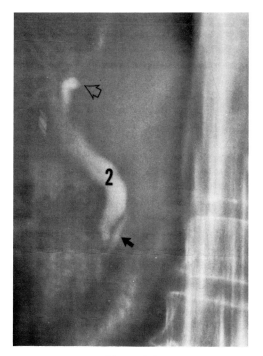

Figure 4-6

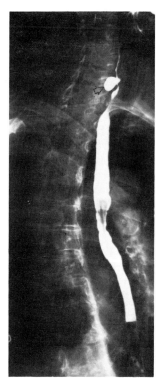

Case MD-1

any area of the body with better definition than ultrasound, but uses x-rays to produce clear static cross-sectional images. Due to cost, these newer modalities are not yet universally available.

MOTILITY DISORDERS

CASE PRESENTATIONS

Case MD-1

This patient came to the hospital without symptoms referable to the gastrointestinal tract. However, for some unknown reason, an esophagram was included in his workup; and an incidental finding was diagnosed. The patient demonstrates a small diverticulum just above the esoph-

agus extending posteriorly in the hypopharynx. This abnormality is believed to occur because the upper esophageal sphincter (cricopharyngeus) fails to relax completely during swallowing and becomes hypertrophied. This increases the tension in the hypopharynx and causes protrusion of the wall of the hypopharynx through a weakness (Killian's dehiscence) in the muscles of the throat, causing a saclike structure to develop. While this patient had no complaints, such diverticuli are frequently symptomatic and occasionally need to be surgically corrected. The open arrow points to the diverticulum that was produced in this patient. Final diagnosis: Zenker's diverticulum.

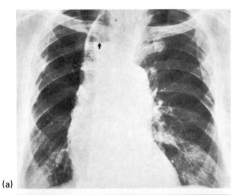

(a)

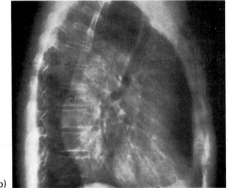

(b)

Case MD-2

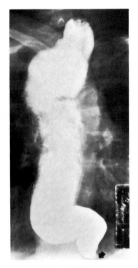

Case MD-3

Cases MD-2 and MD-3

Cases MD-2 and MD-3 demonstrate two patients with the same diagnosis. The chest film (MD-2) is that of a 75-year-old man, who had symptoms of dysphagia. The PA radiograph demonstrates widening of the mediastinum on the right (open arrow). A fluid level is noted (solid arrow) in the upper mediastinum. The lateral film demonstrates forward displacement of the trachea, with a serpiginous shadow (open arrow) coursing down the middle-posterior medastinal area leading towards the diaphragm. There are very few structures in the mediastinum that will show air-fluid levels. An abscess, hiatal hernia, or obstruction of the esophagus are the primary causes. Since this individual demonstrates an elongated structure coursing through the mediastinum, the best or correct answer would be an obstructed esophagus.

The contrast study (MD-3) or esophagram, accompanying the chest films is that of a 66-year-old woman, who also had symptoms of dysphagia. Obviously, the esophagus is dilated and tortuous due to chronic obstruction. It shows small lucencies within the barium compatible with the presence of undigested food and fluid. The most distal aspect of the esophagus is pinched off by an abrupt narrowing, which is causing the obstruction.

These two patients with achalasia have a dysfunction of the lower esophageal sphincter (solid arrow) not allowing the normal opening and closing of the sphincter. While the sphincter does open intermittently, it does not open enough to allow the passage of food, and therefore, causes the proximal obstruction seen on these films. Final diagnosis: Achalasia of the esophagus.

Case MD-4

There is a pathological condition (scleroderma) that affects the muscles and connective tissues of the gastrointestinal tract, as well as the entire body. The film demonstrates several findings in a patient with this disease. The esophagus, which is dilated and atonic, shows no peristalsis because of visceral muscle atrophy. The lower esophageal sphincter is widely patent, allowing reflux of gastric contents and the formation of strictures secondary to esophagitis. Food and fluid and, for that matter, barium may sit in the esophagus for long periods of time without the normal stripping peristaltic waves, which empty the tubular structure.

Similar changes in the remainder of the intestine cause lack of peristalsis, slow motility, and dilated, atonic structures. The small bowel may show dilated loops with thickened folds. The colon, as demonstrated in the adjoining radiograph, demonstrates multiple saclike structures off the lumen of the transverse colon, so-called wide mouth pseudodiverticuli or sacculations (solid arrow). The lung bases may show basilar fibrotic change as the disease progresses. Films of the hands (MD-4c) show atrophy of the soft tissues with soft-tissue calcific deposits (solid arrow). Final diagnosis: Scleroderma (progressive systemic sclerosis).

Case MD-5

The patient in this case demonstrates one of the most common gastrointestinal disorders in man. This disorder is frequently identified on the chest film, as it was in this individual, as a soft-tissue structure above the diaphragm behind the heart frequently containing an air-fluid level. Many of these are asymptomatic

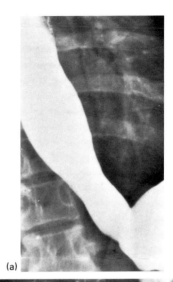
(a)

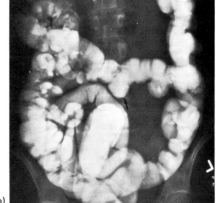
(b)

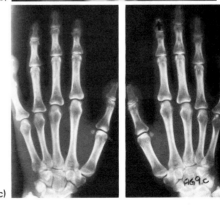
(c)

Case MD-4

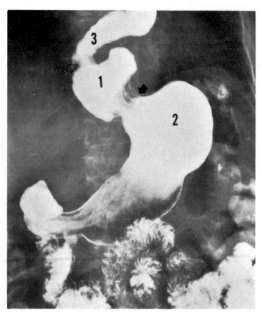

Case MD-5

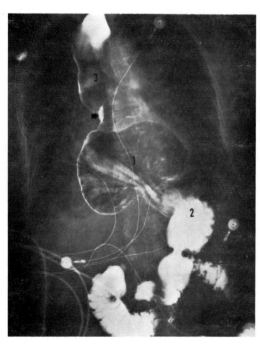

Case MD-6

and found in patients who have a weakened esophageal hiatal opening in the diaphragm. This allows the stomach to herniate or slide back and forth in varying degrees, depending upon the size of the opening. Increased abdominal pressure, which is present in overweight people, tends to increase the frequency of this disorder.

The accompanying radiograph demonstrates a small saclike structure (1) above the level of the left diaphragm (black solid arrow), which is a herniated part of the stomach. The gastroesophageal junction area or lower esophageal sphincter (open arrow) may be either closed or open, but is frequently open, allowing reflux of the gastric contents into the distal esophagus (3), as demonstrated in this case. Note that the stomach (2) is devoid of rugal folds, a finding frequently seen in the aged. Although it can represent atrophy of the gastric mucosa, overdistention of the stomach will stretch and make the rugi disappear as well.

Patients with this type of abnormality may be admitted with chest pains, which are commonly misdiagnosed as angina or myocardial infarction. Because of the reflux associated with the hiatal hernia, fluid will propel itself up the esophagus and into the throat, especially when recumbent. Reflux can be transient and at times difficult to show and can also be present without complications. Surgical procedures may be warranted to correct symptomatic hernias and reflux. Final diagnosis: Sliding hiatal hernia with gastroesophageal reflux.

Cases MD-6 through MD-8

A sequel to reflux of gastric contents into the distal esophagus is seen in the three patients represented here. One of the patients has no hiatal hernia, but reflux does not have to be associated with a hernia. Reflux apparently is due to failure of the lower esophageal sphincter to remain competent or closed, preventing gastric acid from entering the esophagus leading to inflammatory changes. If this occurs, inflammatory change is seen where the acid has irritated the mucosa causing edema, erythema, spasm, and ulcerations of different sizes.

The largest hiatal hernia (1) is seen in MD-6. As the hernia becomes larger, the entire stomach may enter the chest cavity. This hernia (1) is associated with a patent gastroesophageal sphincter and a giant distal esophageal ulcer (solid arrow). The second radiograph (MD-7) shows four images of a small hiatal hernia (1) in different positions with a small ulcer at the level of the gastroesophageal junction area (solid arrows). The final radiograph (MD-8) shows diffuse inflammatory change of the distal half of the esophagus (3) with multiple small ulcerations (open arrows).

As a complication of recurrent esophagitis, scarring will develop causing inflammatory strictures and narrowings of the esophagus, usually involving the distal esophagus. As the esophagus shortens, due to scarring, a second variety of hiatal hernia may occur—the so-called short type of esophageal hiatal hernia—because as the esophagus shortens, the stomach is pulled through the hiatus. The previously mentioned types of hiatal hernias occur with the gastroesophageal junction area above the area of the left diaphragm.

The final form of hiatal hernia is the paraesophageal hiatal hernia. In this form the gastric wall herniates through the hiatus, around the distal esophagus, leaving the gastroesphageal junction area below the left diaphragm. Final diagnosis: (1)

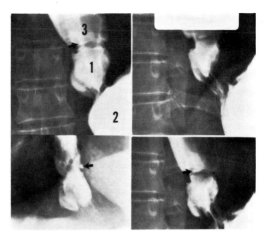

Case MD-7

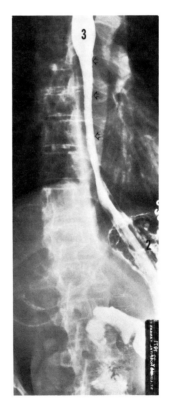

Case MD-8

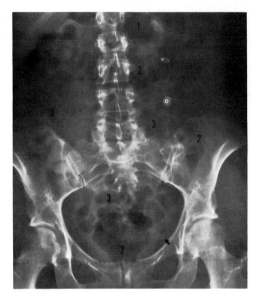

Case MD-9

Esophagitis with esophageal ulceration, with and without hiatal hernia; (2) esophageal stricture.

Case MD-9

This film demonstrates diffuse lucencies throughout the abdomen compatible with intraluminal intestinal gas. Gastric air (1) is identified in the epigastric region, slightly more to the left of the midline. Gas in the colon (2) is identified in the transverse colon, descending colon, and rectal areas. The remaining gas shadows are short segments of amorphous-appearing bowel, which are serpiginous, measuring less than 2 cm in diameter and scattered throughout the abdomen in the paraumbilical region. This represents small bowel intestinal gas. While a person in pain can swallow enough gas to distend the entire GI tract, there are many disorders that paralyze the gastrointestinal tract and inhibit its motility, which give this type of picture. Gas in this type of disor-

der is usually seen distributed throughout the GI tract from the stomach to the anus. At times these loops of bowel will be dilated; if films of the abdomen were taken several minutes apart, the gas shadows would remain in the same place, signifying a lack of movement of bowel. Clinically, no bowel sounds are identified.

The diffuse pattern of gas throughout the abdomen with no specific focal concentrations could represent generalized peritonitis, metabolic bowel inhibition, postoperative bowel inhibition, or any generalized cause that would affect the entire bowel. This pattern can also be seen with a local inflammatory problem, such as acute cholecystitis, pancreatitis, renal stones, or appendicitis. When a local ileus or collection of small bowel gas is identified in a specific location, it helps in differentiating abdominal pain by associating this pattern with organs located in that region. Incidentally noted are three phleboliths or calcifications in the pelvic veins located in the left aspect of the pelvis (solid arrow). They are characteristically circular with dense outer calcification and a lucent center. Final diagnosis: Paralytic or adynamic ileus.

Case MD-10

This film represents an 80-year-old woman who was admitted to the hospital with nausea and vomiting. A nasogastric intestinal tube was inserted into the stomach with the tip lying in the antrum of the stomach. The stomach (open arrows) is dilated and full of secretions and food particles. Barium, given to the patient several days previously, can faintly be seen mixed with the food particles in the stomach, giving a slightly more dense appearance than is seen without the barium. The barium that left the stomach previously is now seen in the colon and

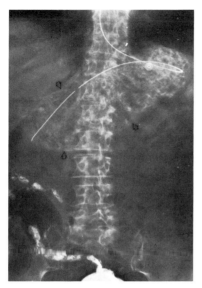

Case MD-10

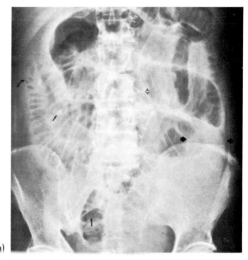

(a)

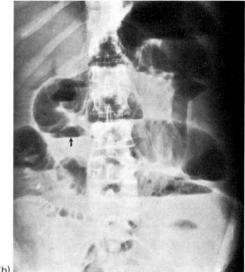

(b)

Case MD-11

rectum. There is a small amount of intestinal gas in the small bowel loops in the left midabdomen and right colon. This pattern is consistent with gastric outlet obstruction. The obstruction may be in the distal antrum, pyloric channel, or even in the duodenal loop. This obstruction is apparently only a partial obstruction, as gas and barium are seen distal to the area of obstruction in the right upper quadrant.

There are multiple etiologies that could be present to give this radiographic pattern. Acid peptic disease with acute ulceration or its complication of scarring and stricture are the most common cause. Neoplasm of the upper gastrointestinal tract would be less likely. Gastrointestinal contrast studies are not necessarily needed for this diagnosis. However, if they were done, it is best that the stomach be emptied of the retained food particles, so that barium can coat the mucosal wall. Final diagnosis: Gastric outlet obstruction.

Case MD-11

This film demonstrates an older female patient, who has had previous surgery, as identified by the shadows of the metallic sutures down the midline just to the left of the spine (open arrow). This patient was complaining of abdominal pain, cramps, nausea, and vomiting. The lucencies seen within the abdomen are multiple dilated loops of small bowel gas. These loops do not retain their serpiginous appearance, which has been previously identified in paralytic ileus, but are elongated and arranged in a pattern, one above the other. Each loop shows its folds. Minimal colonic gas (1) is identified, indicating that this is virtually total small bowel obstruction. While numerous gas-filled small bowel loops are demonstrated in the upper half of the abdomen on the left, there are multiple small bowel loops filled with fluid containing little or no gas (solid large arrows). Loops that contain a large amount of fluid, but very little gas, are demonstrated by small air bubbles in the right midabdomen (solid curved arrow). This is the so called string-of-beads sign identified in small bowel obstruction. The small solid arrow demonstrates undissolved medication in the gut.

The accompanying upright film (MD-11b) of the abdomen shows straight lines (solid straight arrow) crossing the bowel segments in a horizontal fashion. These are loops filled with fluid and air. The fluid gravitates to the most dependent portion of the bowel segment, and the gas localizes superiorly when the patient is upright. These loops are called air/fluid levels, and can be seen both in paralytic ileus and in small bowel obstruction. Note also the valvulae conniventes or folds of the small bowel, which are vertical opaque lines crossing the loop.

The most likely cause of this patient's small bowel obstruction is an adhesion created by the previous surgery, which binds or closes off a segment of small intestine. However, there are multiple causes for small bowel obstruction including neoplasm (either primary in the gut, or secondary), gallstone ileus, stricture formation, hernias with entrapment of

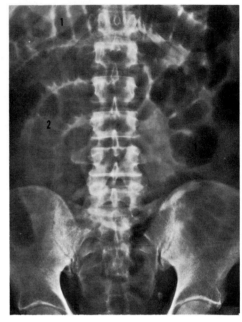

Case MD-12

bowel, and intussesception. Final diagnosis: Complete small bowel obstruction.

Case MD-12

This film represents a 69-year-old man admitted to the hospital with nausea, vomiting, and abdominal distention. The radiograph demonstrates abundant intestinal gas, seen distributed through the GI tract. Colonic gas is identified by its haustra (1). Note that the colonic gas that is present is not dilated nor distended, so there is no colonic obstruction. Distended small bowel loops (2), demonstrated in the right mid abdomen, are elongated with their valvulae conniventes shown. This disproportionate dilatation is compatible with a partial small bowel obstruction.

The earlier a radiograph is obtained of the abdomen in a patient who is acutely obstructed, the greater the chance of seeing gas in the colon even in a patient with complete small bowel obstruction. As the obstruction progresses, the colonic gas disappears and only small bowel gas will be identified. However, in that time period, both small bowel and colonic gas will be seen compatible with a partial small-bowel obstruction. In colonic obstruction, the small bowel may be distended if the ileocecal valve is patent. Final diagnosis: Partial or incomplete small bowel obstruction.

Cases MD-13 through MD-15

The accompanying radiographs in Cases MD-13 through MD-15 are of different patients with the same problem. The small bowel, or for that matter, the colon, will herniate through weaknesses in the abdominal wall, most commonly the inguinal opening. The bowel may extend down the inguinal canal into the scrotal sac. The canal will dilate allowing this to happen, and the bowel will protrude into the sac as abdominal pressure increases with exertion. Hernias can be reduced by manipulation, and the bowel loops forced back into the abdomen through the opening. However, there are times when the hernia cannot be reduced, and the gut becomes incarcerated. The larger the herniated sac, the more likely these bowel loops are to become entrapped, twisted, and closed off from the adjacent intestinal lumen and blood supply. This leads to small bowel obstruction, and can cause necrosis and gangrene of a segment of entrapped bowel.

The initial radiograph (MD-13a) demonstrates an unusual gas shadow overlying the right groin (solid arrows). Gas is scattered throughout the GI tract with minimal dilatation that is compatible with an ileus, but no obvious obstruction has developed. A subsequent barium enema

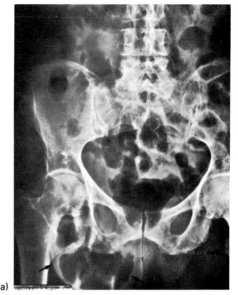

(a)

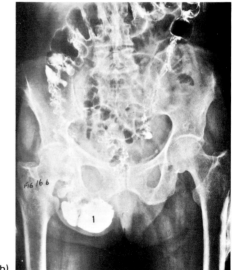

(b)

Case MD-13

(MD-13b) demonstrates the cecum (1) lying in the hernia sac. Since the ileum must find its way through the inguinal canal so that it may enter the cecum at the ileocecal valve, it is easy to see that small-bowel obstruction could occur. The film

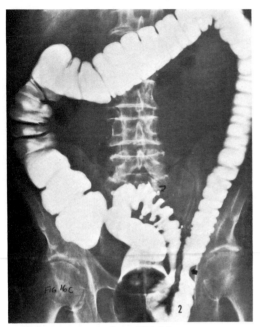

Case MD-14

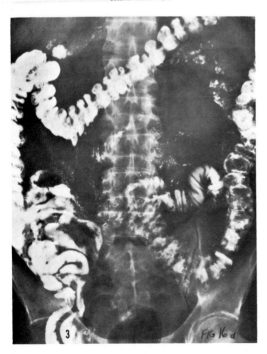

Case MD-15

of another patient (MD-14) demonstrates the sigmoid loop (2) trapped in the inguinal hernia, with narrowing of the bowel (large solid arrow) as it goes through the inguinal canal.

The film of the patient in MD-14 demonstrates several saclike structures (curved solid arrow) extending from the sigmoid colon that have the characteristic appearance of diverticuli. This segment of the sigmoid lacks the usual tubular structure that is normally seen and shows a zigzag lumen, secondary to the muscle hypertrophy seen in diverticulosis. Incidentally, an air-filled balloon attached to the rectal enema tip is used for patients who cannot retain barium during barium enema examination.

The final film (MD-15) demonstrates herniation of the distal small bowel (3) into the right inguinal hernia without proximal small bowel dilatation that would indicate an obstruction. Final diagnosis: Inguinal hernias containing colon and/or small bowel.

Case MD-16

The radiograph in MD-16 is of a 77-year-old man admitted to the hospital with vomiting. The initial radiograph obtained demonstrates air in a distended stomach (1), minimal stool and gas in the rectum (3), and a short dilated segment of small bowel (2) identified because of its valvulae conniventes. There is also a sausage-shaped soft-tissue density lateral to the small-bowel loop. This represents a fluid-filled, dilated loop of small bowel (multiple solid arrows). In the right upper quadrant is a curvilinear lucency, approximately 1 cm wide (solid straight arrows), which extends towards the right diaphragm. There is a round soft-tissue density in the left upper quadrant (curved solid arrows) that represents fluid in the dependent portion of the stomach, the fundus. Incidentally noted are small circular opaque densities in the lower abdomen (straight open arrow). This is a small amount of barium retained in diverticuli of the colon from a previous barium enema examination. Multiple phlebolithlike densities are seen in the pelvis. There is a tubular-appearing calcification in the lateral aspects of the pelvis (long solid arrows). This is arteriosclerotic calcification of the pelvic vessels. The vertebral bodies of the spine, rather than having a square smooth shape, demonstrate calcific spurs (open curved arrow) that are compatible with degenerative osteoarthritic change of the lumbar dorsal spine.

The findings here are compatible with small-bowel obstruction. The only clue to the cause of the obstruction is the air appearing in the right upper quadrant, which is usually homogeneous due to the uniformly dense liver. This is air in the common biliary duct that is never identified unless the gut communicates with the biliary tract abnormally. Most commonly, surgical anastomosis of the biliary system to the gut can explain this. Otherwise, air arrives in the biliary system by a fistulous communication between the bile system and the gut. This is usually due to a gallstone that erodes through the gallbladder wall or bile duct, and into the adjacent bowel, usually the duodenum or small bowel. The gallstone may then pass into the lumen of the intestine, and if small enough, be evacuated from the bowel. However, the gallstone may impact itself at various locations in the gut, causing bowel obstruction. The most common areas of obstruction are in the duodenum or the jejunum or at the ileocecal valve. This patient's radiolucent stone impacted

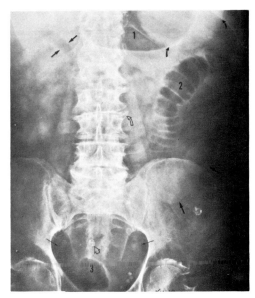

Case MD-16

in the jejunum and is not visualized. Final diagnosis: Gallstone ileus.

Case MD-17

This case is a 65-year-old man with abdominal distention. The radiograph (MD-17) shows abundant intestinal gas. Most bowel gas is colonic in origin (2). Air is seen in the ascending colon, transverse colon, and descending colon, down to the distal aspect of the descending colon. At this point there is a soft-tissue density (curved solid arrows) that represents a carcinoma obstructing the distal colon. Minimal small-bowel gas (1) is identified in the right mid abdomen. If the ileocecal valve is incompetent, it allows gas to reflux into the small bowel and the colon can decompress itself. However, if the ileocecal valve is competent and surgery to relieve the obstruction is not performed, gas will accumulate in the colon distending it to the point of rupture

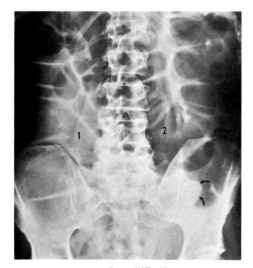

Case MD-17

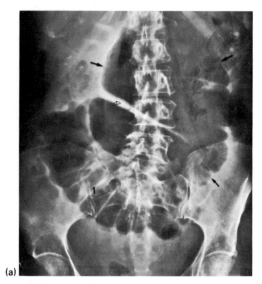

(a)

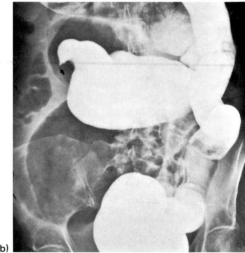

(b)

Case MD-18

(which will usually occur in the cecal area). Nine to 12 cm is the maximum diameter allowed for the cecum to distend before decompression must be done, be it for ileus or obstruction. If the obstruction were more proximal, less colonic gas would be visualized. Note that there is no colonic gas distal to the point of obstruction. The diagnosis is easily made by a barium enema that shows the characteristic appearance of carcinoma of the colon. Final diagnosis: Total colonic obstruction due to carcinoma of the descending colon.

Case MD-18

The radiographs of the next case are of a 60-year-old woman with abdominal distention. The plain film of the abdomen demonstrates a large radiolucent gas shadow in the mid-abdomen. This has a configuration of the cecum, but is dilated and upside down (solid black arrows). Using your imagination, you can see an ileocecal valve area (open curved arrow). Distention of a colonic segment (1) of bowel is seen across the right lower abdomen, manifesting haustral folds. No other colon gas is seen in the abdomen, but small bowel gas (2) is seen scattered throughout the abdomen. There is a slight curvature or scoliosis of the lumbar spine with its convexity to the left, suggesting spasm and contraction of the right iliopsoas muscle. This radiograph has the characteristic appearance of a cecal volvulus.

The cecum and the ascending colon apparently are on a long, free mesentery. They are normally attached to the posterior abdominal wall, but the free unattached segment can now float and rotate, twisting the bowel at its point of attachment in the right gutter. As the cecum enlarges and distends, it will usually float up and point towards the left upper quadrant of the abdomen. A barium enema shows the characteristic "beak" (solid straight arrow) sign of a volvulus or twisting of the bowel. There is an obstruction of the proximal colon at this point, causing the great dilatation seen in the preliminary radiograph. Final diagnosis: Cecal volvulus.

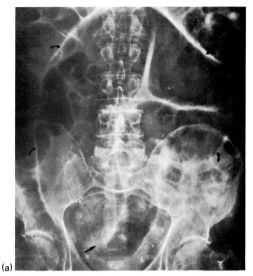
(a)

Case MD-19

This case demonstrates still another kind of colonic obstruction. The preliminary radiograph of the abdomen again demonstrates a large amount of bowel gas. No valvulae conniventes are seen, indicating this is colonic in origin. There is a single loop of bowel gas, centrally located on the film (curved solid arrows), that looks like an upside-down U. Both sides point towards the pelvis as their origin (solid straight arrow). Other bowel gas loops are identified, some of which are apparently small bowel because they retain their characteristic serpiginous character. Colon gas is suggested in the right lateral aspect of the abdomen. The shadows of metallic sutures are seen down the left paramedian area of the abdomen, and there is vascular calcification in the pelvis. Barium enema examination demonstrates another beak-shaped narrowing in the mid sigmoid (solid straight arrow).

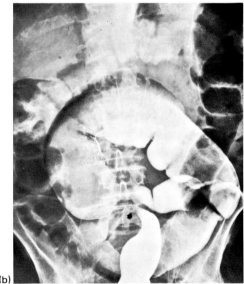
(b)

Case MD-19

This corresponds to the point of obstruction of the colon, and is similar to the cecal volvulus seen on the previous case. However, the point of obstruction, in this case, lies in the sigmoid; this is due to a redundant sigmoid, on a long mesentery, allowing the sigmoid to twist. If you trace the faint barium that was placed in the colon past the point of obstruction, you will note that this outlines the inside of the inverted U, previously described. The colon proximal to the point of obstruction is dilated and distended, and minimal small bowel gas is seen. Although treatment of this condition ultimately is surgery, the surgeons may decompress the bowel by inserting a colon tube through the narrowed area. The deflation of the colon alone may untwist the redundant segment, but it may twist at a future date if the circumstances are repeated. Final diagnosis: Sigmoid volvulus.

INFLAMMATORY DISORDERS

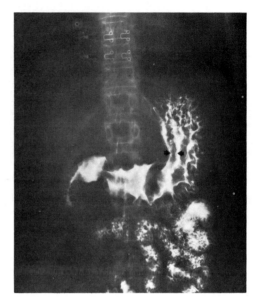

Case ID-1

CASE PRESENTATIONS

Case ID-1

Abdominal pain was the symptom which brought this 44-year-old woman for upper gastrointestinal examination. The radiograph is one of several taken during an upper GI exam. The most prominent finding on the radiograph is the enlargement of rugal folds (solid straight arrows) throughout the entire stomach. Even the duodenal bulb and proximal duodenum exhibit prominent folds. Normally, the rugal folds should be no greater than ½ cm wide. This patient is manifesting an inflammatory condition of the stomach, diffuse hypertrophic gastritis. This is believed due to irritation of the gastric mucosa by a chemical, such as ethanol. There are, however, other pathological conditions that enlarge rugal folds. Lymphoma may present a similar pattern. Ménétrier's disease usually shows enlarged rugal folds in the fundus and body of the stomach. Inflammatory gastritis, resulting from any one of many causes, usually attacks the antrum.

An air contrast exam of the upper gastrointestinal tract in this patient would probably have shown multiple superficial punctate ulcerations throughout the stomach. This patient's upper GI exam was normal, both before and after this study, indicating that this was a benign inflammatory condition, possibly brought on by acid peptic disease or ethanol ingestion. Final diagnosis: Diffuse hypertropic gastritis.

Cases ID-2 through ID-4

The three films of Cases ID-2, ID-3, and ID-4 demonstrate the same disorder, but each film demonstrates a different facet for diagnosing this problem. All of these patients exhibited abdominal pain with blood in the stool. The first radiograph

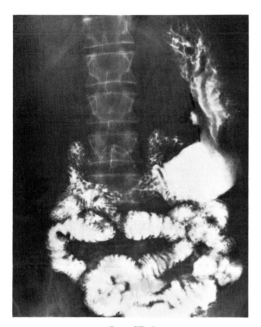

Case ID-2

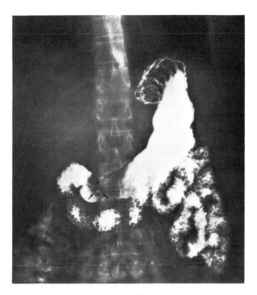

Case ID-3

(ID-2) demonstrates an accumulation of barium (open arrow), which protrudes from the lesser curvature of the stomach lumen (solid straight arrows). This out-pouching or niche is one sign of benign gastric ulcer using conventional techniques. Note the nonspecific irregularity of the ulcer base. Malignant ulceration, or ulceration on the surface of a malignant neoplasm, would have a similar appearance, but the ulcer would be within the lumen of the stomach.

The second radiograph (ID-3) shows a symmetrical smooth lucent halo (solid straight arrows) about a central white density in the antrum of the stomach. The circular opacity represents the ulcer crater, and the lucent ring represents edematous tissue mound about the ulceration. This is a sign of an acute ulceration. However, based upon this single radiograph, it would be difficult to exclude malignant

tissue about the ulceration, rather than edema.

The final radiograph (ID-4) demonstrates a large collection of barium (open arrow) along the greater curvature of the antrum. Rugal folds (curved solid arrows)

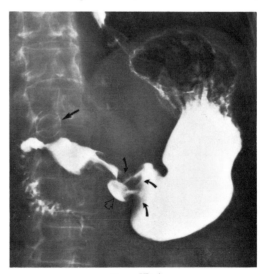

Case ID-4

are seen to radiate towards the ulcer. The smooth, even folds go right up to the ulcer opening, a sign indicative of benign ulcer disease. A malignant ulcer may show radiating folds, as this is a sign of a healing ulcer, but they would stop before the ulcer edge was reached, possibly ending in nodular or clubbed processes. Incidentally noted are two calcific ringed gallstones (solid straight arrow) in their typical location in the gallbladder, which sits on the proximal duodenum anteriorly.

Most gastric ulcers are benign (95%) and are 1/2 cm or less in diameter. They usually lie in the antrum or along the lesser curve. Ulcers occurring along the greater curvature in the fundus have a higher incidence of being due to a malignancy. Older patients have more proximal ulcers than younger people and are therefore more difficult to see. Not always will the ulceration be found, especially if superficial; and, therefore, secondary signs of acid-peptic disease have been delineated. These include deformity, heavy mucosal folds, pylorospasm (spasm of the pyloric canal), and hypertrophy of Brunner's glands (submucosal duodenal glands). Final diagnosis: Benign gastric ulcer.

Case ID-5 through ID-8

The radiographs of Cases ID-5 through ID-8 demonstrate the same pathological condition. There is an accumulation of barium in a circular fashion (solid straight arrow) in the duodenum, but at different locations. Similar symptoms, such as GI bleeding or postprandial epigastric pain, were present in each case, despite the location of the ulcer. The largest ulcer (ID-5) is located at the apex of the duodenal bulb, and shows radiating folds (curved solid arrows) similar to those seen with gastric ulceration. The second radiograph

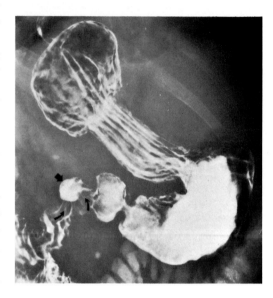

Case ID-5

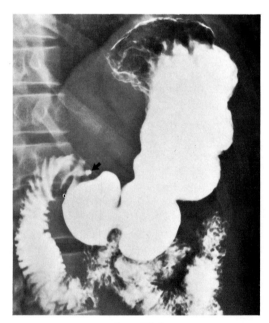

Case ID-6

(ID-6) shows a small ulceration at the base of the duodenal bulb (solid straight arrow). The entire bulb is deformed with enlarged folds secondary to edema. Had the ulceration been nearer the pyloric channel, gastric outlet obstruction might have occurred. The third radiograph (ID-7) demonstrates a faint ulceration (solid straight arrow) in the mid portion of the duodenal bulb with radiating edematous folds leading towards the ulcer crater. Note the prominent rugal folds that can be seen in acid-peptic disease, whether or not an ulceration is found. The fourth film (ID-8) demonstrates a postbulbar ulcer, an ulcer beyond the bulb (straight solid arrow) These ulcers commonly cause spasm and changes on the opposite wall of the ulceration.

The radiographic deformity of the duodenum is very much dependent upon the depth of ulceration itself. If the ulcer is superficial and involves only the mucosa, there may be little or no deformity of the bulb. However, if the ulcer penetrates the muscle of the duodenum, one would expect the muscle to contract and produce a sharp indentation all the way around the bulb at the site of the ulcer. This is the origin of the classical cloverleaf deformity, which may scar in this configuration. It also explains the puckering seen on the opposite wall of the duodenum or stomach in patients with active ulcer disease.

Gastric and duodenal peptic ulcers have a high incidence in our population. Treatment is usually medical, and the resultant healing of the ulcer crater may produce: (1) no change if superficial, (2) slight deformity secondary to scarring, or (3) marked deformity of the segment involved with stricture formation. Complications of ulcers include perforation, bleeding, penetration into the pancreas

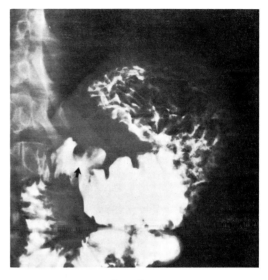

Case ID-7

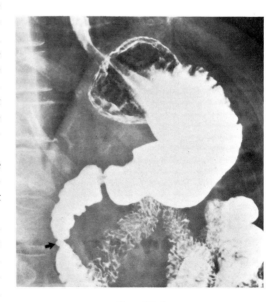

Case ID-8

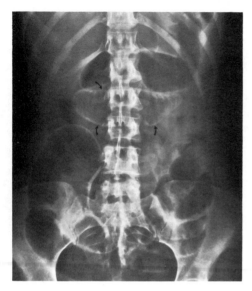

Case ID-9

causing pancreatitis, and stricture formation leading to obstruction. Final diagnosis: Benign duodenal ulceration.

Cases ID-9 through ID-12

The patient in Case ID-9 experienced
acute abdominal pain. When he was examined, his abdomen was tender and

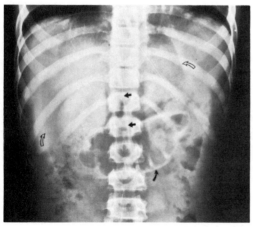

Case ID-10

rigid like a board. The patient was seen
in the emergency room, and the most
common x-ray of the abdomen, the KUB,
was obtained. The film demonstrates dilated small bowel loops throughout the
abdomen. Note the valvulae conniventes.
In the mid portion of the abdomen there
is a segment of bowel, in which you not
only see the inner wall of the bowel, but
also the outer wall of the bowel (curved
solid arrows). This signifies air outside
the bowel or pneumoperitoneum, most
likely from a perforated viscus, i.e., gastric or duodenal ulcer.

A more subtle finding of free gas in the
abdomen is a faint radiolucent density in
the abdomen, the edge of which is seen
overlying the liver (open curved arrow).
This is perhaps better seen on the second
radiograph (ID-10) in a different patient
with similar problems, and is the so-called
football sign (curved open arrows). This
sign is produced by free intra-abdominal
air accumulating under the anterior abdominal wall when the patient lies on his
back. Note that in this second individual
the outer bowel wall (curved solid arrow)
can also be identified, but a third radiographic sign of pneumoperitoneum is
also seen. An opaque line is seen traversing the lower dorsal, upper lumbar spine
area (solid straight arrows). This represents the falciform ligament from the liver
area going towards the umbilicus and is
surrounded by air, allowing it to be visualized. This is a less frequent sign. Note
the nasogastric tube directed from the
chest into the left upper quadrant of the
abdomen.

Definite proof of free intra-abdominal
air can be obtained by two means. An
upright film of the abdomen or of the
chest will allow free intra-abdominal air
to flow upwards, limited by and lying

under the diaphragms. The film in case ID-11 demonstrates lucencies beneath both diaphragm leafs (curved solid arrows) compatible with pneumoperitoneum in this patient with a perforated ulcer. Many of these patients may not tolerate being upright to show the more classical findings of air beneath the diaphragms, and therefore, the left lateral decubitus film will be needed. This film (ID-12) obtained after laying the patient on his left side for about ten minutes, demonstrates even small quantities of free intra-abdominal air accumulated against the right lateral abdominal and chest wall. The liver edge can be identified (short, straight solid arrow) pulled away from the abdominal wall by gravity, and an air fluid level (long straight solid arrow) is seen signifying free intra-abdominal fluid, as well as air in the abdomen. The right diaphragm leaf (curved solid arrow) is identified.

Final diagnosis: Duodenal perforation with pneumoperitoneum (free intra-abdominal air).

Case ID-13

Normally, minimal amounts of fluid are present in the abdominal cavity, which lubricate bowel loops. There are many pathological conditions that may increase the amount of fluid floating free in the abdomen. Perforation of a hollow viscus or organ will not only spill intestinal gas into the peritoneal cavity, but will also soil the cavity with intestinal contents and fluid. Peritoneal fluid or ascites can also be produced by malignancy, either primary or secondary (metastatic), which involves the peritoneal lining of the abdomen causing weeping of fluids into the peritoneal cavity. Inflammatory conditions throughout the abdomen (e.g., ap-

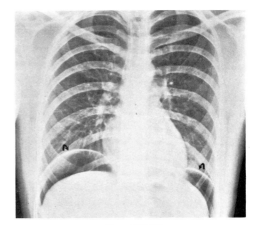

Case ID-11

pendicitis, diverticulitis, and abscess) will irritate the peritoneal lining by producing copious fluid. Cirrhosis of the liver creates an obstruction of the flow of blood from the gut into the liver, with weeping of the wall of the gut and liver producing ascites in patients with low serum protein levels. Right-sided heart failure can cause similar findings, as can bleeding in the abdominal cavity.

A radiograph of the abdomen in a patient with ascites is usually diffusely hazy, which is demonstrated in Case ID-13a. Intestinal gas is identified in the stomach,

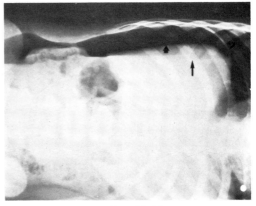

Case ID-12

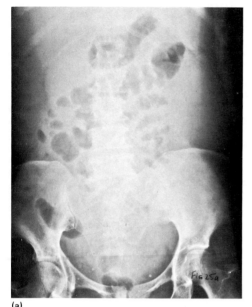

(a)

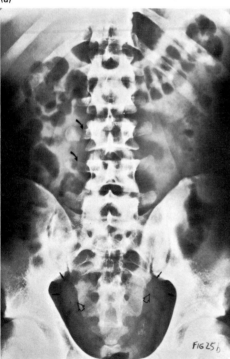

(b)

Case ID-13

colon, and small bowel, but it is situated near the midline. This is because gas within the lumen of the bowel will rise to the highest point of the abdomen. When the patient is lying on his/her back, the highest point of the abdomen is near the midline and anterior abdominal wall. Fluid will gravitate to the dependent portions of the abdomen in that patient, i.e., the flanks or gutters and pelvis. Also note that there is separation of the bowel loops from each other by free floating fluid.

Not always will fluid in the abdomen be enough to demonstrate the above radiographic pattern. Small amounts of fluid can be seen in the dependent portions of the pelvis (ID-13b) below the pelvic brim and above the bladder that is outlined in fat (open arrows). These triangular-shaped densities (small solid arrows) have a characteristic appearance of dog ears and have been named appropriately. Incidentally noted are fractures of the right transverse processes of the third (L3) and fourth (L4) lumbar vertebra (solid curved arrows). Final diagnosis: Ascites (free intra-abdominal fluid).

Cases ID-14 and ID-15

When a patient has an inflammatory process in the abdomen that goes undetected or undiagnosed, a complication may be the formation of an abscess within the abdominal cavity. These abscesses tend to localize in the dependent gutters and recesses of the abdomen and beneath the leaves of the diaphragm. The patient is admitted with spiking fevers without definite complaints localizing this abnormality.

Subtle changes on the chest film may signify an intra-abdominal process beneath the diaphragm. The radiographs presented here are of two such patients

(ID-14 and ID-15). The PA and lateral radiograph of the chest shows what appears to be a right diaphragm, flattened, and elevated above the left diaphragm. The right costophrenic angle is blunted, as is the posterior sulcus. Both of these findings suggest free intrapleural fluid or pleural effusion. Subdiaphragmatic processes, such as a subphrenic abscess, will cause sympathetic accumulation of pleural fluid above that leaf of the diaphragm. Segmental atelectasis in the lung base may also occur. Close observation in this patient, however, discloses multiple lucencies (solid straight arrows) beneath the right diaphragm area. Normally the liver, which lies beneath the right diaphragm, creates a homogeneous soft-tissue shadow without gas shadows present. A second example of abscess air (solid straight arrows) beneath the right diaphragm is presented in Case ID-15b, which is more distinct, with an air fluid level, indicating this to be a loculated pocket, i.e., abscess. Final diagnosis: Right subphrenic abscess.

Cases ID-16 and ID-17

Patients with cholecystitis usually are admitted with epigastric or right upper quadrant pain, radiating around the right lateral aspect of the abdomen or to the right shoulder blade area. This is usually associated with nausea and vomiting, and may be accompanied by a fever, with physical findings of tenderness in the right upper quadrant. Radiographic examination of the abdomen is usually normal.

However, when findings are present, they may be in the form of an ileus, either diffuse or perhaps localized to the right upper quadrant. The film of Case ID-16

(a)

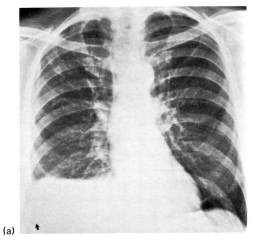

(b)

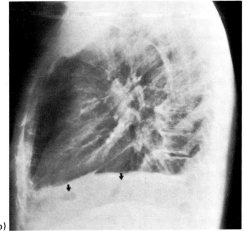

Case ID-14

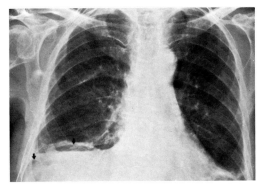

Case ID-15

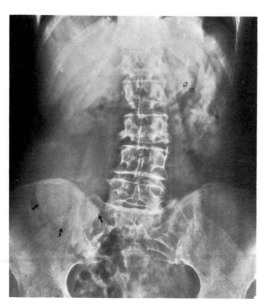

Case ID-16

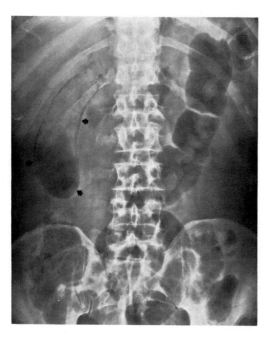

Case ID-17

demonstrates small-bowel gas in the lower abdomen, that is compatible with an ileus. However, it by no means indicates a gallbladder problem in that location. The film demonstrates good rugal folds (open arrows) in the small amount of gas contained within the stomach. Note the rounded soft-tissue density (short black arrows) lying over the right iliac crest. This is actually a gallbladder distended with mucus and pus in a patient with empyema of the gallbladder. No stones or abnormal calcifications are seen in the gallbladder. If stones are present, they are radiolucent, which is the most common presentation of gallstones.

The radiograph of Case ID-17 demonstrates an unusual appearance of an acute inflammatory process involving the gallbladder. The gallbladder is so inflamed that it has undergone necrosis with the production of gas by the bacteria that are present. This gas is seen not only as a round lucency within the gallbladder lumen, but is also seen in the wall of the gallbladder outlining the entire structure (short solid arrows). This is an acutely inflamed gangrenous gallbladder. Usually, an acute gallbladder attack will prevent the gallbladder from visualizing on an oral cholecystogram. This is because the inflamed gallbladder neck is obstructed by edema or a stone, so contrast can't enter. Chronic cholecystitis is different in that visualization of the gallbladder may occur when the contrast is given. Sometimes it takes two successive days of gallbladder pills to visualize a gallbladder. Thirty percent of these people may still be normal. If no visualization occurs, ultrasonography can display the gallbladder and its lumen wall, and some institutions do this study first.

Final diagnosis: (1) Cholecystitis of the

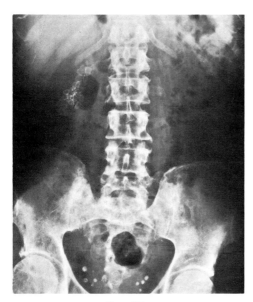

Case ID-18

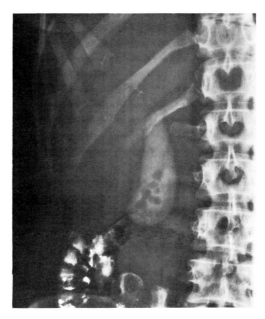

Case ID-19

gallbladder with empyema. (2) Emphysematous cholecystitis.

Cases ID-18 through ID-21

There are multiple appearances of gallstones. Most gallstones, 70% to 80%, are radiolucent and cannot be identified on a plain radiograph of the abdomen. The remaining small number of gallstones can appear as single or multiple calcific shadows in the right upper quadrant (ID-18). They may be either circular or multifaceted in character, or possibly even laminated. Despite their presence on preliminary radiographs, gallstones, not infrequently, are asymptomatic.

To demonstrate nonopaque gallstones, contrast material must be given and secreted into the bile so that stones in the lumen of the bile system can be outlined by the contrast material. Frequently only a few stones are seen, as is demonstrated by our first oral cholecystogram (ID-19).

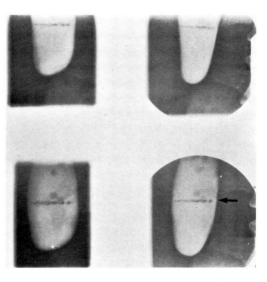

Case ID-20

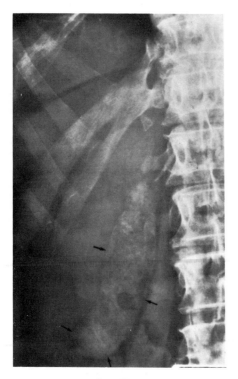

Case ID-21

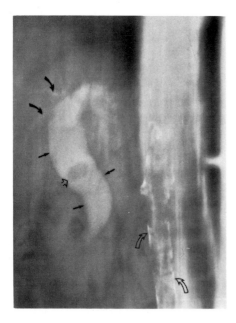

Case ID-22

At least six 1 cm intraluminal lucencies are noted compatible with calculi. In the upright position these will settle to the most dependent portion of the gallbladder, and are easily recognized. Occasionally, these gallstones may be small and of a specific gravity lighter than contrast, so that they float in a horizontal line (straight solid arrow) across the body of the gallbladder as is demonstrated in case ID-20.

The final radiograph (ID-21) demonstrates a faint outline of the gallbladder (solid straight arrows) with thousands of sandlike stones within it. Note that as on most of the radiographs, the kidney and liver edges are well visualized. The formation of gallstones is not well understood. The lipogenic environment of the gallbladder is apparently important for their construction, perhaps with the initial formation of a central nidus. Abnormal concentrations of compounds, such as cholesterol, calcium, and bilirubin in the bile fluid, intensify the rate of development of these calculi. Final diagnosis: Gallstones (cholelithiasis).

Case ID-22

Case ID-22 is an 80-year-old woman who had her gallbladder removed many years ago. Following gallbladder surgery, she remained symptomatic with recurrent bouts of cholecystitis-like symptoms. Jaundice gradually developed, and the patient was hospitalized for evaluation of biliary tract disease.

Since the patient has no gallbladder, an oral cholecystogram exam cannot be used. This is because that study needs the gallbladder to absorb water and concentrate the bile and contrast material, allowing the contrast to be visualized by x-ray film. This patient is ideal for intravenous biliary tract visualization with aqueous contrast material (Cholografin) since her bilirubin is below 3 mg%. The radiograph presented is a body section x-ray film or tomogram of the right upper quadrant during an intravenous cholangiogram (IVC). It demonstrates contrast material within the lumen of a dilated common bile duct (solid straight arrows). Normally, the common bile duct should be less than 10 mm in diameter. Proximally, faint fingerlike projections are seen radiating from this dilated duct. These are intrahepatic biliary ducts (curved solid arrows). In the midportion of the dilated biliary duct there is a 1 cm lucency (open straight arrow) compatible with a calculus. This stone either developed in this duct causing obstructive bile duct symptoms, or was inadvertently left behind when the gallbladder was removed. While the calculus is seen in the midportion of the duct, in the upright position, it settles to the inferior or lower aspect of the duct occluding its lumen. Partial obstruction of the duct occurs giving rise to the patient's symptoms. Incidentally noted is irregular, but linear, calcification in the abdominal aorta (curved open arrows) close by. If this patient's bilirubin had been too high, no opacification of the ducts could have been obtained by an IVC and other modalities, such as ultrasound or CT body scanning, would be needed. Final diagnosis: Bile duct calculus causing obstructive changes in the biliary system.

Case ID-23

As with cholecystitis, other inflammatory conditions in the abdomen may show a normal abdominal film or an ileus-type pattern. Pancreatitis is a similar process that produces few radiographic signs. When these signs are present, specific changes should be looked for. A localized ileus in the left upper quadrant or upper abdomen should suggest pancreatitis. The

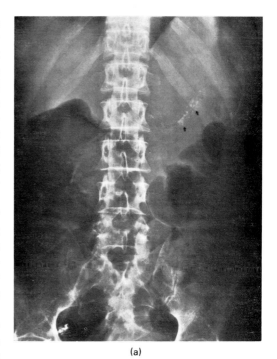

(a)

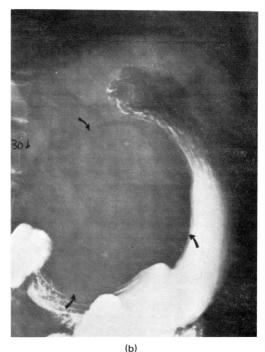

(b)

Case ID-23

most classical radiographic sign of pancreatitis is the visualization of faint small calcifications, which stud the pancreas. The pancreas lies across the upper lumbar vertebral bodies, with its tail directed towards the left upper quadrant and hilus of the spleen. Therefore, these calcifications will usually lie in a diagonal position across the left upper quadrant and midline.

When calcifications are noted, the patient has had recurrent bouts of pancreatitis or inflammation of the pancreas. When pancreatitis develops, pancreatic enzymes, which normally digest food, will destroy the pancreas and result in these calcifications (ID-23a, curved solid arrows). Note also the calcification-like densities seen overlying both hips. These densities are usually explained by intramuscular injections. Either the injections were of the heavy metal type, such as bismuth, which was once used in the treatment of syphilis, or they are injections that have produced local fat necrosis, and the fat necrosis has calcified. In either event, soft-tissue buttock calcification usually means previous intramuscular medication.

A complication of pancreatitis is the formation of walled-off products of pancreatic enzyme digestion in the inflamed area. These pseudocysts can be of various sizes, but when large will distort the adjacent organs. The film in case ID-23b shows a large pseudocyst of the pancreas (curved solid arrows), which causes indentation of the lesser curvature of the stomach, pushing the stomach forward and laterally. This is because the pancreas lies posterior to the stomach and within the duodenal loop, thereby also distorting the duodenal loop. Final diagnosis: Pancreatitis with pancreatic calcifications and pseudocyst formation.

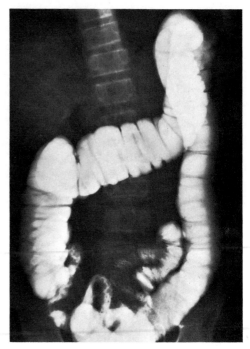

Case ID-24

Cases ID-24 through ID-26

A typical history for the patients represented in these cases is recurrent abdominal pain with chronic diarrhea. These patients are usually teenagers or young adults, although the disease may progress into middle-aged persons. Usually, the diagnosis is made by a barium enema exam that typically shows the terminal ileum to be spiculated, nodular, spastic, and amorphous, with loss of normal folds. This appearance is produced by ulceration of the mucosa with edema and inflammatory reaction. Similar changes are demonstrated in case ID-24. These changes are findings compatible with inflammatory disease of the small bowel, called granulomatous enterocolitis or Crohn's disease. Its cause is unknown but felt to be viral or bacterial in origin.

While Crohn's disease may involve any

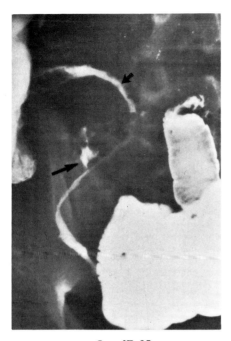

Case ID-25

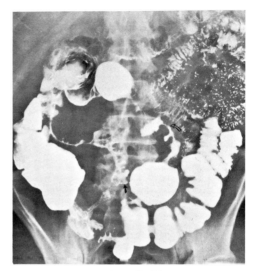

Case ID-26

part of the gastrointestinal tract, it most commonly involves the distal small bowel or terminal ileum. Changes in this structure are the changes that are seen in other organs that are involved. Occasionally, the terminal ileum will be so spastic that it will become very narrow; and only a small amount of barium may be refluxed into the terminal ileum. When this occurs, only a narrow channel of barium is identified, the so-called string sign (ID-25, straight short solid arrow). As the disease progresses, the bowel wall becomes markedly thickened secondary to chronic inflammation, which leads to further narrowing. A complication, and often a diagnostic entity that occurs in Crohn's disease, is the formation of sinus tracts and fistulae (straight long black arrow). The inflammatory process will not only involve the intestinal segment, but will also involve the adjacent mesentery,

which houses edema and inflammatory reaction, separating the bowel loops and making the loops easily identifiable.

As the disease progresses, scarring produces stricture formation (ID-26, open curved arrow). Characteristically, since the disease is segmental in distribution, multiple, inflamed, or strictured areas will be seen at varying intervals in small bowel loops creating a sausage-link configuration to the bowel. The areas between the inflammatory or strictured process may be entirely normal intestinal wall, but it is usually dilated due to the obstruction that was created. Furthermore, Crohn's disease characteristically may be eccentric, involving only one side of the bowel wall. When this occurs, the side opposite the inflammatory process will be changed into a series of sacs or folds called pseudodiverticuli (solid straight arrow). Final diagnosis: Crohn's disease of the small bowel and terminal ileum.

Case ID-27

This patient is a 24-year-old woman with anemia and GI bleeding. While most

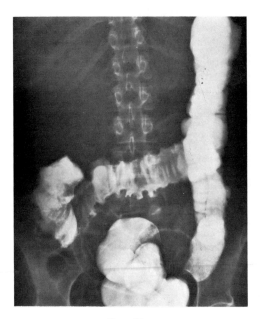

Case ID-27

patients with granulomatous colitis do not bleed, bleeding will occasionally occur. These patients will usually present with recurrent problems of right lower quadrant or lower abdominal pain, chronic diarrhea, and occasionally fever. Keeping in mind the changes that were discussed with Crohn's disease of the small bowel, one can predict the changes that occur in the colon.

The accompanying radiograph shows segmental involvement of the colon with areas of irregularity. These are seen in the transverse colon and distal descending colon. The irregularity represents edema of the bowel wall with mucosal ulceration. Notice the presence of diverticuli along the inferior aspect of the transverse colon. Also, in the distal descending colon, only the left lateral aspect of the colon is involved. This is a classical picture of the eccentrical involvement seen in Crohn's disease. The fact that the rectum is spared from the disease favors the diagnosis of

Crohn's disease. The terminal ileum is not filled with barium, a factor that may be important in this diagnosis, as inflammatory changes around the ileocecal valve will make the valve area inflamed and edematous, not allowing contrast to be refluxed into the distal small bowel.

At times it is difficult to distinguish radiographically between granulomatous colitis and ulcerative colitis (UC) of the colon. If a moderate to long segment of the distal small bowel is involved, the diagnosis is Crohn's disease. However, when the terminal ileum is not involved, it makes the differentiation more difficult. Even the pathologist may have trouble distinguishing the two, but remember that ulcerative colitis involves only the mucosa and submucosal areas of the colon, while Crohn's disease involves the entire thickness of the bowel wall and the mesentery. Through an endoscope, Crohn's disease would show ulcers scattered throughout the colon with the intervening colon mucosa normal. Ulcerative colitis, on the other hand, would show diffuse ulceration with a granular-appearing mucosa with no intervening normal mucosa. Final diagnosis: Granulomatous colitis (Crohn's disease of the colon).

Cases ID-28 through ID-31

Each radiograph in this series will present a different patient with the same disease process, but show different radiographic characteristics. The first radiograph presented (ID-28) shows a pattern similar to the previous case. There is irregularity of the transverse colon, splenic flexure, and descending colon. This irregularity is produced by deep ulcerations of the bowel in ulcerative colitis (UC). The solid straight arrow shows a prominent ulcera-

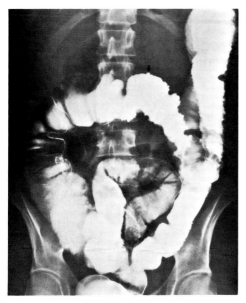

Case ID-28

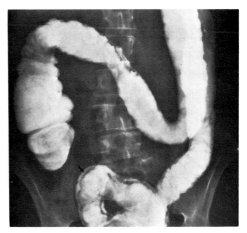

Case ID-29

tion on the superior aspect of the mid transverse colon. This is a collar-button-type ulceration, which was formerly considered characteristic of UC. This ulceration extends through the mucosa and submucosa and undermines those areas. Many of these ulcers can be seen along the wall of the left colon. Note that both sides of the colon wall are involved—without skip areas. In this case the rectum is not involved, which is unusual for UC as this is the most common area of involvement. Haustral folds are still present and the colon is of normal length, indicating that this is an early stage of UC. This disease, like Crohn's disease, is a chronic process with recurring acute exacerbations leading to scarring.

The second radiograph (ID-29) is in a similar stage or phase of UC. Note, the colon is involved from the ascending colon to the rectum. Haustral folds are not seen, but there is a lucent line on the outer margin of the lumen of the colon. It is best seen in the sigmoid colon (solid straight arrow). This radiolucent structure represents debris from the diffusely ulcerated colonic mucosa. Ulcerations are so diffuse and small that they are not radiographically visualized.

The film in case ID-30 shows the results of ulceration of the mucosa, producing polypoid or round lucent structures

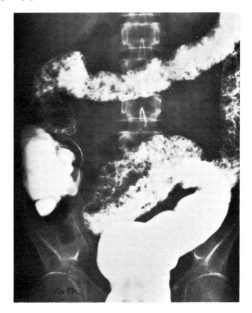

Case ID-30

throughout the colon. These are heaped areas of normal or inflamed mucosa between the ulcerations, and are referred to as pseudopolyps since they are not true neoplastic growths. This is a florid case, and as one might expect, the pseudopolyp formation may be at various stages (either focal or diffuse). Again note that the colon is of normal length, but haustra are lacking. The enema tip that was placed in the rectum had a balloon on it. This should be inflated by the radiologist since it is a hazardous procedure in patients with UC. Note that the lucency produced by the balloon does not extend to the lateral wall of tbe rectum. People with UC, inflammatory bowel disease, or any scarring processes in the rectum will fibrose and shrink the rectum. If a balloon is inflated and stretches the tight rectum, the rectal wall may tear, extravasating barium into the perirectal tissues.

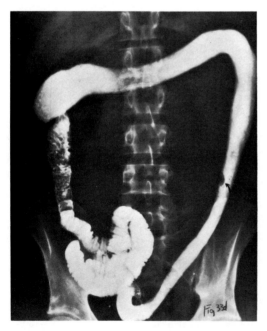

Case ID-31

The fourth patient (Case ID-31) with UC demonstrates the chronic form of the disease. The mucosa is completely effaced or eroded and scarred. The haustral markings are completely absent. The colon is short; and as the colon scars and shortens, its redundancy disappears, with the flexures and component segments easily recognized. The ileocecal valve is scarred in the open position, so there is easy filling of the distal small bowel. At times, inflammatory change may involve the terminal ileum (referred to as backwash ileitis). Incidentally, there is a 1 cm elliptical polyp (solid curved arrow) seen in the mid descending colon that represents an adenomatous or neoplastic polyp and not a pseudopolyp as previously seen. This is an important finding as patients with chronic ulcerative colitis (CUC) have an increased incidence of carcinoma of the colon, and probably should undergo prophylactic colectomy after ten years with the disease. Inflammatory polyps can also be found. Final diagnosis: Ulcerative colitis.

Cases ID-32 and ID-33

Both of these patients have had CUC for differing periods. What is represented here are two of the complications that are seen in CUC.

The first individual with CUC is an 85-year-old woman. In her case, the CUC is radiographically manifested by a loss of haustral folds, shortening of the colon, wide-open ileocecal valve, and filling of the distal small bowel. However, in the proximal descending colon area (solid straight arrows) is an irregular, more narrowed segment of colon. The lowest arrow shows a lucency within the lumen of the mid descending colon compatible with soft tissues encroaching on the lumen.

This segment is characteristically rather long in appearance and represents neoplastic involvement of the proximal descending colon in this patient. The neoplastic involvement of the bowel may take many forms. Frequently they are polypoid or fungating, but can also be annular in appearance (all three will be discussed in the chapter on neoplastic changes). Furthermore, they may appear with an area of narrowing, much like a stricture, but in reality it will be a diffuse, infiltrating, fibrosing-type carcinoma. The strictures are easily recognized, but the benign and malignant ones cannot be distinguished, and therefore must be biopsied.

The second case (ID-33) is in a very toxic condition of the disease. This individual, who is 37 years old, is extremely sick clinically with fever, tachycardia, malaise, nausea, and vomiting. His abdomen is distended and tender. The radiograph demonstrates abundant gas in the transverse colon, with gas seen in segments in the ascending colon and the sigmoid colon. Minimal small-bowel and stomach gas is identified. Note the margin of the ascending colon. The outline is irregular, showing small bumps and lumps (straight solid arrows), that represents edema of the bowel wall. The transverse colon is markedly dilated due to involvement of the myoneurenteric plexus. Relaxation of the colon results, and air will collect in this atonic segment. In actuality the entire colon is involved with the inflammatory process, but the ascending and descending colon lie in the gutters, and are more filled with fluid than with gas. The transverse colon, being anterior, is distended with gas. This individual manifests a toxic megacolon, which was once believed to be seen only in UC, but is now known to exist in Crohn's disease as well. Since the

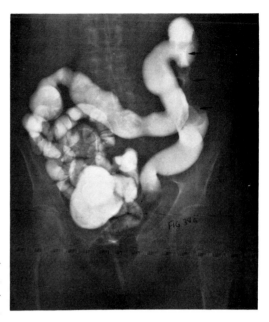

Case ID-32

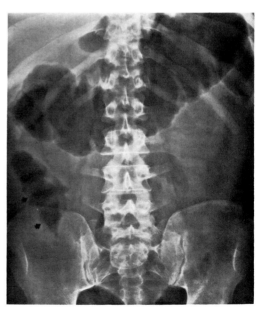

Case ID-33

bowel is markedly inflamed and stretched due to the gaseous distention, a barium enema must not be done as the bowel wall is thin and may perforate. In fact, the patient may perforate anyway, which is one of the signs watched for in patients in such a toxic condition. Final diagnosis: Chronic ulcerative colitis associated with carcinoma of the colon and toxic megacolon.

Case ID-34 through ID-38

The radiographs for these cases demonstrate the most common inflammatory condition in the abdomen. These patients all had appendicitis. The first pair of radiographs represent a KUB and upright abdomen. The supine radiograph (ID-34) shows scoliosis of the spine with the greatest convexity pointing towards the left, indicating spasm, irritation, and contraction of the right iliopsoas muscle.

Bowel gas is seen throughout the GI tract, suggesting an ileus, as not only the stomach (1), duodenum (2), and small bowel (3) is seen, but also colonic gas (4) is seen down to the level of the anus. There is slight dilatation of all the segments, but the small bowel has retained its serpiginous or snakelike character, indicating that this is an ileus, rather than an obstruction. It would have been helpful if the ileus were more localized to the right lower quadrant, which would pinpoint an inflammatory process in the area of the appendix. Note the homogeneous opacity in the right lower quadrant and upper pelvis (multiple solid arrows). This is frequently seen in appendicitis, and represents inflammation and/or abscess formation in the area of the appendix. The upright film (ID-35) shows multiple air/fluid levels in the small bowel, which is minimally dilated.

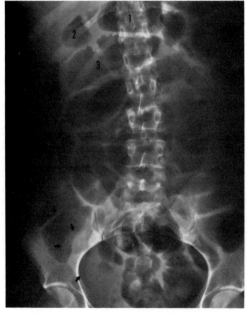

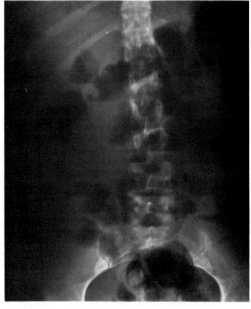

Case ID-34   *Case ID-35*

Even more helpful would have been the visualization of a calcific density in the right lower quadrant, that would have indicated an appendicolith. The film in case ID-36 shows an appendicolith (solid short straight arrows) but no other changes. These structures frequently overlie the bony pelvis and sacrum, making it difficult to visualize. In this patient the acetabulum and femurs have radiolucent lines in the bony structures with adjacent sclerotic borders. These lines represent the epiphyseal plates (solid straight long arrows) or the growing parts of the bones in this child. These lines will disappear when growth ceases.

The pathogenesis of appendicitis is the occlusion of the lumen of the appendix with inflammation distal to the occlusion with or without perforation. This inflammatory process is usually easy to recognize clinically. At times, especially in older persons, appendicitis will show an unusual clinical pattern. The patient may show laboratory evidence of infection but have atypical pain and few if any localized signs. At this point a barium enema may be helpful and offer no extra risk. The first barium-enema radiograph (ID-37) demonstrates deformity of the cecum (4) and terminal ileum (3). There is a soft-tissue mass extrinsic to the cecum and terminal ileum (solid straight arrow) that produces scalloping and elongation of the folds of the bowel. The terminal ileum is displaced slightly towards the midline. This combination of radiographic signs is characteristic of an appendiceal abscess. The subsequent barium-enema radiograph (ID-38) shows what may happen if the abscess is not surgically corrected or cured by antibiotics. Multiple sinus tracts (solid straight arrows) lead from the abscess cavity to the ascending colon and terminal

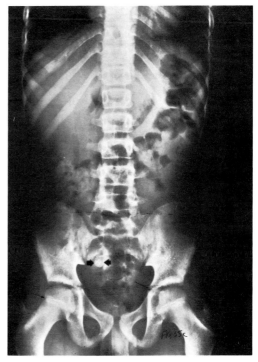

Case ID-36

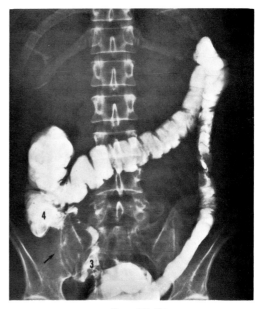

Case ID-37

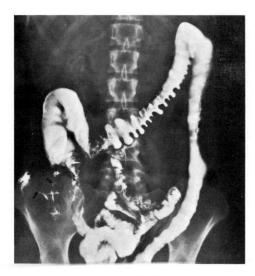

Case ID-38

ileum, but also to the skin. Final diagnosis: Appendicitis associated with appendicolith and abscess cavity with fistula formation.

Case ID-39

This case is a 63-year-old man with left lower quadrant abdominal pain and fever. This is a frequent presentation for patients

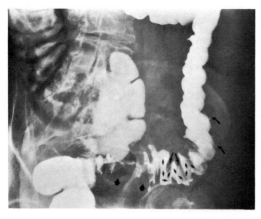

Case ID-39

with diverticulitis. This inflammatory condition of the abdomen is common and is usually seen in older adults. Diverticulosis and its companion disease, diverticulitis, are diseases apparently limited to the Western world. This developmental disease process represents a whole spectrum of clinical and radiographic presentations.

Initially, the patient may complain of diarrhea and constipation, which may alternate with each other. Clinically, he/she is suspected of having functional bowel disease or spastic colon. When a barium examination is performed, the colon may be irritable and spastic, but shows no other abnormality. The spasm is radiographically represented by contractures of the lumen of the colon, which may be intermittent during the fluoroscopic examination. The barium may flow rapidly to the cecum. The patient may show signs of muscle hypertrophy in the colon (solid straight long arrows), which is due to chronic increase in muscle tension of the bowel. It is best seen in the sigmoid as a sawtooth-type pattern or zigzag intestinal lumen (small solid straight arrows). As the syndrome progresses, small saclike structures (solid curved arrows) will protrude from the colon lumen at areas of weakness in the bowel wall. The weakest area is that where the vessels penetrate the bowel wall to feed the colon. These diverticuli are characteristically round when completely filled with barium, but may show irregularities or odd shapes when the diverticulum contains wastes. The base of the diverticulum is narrow, which is in contrast to the pseudodiverticula or sacculations seen in scleroderma. Most of the diverticula occur in the left colon, especially the sigmoid.

Not infrequently, a diverticulum may

rupture, allowing the contents of the intestine to leak into the surrounding mesentery. This results in a localized abscess about the bowel wall. The diverticulum rarely ruptures into the peritoneal cavity with perforation of the bowel and free intra-abdominal air. As the inflammatory process evolves, many radiographic changes take place. Usually only a limited segment of bowel will be involved, which will show narrowing and deformity (short solid straight arrows) with lack of complete distensibility. Lack of distension is usually due to spasm and the adjacent abscess that indents the lumen and surrounds the gut wall, not completely encircling it. Nodularity and spiculation due to the inflammation and edema in the bowel segment are identified. Occasionally, barium will extravasate from the lumen of the intestine into the abscess cavity, which is the sine qua non of diverticulitis. Unfortunately, since there is incomplete distention of these inflamed segments, the radiologist cannot always differentiate this process from carcinoma of the colon. Therefore, when the patient's symptoms subside, a repeat barium enema will usually visualize this involved segment with less acute deformity, signifying that this was an inflammatory process.

Ultimately, as this disease recurs or if the initial inflammatory process was vigorous, extensive fibrosis and scarring will occur. This causes further narrowing and deformity, often leading to obstruction. Segmental resection of the bowel may be necessary to improve the condition. In addition to obstruction and inflammation, another complication of diverticulosis and/or diverticulitis is GI bleeding. This may appear as a chronic anemia or as an acute exsanguination with the patient hypotensive. Waste matter and/or inflammation will erode into the mucosa of a diverticulum, and into an adjacent or underlying vessel. It is noteworthy that most of the severe bleeding from diverticuli apparently comes from the right colon and must be diagnosed by an arteriogram. Segmental resections of the right colon performed blindly without locating the bleeding site have improved the prognosis of the disease. Final diagnosis: Diverticulosis syndrome (spastic colon, diverticulosis, diverticulitis).

NEOPLASMS OF THE BOWEL

CASE PRESENTATIONS

Case N-1

This is a 56-year-old woman, who was admitted to the hospital with dysphagia. Because of this complaint an esophagram was obtained, which demonstrates the pathological entity presented in this case. The distal esophagus shows abrupt narrowing just above the left diaphragm. The

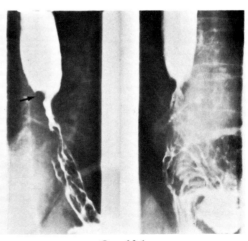

Case N-1

narrowed segment is irregular in outline and enters into a small hiatal hernia of the stomach. A protrusion of soft tissue or shelf (solid straight arrow) indents the dilated barium column above the rigid, narrowed area. These findings are compatible with neoplastic involvement of the distal esophagus.

Carcinoma of the esophagus more commonly involves the distal two thirds of the esophagus than the proximal one third. This is usually a squamous-cell variety of carcinoma, although adenocarcinoma of the stomach does exist at the junction of the esophagus with the stomach, with growth into the distal esophagus. A neoplasm involving the esophagus can appear in many forms, including a polypoid, fungating mass within the lumen, stricture formation as in this case, ulceration of the mucosa, or just simply irregularity along the wall of the lumen. Endoscopy must be performed as it is difficult radiographically to distinguish these forms from esophagitis and its complications.

Carcinoma of the esophagus spreads rather easily in the mediastinum as there is no outer fibrous wall to the esophagus limiting the growth of the cancer. Metastasis in mediastinal nodes is common. Surgery on the esophagus can be performed, but it is much easier when the carcinoma is distal. Final diagnosis: Carcinoma of the distal esophagus.

Cases N-2 and N-3

The two radiographs presented here demonstrate three appearances of malignancy of the stomach. Both of these patients are elderly women with anemia. The first radiograph (N-2) demonstrates a large, round soft-tissue density in the fundus and upper body of the stomach (solid

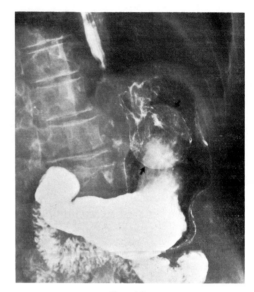

Case N-2

straight arrows). This is one of the common forms of gastric carcinoma, appearing as an intraluminal fungating type mass. Note that the rounded, soft-tissue density does extend into the upper medial aspect of the stomach, and could have easily obstructed the distal esophagus as it enters the stomach. Note also the relative absence of rugal folds as atrophy of the gastric mucosa is associated with a high incidence of carcinoma of the stomach.

The second radiograph (N-3) shows not only rugal atrophy, but two other common manifestations of carcinoma of the stomach. Ulceration of the antrum is identified by persistent accumulation of barium along the greater curvature (solid straight arrow). As previously indicated during the discussion of benign gastric ulcers, this ulceration should lie along the surface of a neoplastic mound of tissue. As the tissue grows, it outgrows its blood supply, creating ulceration of its surface which

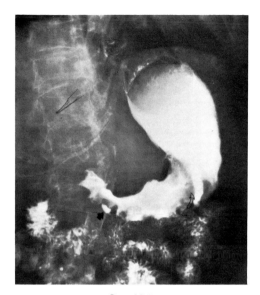

Case N-3

declining in our country, although it is still very high in Japan.

Of incidental note on the second radiograph are the black stringy lines that point towards the gastroesophageal region. These represent static electricity produced as the film is taken from the cassette for developing. Final diagnosis: Carcinoma of the stomach.

Cases N-4 and N-5

These two cases show the same disease process involving the stomach. The rugal folds of the greater curvature of the stomach are markedly enlarged (solid straight arrows). When seen in profile, they appear as thumbprints along the outline of the stomach. When seen en face they are visualized as large lucent lines coursing through the stomach. Notice the normal rugal folds in the antrum of the stomach for comparison. These abnormal rugae are frequently associated with ulceration, and can occur focally or in multiple areas. This

may then bleed. The same radiograph demonstrates a third common manifestation of carcinoma of the stomach. While the tumorous tissue may not grow into the lumen or ulcerate, it may infiltrate the stomach wall, causing rigidity and deformity with lack of distension of the region of the stomach involved. The curved open arrow shows a narrowed, deformed junction of the body and antrum of the stomach and prominence of rugae created by the infiltrating tumor. During fluoroscopy, this region did not change its contour despite palpation. When the tumor affects the pyloric channel, barium will empty rapidly from the stomach. This occurs characteristically in linitis plastica or diffuse infiltration of the stomach. Tumors of the stomach that are as extensive as the two shown here are usually incurable, and probably have metastasized to regional lymph nodes or liver by the time they are found. Fortunately, the incidence of cancer of the stomach is

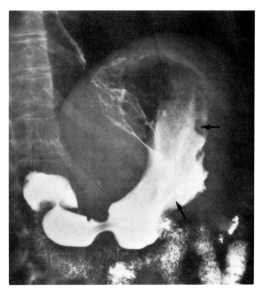

Case N-4

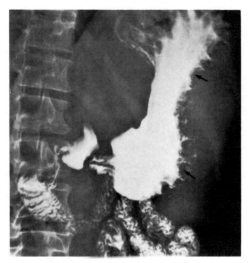

Case N-5

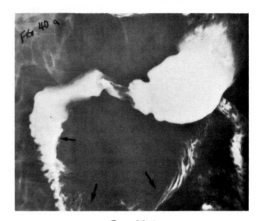

Case N-6

appearance of lymphoma is difficult at times to differentiate from carcinoma.

The stomach is one of the most common locations in the GI tract for lymphoma. The ileocecal area and small bowel are other favorite sites for this disease. In general we expect lymphoma to appear as enlarged lymph nodes in the hilar and mediastinal structures with splenic enlargement. While lymphoma is a malignant process, it has a relatively high cure rate dependent upon the cell type and location. Surgery, radiation, and chemotherapy, alone or in combination, are the treatments for this disorder. Final diagnosis: Gastric lymphoma.

Cases N-6 and N-7

The radiographs accompanying this discussion represent two 60-year-old men with jaundice, one of whom was believed to have hepatitis. Normally, the pancreas lies within the duodenal loop behind the stomach. As the pancreas enlarges, it will widen the duodenal loop (N-6, solid straight arrows). The stomach is displaced forward and upward, and the duodenal loop to the right and downward. It will indent adjacent organs extrinsically, creating a deformed, narrowed appearance. If the mass is well defined and encapsulated, no mucosal involvement will be found. Both pancreatic carcinoma and pancreatitis with edema or pseudocyst formation can present a similar appearance. As the tumor infiltrates the surrounding tissues, it will infiltrate the duodenum, and produce a spiculated appearance in the duodenum (N-7, open arrow). Nodular indentations (N-7) are seen along the medial aspect of the second portion of the duodenal loop as the tumor enlarges (solid straight arrows). These radiographs demonstrate a mass located in the head and body of the pancreas. Not all the pancreatic masses occur in that area and may be localized in the body or tail of the pancreas, even near the hilus of the spleen. Characteristic extrinsic displacement will be encountered with each mass location.

Coursing through the head of the pancreas is the common bile duct, which will

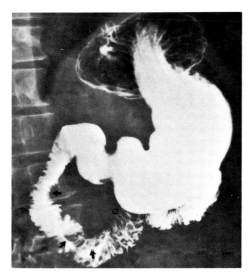

Case N-7

empty bile into the duodenum at the duodenal papilla. As a tumor mass in the
head of the pancreas enlarges and infiltrates the adjacent structures, it may also
deform, narrow, and obstruct the common bile duct, causing jaundice. This was
true in the patients in these cases. Occasionally, a large common bile duct will be
seen, making a linear indentation near the
duodenal bulb apex; but this is not identified on these radiographs. Further evaluation of the pancreatic area could be
accomplished with ultrasound and CT
scanning. Endoscopic retrograde cholangiopancreatography (ERCP) can also be
done.

Cancer of the pancreas, unfortunately,
usually defies diagnosis until the disease
is widespread and usually inoperable.
This is because the pancreas has no fibrous capsule that might hinder the
growth of the tumor, and is located in an
area that is difficult to image. It spreads
easily to adjacent structures and lymph
nodes. By the time the radiographic
changes involve the stomach and duoden-

um, the patients are usually inoperable.
Hopefully, newer techniques in radiography, such as computerized body scanning
and ultrasound, will help make the diagnosis earlier. Final diagnosis: Carcinoma
of the head of the pancreas.

Case N-8

This patient is a 54-year-old woman
with rectal bleeding. This is a common
manifestation of this disorder. The radiograph (N-8a) demonstrates multiple, intraluminal densities within the colon
(curved solid arrows). The solid arrows
represent adenomatous polyps in a full
column type barium enema. While only
three polyps are pointed out on the initial
radiograph, multiple black lucencies are
seen throughout the colon, compatible
with multiple polyposis. More commonly,
only a single polyp is found. These polyps
usually appear as a round or lobular density in the lumen of the colon. They may
be attached to the wall of the colon by a
stalk (pedunculated polyps), or will have
no stalk (sessile polyps). These polyps
may vary in size. The larger the polyp,
the greater the incidence of carcinomatous
change. If the polyp is sessile, rather than
pedunculated, the incidence of carcinoma
also is increased.

Most polyps are neoplastic transforma-
tions of the mucosa. But some are inflammatory or hamartomatous in origin, rarely
associated with polyposis syndromes.
Most polyps manifest themselves by
bleeding. This occurs because the surface
of the polyp is eroded or abrased by
passing waste material exposing the underlying vessels. Carcinomas develop
from adenomatous polyps. Polypectomy
can be done through an endoscope or
surgical segmental resection. Prophylactic
colectomy may be used to control the

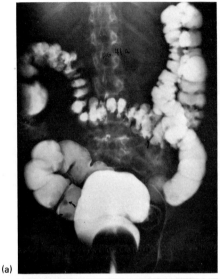

(a)

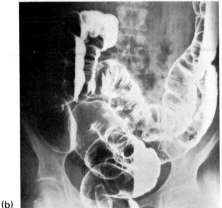

(b)

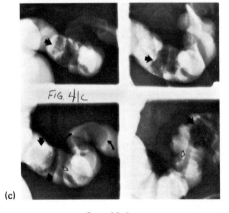

FIG. 4|c

(c)

Case N-8

development of the carcinoma that occurs in some of the polyposis syndromes.

The second radiograph (N-8b) in this case represents a common technique, which is gaining favor in diagnosing mucosal lesions of the colon. This is an air contrast barium enema examination of the colon. It uses a small quantity of special thick, tenacious barium, which coats the surface of the mucosa. Then the colon is distended with air. A double contrast effect is obtained, and the mucosa of the colon can be well outlined. Note the easily identified sessile colon polyps (curved open arrow) using this technique.

The film in N-8c demonstrates a 2 cm intraluminal filling defect (solid straight arrow) in the mid portion of the sigmoid colon. Its surface is slightly irregular in outline, with white streaks through the mass compatible with barium lying in the crevices of its surface. There is movement of the polyp in the sigmoid as demonstrated by its altered position in the four spot films. There is a 2 cm by ½ cm stalk (open arrow) attaching the neoplasm to the surface of the colon. Nearby is a 2 cm eliptical lucency (curved arrows), an air bubble, easily confused with this stalked polyp. Final diagnosis: Colon polyps.

Cases N-9 through N-12

This is a series of patients with carcinoma of the colon. Two centimeter or slightly larger intraluminal densities (solid straight arrows) are seen in the colon of Case N-9 (a and b). One is located in the cecum. Two other lesions are seen in the same patient, one in the transverse colon and one in the rectum. These intraluminal densities have no demonstrated stalk and are sessile. As a polyp approaches 2 cm, the risk of carcinomatous change approaches 50%. Therefore, these require polypectomy.

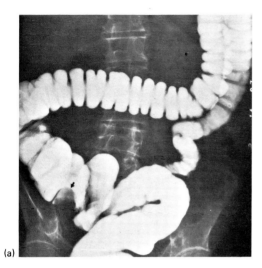

(a)

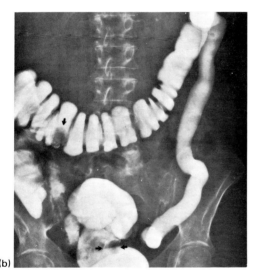

(b)

Case N-9

Polypoid carcinoma may occur at any level in the colon, but it occurs predominantly in the right colon. Carcinomas of the right colon are usually fungating soft-tissue masses that do not obstruct the liquid fecal stream until they are very large. It is not until the more distal colon is reached that water has been removed from the stool, and the feces become solid. The other common form of carcinoma of the colon is the plaque or constricting mass of soft tissue around the circumference of a short segment of colon, the so-called "napkin ring" or "apple core" deformity (Case N-10 and N-11, short straight arrows). This type of deformity is more frequent in the left colon, creating obstruction of the solid stool, leading to constipation and obstructive symptoms. Case N-10 shows diverticuli (curved open arrows).

The most frequent sites for carcinoma of the colon are in the cecum and rectosigmoid areas. In the cecum these tumors tend to bleed, with the patient showing a chronic anemia. Tumors of the rectosigmoid area are similar, but also tend to obstruct, and the patient is admitted with a distal colonic obstruction. It is not uncommon for a patient with carcinoma of the colon to have a polyp or second carcinoma elsewhere in the bowel, as demonstrated by the patient with two lesions. In this patient the density in the transverse colon was a benign adenomatous polyp, while the one in the rectum was a carcinoma.

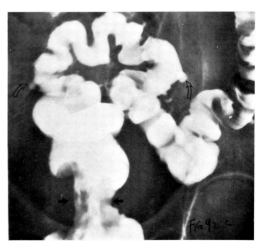

Case N-10

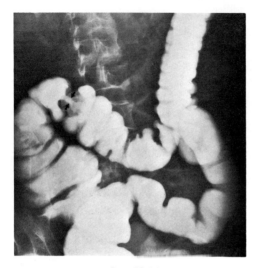

Case N-11

in this patient—characteristic for this type of lesion. Also note the white, stringy densities on the papillary surface of this mass, which represents barium in the crevices of this tumor. This patient had a large villous adenoma of the colon, which is a premalignant lesion showing frond-like surfaces, entrapping barium. It is also so soft that stool will pass by it without obstruction, and is so soft it is easily diagnosed as stool when palpated, unless it is of considerable size. Final diagnosis: Neoplasms of the colon.

MISCELLANEOUS GI DISORDERS

CASE PRESENTATIONS

Case GI-1

The final radiograph (N-12) in this series demonstrates a huge, fungating neoplasm of the rectum (straight solid arrows). Of interest is the considerable size of the lesion. Something of this size in the rectosigmoid area would often obstruct the bowel, but no obstruction was present

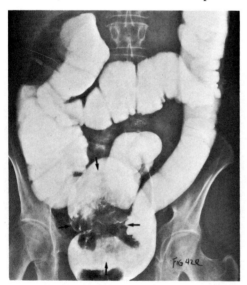

Case N-12

This patient is a 46-year-old woman, who had a carcinoma of the colon resected many years ago. Note that the upper abdomen is devoid of gas, especially on the right. The gas shadows that are present are scattered throughout the GI tract with no dilation. The stomach and colon are displaced inferiorly (curved arrows). This signifies that there is an enlarging mass in the right upper quadrant pushing the stomach, colon, and other gas shadows into the lower abdomen. Although this could be an inflammatory or neoplastic mass, liver enlargement is the logical diagnosis.

Note the faint calcifications (solid straight arrow) in the right mid abdomen, occurring in a round focus in three different areas. These represent calcifications in metastatic foci in the liver. This is an infrequent finding in carcinoma of the colon that has metastasized to the liver. It

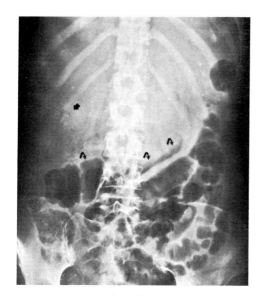

Case GI-1

This patient is a 61-year-old woman with chronic lymphatic leukemia. As in many of these patients, lymphadenopathy and splenomegaly are encountered. Enlargement of the spleen occurs due to leukemic infiltration.

Normally, the spleen lies above the edge of the costal margin in the left upper quadrant. It is seen as a homogeneous density beneath the left diaphragm and

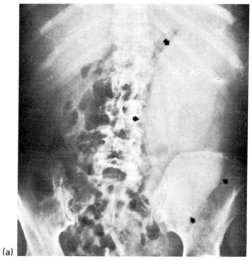

(a)

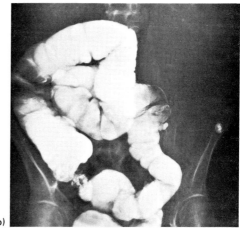

(b)

Case GI-2

is seen in mucinous carcinomas of the bowel.

The liver is a homogeneous structure normally lying in the right upper quadrant, rarely extending below the iliac crest or across the midline radiographically. As it enlarges it does so frequently more to the anterior than to the posterior, causing the displacement of gas shadows seen in this case. The stomach, which is anterior and to the left of the midline, is displaced posteriorly and to the left, or downwards as is the duodenum, which may be seen across the midline to the left. Other gas shadows of both small bowel and colon are pushed inferiorly, and the right kidney, even though retroperitoneal, may be pushed downward and medially. Unless significant displacement of organs and gas shadows is seen, liver enlargment is difficult to diagnose. Final diagnosis: Hepatomegaly secondary to calcified colonic metastasis.

against the left upper lateral abdominal
wall. As the spleen enlarges, the adjacent
bowel will be displaced in a manner similar to that seen in liver enlargement. The
left kidney may be depressed downward
and medially. The stomach, small bowel,
and colon will be displaced downward
and medially (GI-2a straight solid arrows).
If barium is placed in the colon, displacement of the colon is observed (GI-2b).

There are many causes for splenomegaly. It is commonly seen in patients with
cirrhosis. This scarring of the liver obstructs the flow of blood entering from the
gut and produces portal hypertension.
Blood must then be rerouted so that it
may return to the heart. The blood is,
therefore, redistributed through the collateral circulation, which involves congestion of the spleen, stomach, and esophagus. Lymphoma, like leukemia, will
enlarge the spleen. Hemorrhage into or
around the spleen will enlarge the splenic
shadow. The clinical history of trauma or
associated rib fractures will usually differentiate this problem from other clinical
entities. Mononucleosis, congenital stor-
age diseases, and idiopathic reasons also
cause splenic enlargement. The spleen
may need to be removed in these individuals to prevent splenic rupture. Final diagnosis: Splenomegaly.

Case GI-3

This patient is a 66-year-old man with
bleeding from his gastrointestinal tract.
Radiographic evaluation of the esophagus
during an upper gastrointestinal study
demonstrated the reason for his bleeding.
There are longitudinal nodular folds seen
in the distal esophagus. These frequently
appear as tortuous or serpiginous worm-
like structures causing lucencies in the

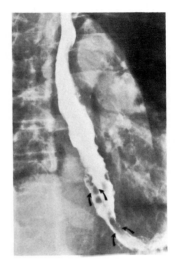

Case GI-3

distal esophagus. Similar densities may
be located at the fundus of the stomach.
These structures (curved solid arrows)
represent esophageal varices.

Varices are dilated tortuous veins,
which may occur at several places in the
gastrointestinal tract. When these vessels
become abraded or lacerated, they often
bleed massively. When they occur in the
esophagus, endoscopy will confirm their
presence, but radiographic visualization
is diagnostic.

There are many causes for esophageal
varices. During the discussion of splenomegaly a cause for esophageal varices was
alluded to. Blood that cannot enter the
liver from the gut is commonly rerouted
to anastomotic channels in the area of the
stomach and spleen. From here vessels are
seen anastomosing with other large venous trunks around the esophagus and
stomach, ultimately entering the caval
system in the chest via the azygous system. Because of this increased flow of
blood into the smaller venous channels,
the vessels become enlarged and tortuous,

and are seen radiographically. The esophageal varices demonstrated in this case represent "uphill" varices produced by obstruction of the flow of blood from the gut to the heart. "Downhill" varices, which occur in the upper aspect of the esophagus with a similar appearance, appear in people with obstruction of the superior vena cava, with collateral blood supply flowing from the upper extremity and head towards the heart through the esophageal venous plexus. Final diagnosis: Esophageal varices.

Case GI-4

This patient is a 71-year-old man, who was complaining of abdominal distension. The initial radiograph of the abdomen of this patient was unremarkable, as it frequently is for this abnormality. Ileus, pseudo-obstruction, especially distal colonic obstruction, are changes on the plain film of the abdomen that are frequently seen in patients with ischemic bowel disease. Many of the patients either go on to necrose their entire gut or, more commonly, their symptoms improve without radiographic changes.

The second radiograph (GI-4a) obtained on this patient did show gas throughout the GI tract, with slight dilatation of the transverse and descending colon. Small-bowel gas is also noted, and there is air in the rectum. All of these findings are compatible with an ileus. There is, however, nodularity along the wall of the transverse colon (curved solid arrow) compatible with bowel-wall edema and/or hemorrhage. This is highly suggestive of ischemic colitis in this elderly patient. Barium enema examination (GI-4b) in this individual shows a contracted, small colon due to spasm and bowel-wall edema and hemorrhage. Multiple thumbprint-type

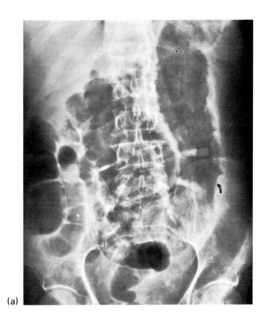

(a)

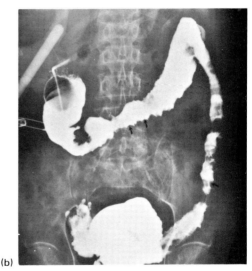

(b)

Case GI-4

indentations or nodularity are seen along the bowel edge (solid straight arrows) compatible with intramural or bowel-wall hemorrhages. The patient underwent a colostomy to put the bowel at rest. A catheter with an inflated balloon was inserted into the colostomy for visualization of the colon during the barium enema.

The reason for an ischemic gut is vascular obstruction—arterial or venous. This can occur because of occlusion of a major arterial branch, such as the superior mesentery artery, which would affect the entire small bowel and right colon; or it may involve any segmental portion of this distribution. A frequent area of involvement is the splenic flexure, which may undergo scarring and stricture formation—as with any inflammatory process. Occasionally, no occlusion is found; and this is felt to be due to reduced perfusion during a hypotensive episode. Final diagnosis· Ischemic colitis.

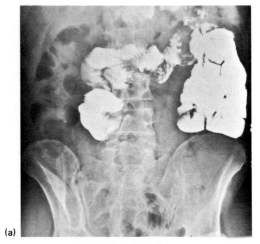

(a)

Cases GI-5 and GI-6

These two patients were admitted to the hospital for chronic diarrhea. They are both in the 50-year age group and demonstrated similar radiographic findings. The workup for chronic diarrhea includes radiographic examination of the duodenum, small bowel, and colon. At the same time laboratory tests are undertaken to rule out parasitic inflammation, malabsorption, and other digestive disorders involving the pancreas and gallbladder.

The first radiograph (GI-5a) demonstrates loss of the usual feathery jejunal folds that are normally visualized in the left upper quadrant. These loops have an amorphous appearance without the identification of normal folds. As the examination is continued, dilated loops of small bowel are observed in the distal jejunum and ileum (GI-5b). There is also a suggestion of an intussusception in the right mid abdomen involving the ileum (solid straight arrows). The final radiograph (GI-6) demonstrates, in the second patient, dilated small-bowel loops, but the folds

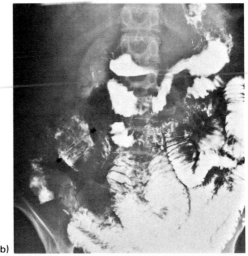

(b)

Case GI-5

are not sharp nor distinct as one might expect. Before the introduction of well-suspended barium, barium would tend to drop out of suspension, causing segmentation of the small bowel and flocculation of barium throughout the GI tract. This is not identified on these radiographs. With the additives in barium keeping the barium in suspension now, only dilatation of the small bowel is noted.

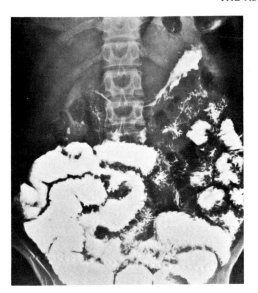

Case GI-6

The puttylike amorphous-appearing jejunal loops in the left upper quadrant are due to villus atrophy. The villi are the undulant mucosa lying on the valvulae conniventes. The indistinct folds in the last case probably represent large amounts of mucous and secretions within the small bowel, and as the barium proceeds through the GI tract, poor coating of the mucosal lining results. Proof of these changes is obtained by a small-bowel biopsy, which is done by passing a tube through the stomach and into the distal aspect of the duodenum, where a small piece of tissue of the proximal small bowel is obtained. These patients may be cured of their disorder by elliminating gluten, a wheat product, from their diet. Both of these patients exhibited the findings of nontropical sprue. Final diagnosis: Nontropical sprue (gluten sensitive).

5

Genitourinary Tract

NORMAL EXCRETORY UROGRAM

One of the best ways that the internal structure of the urinary tract can be visualized radiographically is by injecting iodinated aqueous contrast material. This is usually injected into the antecubital vein rapidly, so that high blood levels can be reached. The contrast material flows through the venous system to the heart and is then dispersed throughout the body in the arterial system, ultimately being filtered by the kidney. Most of the contrast material is eliminated from the blood in the first hour, and usually all of it will be eliminated within the first day. This technique demonstrates urinary excretion of contrast material and, only indirectly, renal function.

During an excretory urogram (intravenous pyelogram, IVP) at our hospital, a series of radiographs are taken in sequence for what we feel gives the best definition of the urinary structures. A 30-second radiograph (Fig. 5-1a) is taken after initial preliminary radiographs. This "blush film" demonstrates contrast material in the finer arteries and capillaries of the kidney as well as the renal tubules (nephrons) before the contrast material has had time to appear in the collecting system. This radiograph defines the margins of the kidneys (solid straight arrows), as well as their size. It will "blush" other organs as well, including the spleen and liver (curved arrows). Occasionally blood vessels will be identified when the film is exposed too early. Note the 3 mm calcification overlying the right kidney (curved open arrow). This represents a calculus lying within the collecting system of the right kidney.

The next radiographs in sequence during the IVP are tomograms. These are longitudinal laminar sections of the body. This x-ray technique visualizes only millimeter to centimeter thicknesses of the body. The single accompanying tomogram (Fig. 5-1b) does show a very excellent outline of the left kidney (short solid arrows). The right kidney is not as well seen because it is not lying in the same plane as the left kidney. Incidentally noted is the tip of the spleen (curved solid arrow). An indentation along the lateral aspect of the left kidney is identified, which is a normal congenital variation. Since the kidneys lie posteriorly in the abdomen, other structures in the same plane will be visualized. Pedicles of the spine (open arrow) and other structures of the spine are well outlined.

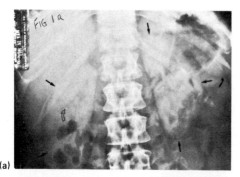

(a)

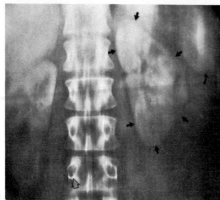

(b)

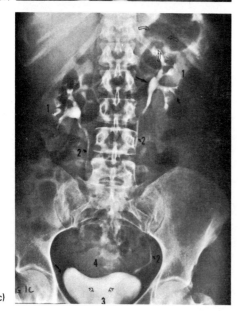

(c)

Figure 5-1

The functioning unit of the kidney is the nephron. The nephrons of the kidney are in the renal parenchyma, which extends from the outer margin of the kidney to the caliceal structures or collecting system (curved open arrows). The renal sinus area of the kidney is where the caliceal structures are found and is surrounded by fat. The renal hilus is where the renal artery and vein enter the kidney, and where the renal pelvis extends out joining the ureter.

At this point the contrast material has yet to reach the collecting system. Subsequent radiographs will show the contrast material in the collecting system as contrast media and urine leave the collecting tubules in the renal papilla and empty into the caliceal structures. The last radiograph (Fig. 5-1c) demonstrates contrast in this collecting system. The collecting system of the kidneys (1) is made up of several anatomical structures. The funnel-shaped small curvilinear densities in the periphery of the kidneys (short solid arrow) lead to larger draining canals. The small cups are called minor calices, and larger ducts are called major calices. There are approximately a dozen minor calices in each kidney, with two to three major calices being formed by those small structures. The major calices then will form a larger funnel-shaped structure, the renal pelvis (long solid arrow). This forms a reservoir for the collection of urine and contrast material before this fluid enters the ureter (2). Once the contrast material and urine enter the collecting system, only drainage is important—kidney excretion has been completed.

The ureters run from the upper lumbar area in the retroperitoneal space to the pelvis, coursing over the iliopsoas muscle. Proximally they take a symmetrical course on either side of the lumbar spine, usually extending close to the bony structures, and more medial and close to the midline than the kidneys. They are normally medial to the tip of the transverse processes of the lumbar spine. When the ureters reach the pelvic brim, they then take a lateral course in the pelvis before extending anteriorly to enter the bladder at the ureterovesical (UV) junction area. The ureters are not just a duct system; they do have a muscular wall, which undergoes peristaltic action from the level of the renal pelvis to the level of the bladder. Therefore, one will see the ureter in segments during an intravenous pyelogram (IVP) unless an abnormality such as atony or obstruction is present.

The ureter courses through a short segment of bladder wall before it enters the lumen of the bladder at the ureteral orifice. While no valve is present within the ureter itself, its course through the bladder wall in an oblique fashion forms a valvelike mechanism, which prevents urine refluxing from the bladder back into the ureter. Normally, only antegrade flow of urine will be present. Reflux does occur abnormally and will be discussed.

The final collecting place for urine and contrast material is the bladder (3). This is a smooth, rounded structure sitting in the most anterior-inferior aspect of the soft tissues of the pelvis. Its shape will change depending upon the quantity of urine and contrast material in the bladder when the film is taken. When the bladder is full, it ultimately will be visualized as a large, round, balloon-shaped structure extending out of the pelvis. The only anatomical structure visualized within the bladder is the interureteric ridge (short straight open arrows). The ureteral orifices open at the lateral edges of this ridge.

This ridge forms the superior edge of a triangle-shaped base in the bladder called the trigone. The inferior point of the triangle is the outlet of the bladder or the uretheral opening. Note that the interureteric ridge sits at the level of the ischial spines (large solid curved arrow). If the ureteral orifices enter the bladder in a position lower than this, a cystocele or pelvic floor relaxation is suspected. Note the soft-tissue shadow (4) sitting above the bladder causing a slight indentation to the superior aspect of the bladder. This represents the uterus in a female pelvis. Also note the faint round densities in the right aspect of the pelvis, some of which overlie the bladder and some of which are just above the right superior lateral aspect of the bladder. These are phleboliths lying in the veins of the pelvis, quite often simulating ureteric stones. One should note the abundant gas throughout the abdomen, which can obscure the kidney outlines and other structures in the urinary system. This is why tomograms are so helpful in delineating the outline of the kidneys and collecting system when looking for masses.

For the urine and contrast to leave the body, it must pass through a short canal, the urethra. This is not normally identified on an excretory urogram as there is a sphincter at the outlet of the bladder which retains contrast material in the bladder until it is voided. A urethrogram is needed to visualize this structure.

CONGENITAL DISORDERS

Case Presentations

Case CD-1

The first case is a 25-year-old woman with recurrent urinary tract infections.

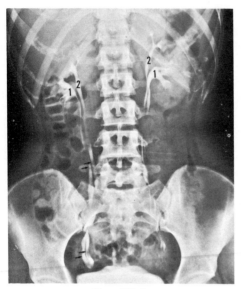

Case CD-1

This is a common symptom in young women, with many etiologies. The single x-ray taken from this urogram demonstrates a common congenital malformation of the urinary system. There has been duplication of the collecting systems of both kidneys. The collecting system of the upper pole of the kidneys has a different renal pelvis (1, 2) from the collecting system of the lower pole of the kidneys, and also different ureters (solid arrows). These extend all the way down to the bladder; and therefore, she has a complete duplication of the collecting system. More commonly, the ureters join somewhere between the renal pelvis and the bladder. This means two proximal ureters and one distal ureter on the same side.

Although the collecting systems in this patient otherwise appear normal, there are associated problems that occur with this congenital disorder. These are recurrent infection and obstruction. Since there are two ureters entering the bladder at different locations, one or both of the entrances of the ureters into the bladder may be abnormal. The ureter from the lower pole of the kidneys usually inserts laterally in the bladder wall and may have a wide open orifice, which will allow urine to freely reflux up the ureter. The ureter from the upper pole of the kidney usually extends distally beyond the orifice of the lower pole ureter, and enters the bladder in a lower medial aspect, going through structures that ureters do not usually pass. This occasionally causes extrinsic narrowing leading to obstruction. When there are two proximal ureters and only one distal ureter, the distal ureter usually enters the bladder in a normal position so that the normal valve mechanism will be present in the bladder wall. If this were not the case, reflux would occur in the distal ureter, and then up both limbs of the proximal ureter into the kidney. Occasionally, the ureter from the upper pole of the kidney will insert in a structure other than the bladder, such as the vagina or urethra. This will lead to continuous wetting.

While medical means may correct the inflammatory aspects for the patient, these anomalies can cause recurrent problems and surgery may become necessary. If reflux continues, or continual wetting is a problem, or even if obstruction is present, the ureters can be reimplanted into the bladder. During this procedure the ureters are put into an oblique tunnel in the bladder wall, which will create the valve mechanism needed to prevent reflux. Final diagnosis: Duplication of the collecting system (congenital).

Case CD-2

The next case demonstrates another congenital anomaly which may lead to recurrent infections, obstruction, and stone formation, not to mention the easy access of the kidneys to trauma. When the kidneys develop in the embryo, they lie in the pelvis and ascend in the retroperitoneal spaces to their normal positions in the flank areas. The renal pelves are anterior in location, at first; as the kidneys ascend, the kidneys rotate with the renal pelves facing medially. As one would expect, abnormalities during this developmental stage can produce many congenital anomalies, one of which is shown on the accompanying radiograph.

This radiograph (CD-2) demonstrates a cystoscope (1) in the bladder with ureteral catheters in the distal ureters (open curved arrows). Contrast material has been injected through these catheters to outline the collecting systems of the kidneys (a retrograde pyelogram). The renal pelvis (2) appears in a more lateral position than the previously noted normal renal pelvis. Furthermore, the long axes of the kidneys are directed from the upper quadrants towards the midline (dotted line) rather than from the midline down towards the lower quadrants as in normal individuals. Other than the calices showing slight dilatation, no pathological abnormality is seen. The lower poles of the kidneys appear to join, or at least meet, near the midline (solid arrow) over the spine. This junction can either be a fibrous union or a joining of the parenchyma of the lower poles. This is easily demarcated at surgery and can be divided if need be.

This anomaly represents the so-called horseshoe kidney—actually two separate kidneys that fuse during ascent into the normal position in the retroperitoneal spaces. Because the ureters must go over the renal parenchyma anteriorly, this anomaly can cause obstruction at the renal pelvic ureteric junction, leading to hydro-

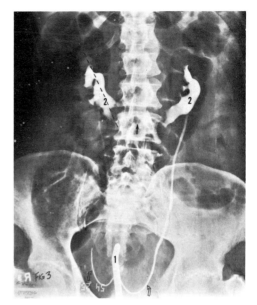

Case CD-2

nephrosis or dilatation of the collecting system. The hydronephrosis may then lead to urinary stasis, which can secondarily lead to inflammation, scarring, and atrophy, as well as stone formation.

Since the kidneys meet in the center of the abdomen over the spine, the kidneys can be easily damaged or ruptured from blunt abdominal trauma. Therefore, these patients are encouraged not to undertake activities that would increase this risk, such as contact sports. Final diagnosis: Horseshoe kidney.

Case CD-3

This is a 23-year-old woman with abdominal pain and fever. During her evaluation in the hospital, an excretory urogram was undertaken to find the source of her symptoms. This patient represents a variation of the horseshoe kidney, which was previously presented. As the kidneys ascend, many variations of abnormal

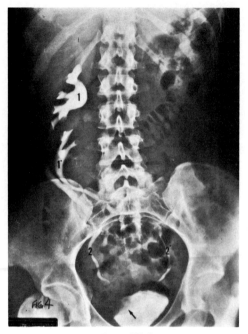

Case CD-3

When attached, this is called a fused anomaly; when unattached, an unfused anomaly. This pattern of abnormal ascent and position of the kidney is called crossed renal ectopia, with ectopia meaning located in an abnormal position. Note that bowel goes into the left renal bed where the left kidney should have been. The left kidney can be easily palpable in the right mid abdomen, and may appear as an abdominal mass. This abnormality is a good indication for an IVP as a surgeon would not like to take out a pelvic or abdominal mass and find out that it is nothing more than an ectopic kidney. Note on the radiograph the lucency in the right superior aspect of the bladder causing distortion of the bladder. This is due to adjacent stool in the cecum (solid arrow). Final diagnosis: Crossed renal ectopia.

alignment or development can occur. The horseshoe kidney is just one example, and this case is a second. When the kidney does not ascend and remains in the pelvis, it usually overlies the sacrum and is called a pelvic kidney. These can be found anywhere adjacent to the spine, up to and including their normal retroperitoneal position.

The radiograph (CD-3) represents a normal right kidney position (1) with an abnormal left kidney position (1'). The right kidney ascended normally, but the left kidney ascended initially on the left as can be deduced because the left ureter (2') is in the normal position in the pelvis. However, as the kidney ascended above the pelvis in the lumbar region, the left kidney proceeded to ascend towards the right. The left kidney can be attached to the right kidney or separate.

URINARY STONES AND OBSTRUCTIVE DISORDERS

CASE PRESENTATIONS

Case US-1

This patient is a 31-year-old female who has recurrent abdominal pain. The initial radiograph (US-1a) shows four ½ cm calcifications overlying the renal areas (small solid curved arrows). Outlines of the kidney edge (open arrow) and liver edge are identified. To definitely show that these calcifications are within the kidney, an oblique radiograph (US-1b) can be obtained as in this case. Note that although there is a change in body position, the renal stones or calculi stay within the boundaries of the kidney (open curved arrows).

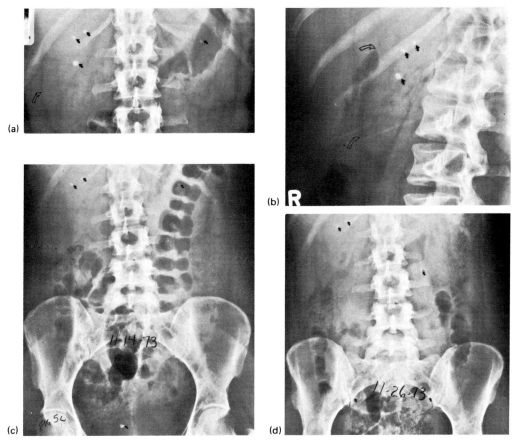

(a)

(b) R

(c)

(d)

Case US-1

The formation of calculi in the urinary system is not completely understood. It is, however, known that a small nidus is usually made either by inflammatory cells or debris that is in the urine. Calcium may then be deposited around this central core, and built layer upon layer with the formation of various sizes and configurations of stones. Most (80%) stones in the urinary system are calcified and opaque to x-ray. The other 20% of stones, usually uric acid stones, are nonopaque. Cysteine stones are faintly opaque to x-ray. While inflammation probably plays the greatest role in the formation of stones, elevations in chemical products in the urinary system can create a saturated environment favoring the formation of stones. This apparently is a mechanism for uric acid stones.

Stones can form in any structure where there is stasis of fluid that contains an environment compatible with the nidus and subsequent stone formation. This condition can occur in the renal tubule, usually the collecting tubule, or in the collecting system, usually the calix, and less frequently in the renal pelvis. Most commonly stones are seen in the fornices or corners of the minor calices and remain there until dislodged to be passed with the flow of urine.

When the patient passes a stone, it will enter the ureter at the ureteropelvic junction, which is a common site for impaction due to the abrupt change in the caliber of the channel. If the stone is small enough to be passed through the ureteropelvic junction, it will by peristalsis and urinary flow proceed down the ureter until the lumen narrows again. This is usually where the ureter passes the bony pelvic rim at the edge of the sacrum. The stone may stop here temporarily or permanently, but more commonly will pass into the distal ureter to the third and most common area of stone obstruction, the ureterovesicle-junction area. The stone will then, if small enough, pass into the bladder where it is easily passed out of the bladder and into the urethra.

A stone that is not small enough for passage into the ureter can lead to obstructive changes and inflammatory scarring; it may need to be removed surgically. Similarly, if the stone is impacted in the ureter at any level, surgical assistance will be needed. Most stones, however, pass with medical management.

The radiograph in US-1c is of the same patient, approximately two weeks later. She passed the lowest stone in the right renal collecting system into the distal ureter, where it is lodged at the right ureterovesicle-junction area (small curved arrow in pelvis). A subsequent radiograph (US-1d) shows that the patient has passed the distal right ureteric stone, but has now proceeded to drop the left renal stone into the most proximal portion of the left ureter at the ureteropelvic junction (small curved arrow on the patient's left). This stone also passed without surgery and without complications. The small curved arrows

near the date in the pelvis show the place at the pelvic brim where stones will hang up because of extrinsic narrowing. Final diagnosis: Renal stones with migration into the ureters.

Case US-2

This is a 56-year-old male with a mass in the right upper quadrant. An excretory urogram was obtained because of the possibility that this mass was renal in origin. The film demonstrates extensive calcification bilaterally in the kidney areas. Note that the calcification appears laminated or layered in places. The calcification is rounded and is taking the configuration of the collecting system, i.e., the major and minor calices. This type of urinary calcification is called a staghorn calculus. It starts with small calcifications and grows by layers until it fills either part of

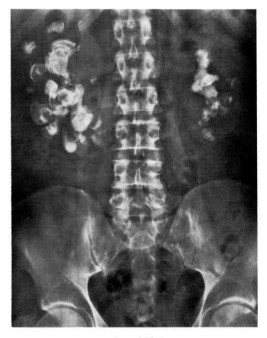

Case US-2

or the entire renal collecting system. Only fragments of this large calculus can be passed, and if removal is necessary, the remainder of the large calculus must be removed by surgery, sometimes along with the affected kidney.

This patient's mass was due to an enlarged kidney, which was infected and showed the effects of chronic obstruction due to this calculus. Even if this kidney had been cleaned of calculi earlier, the calcification probably would have reformed because of the environment in this patient's urine. Occasionally, this environment can be altered by medical therapy; or at least the environment can be improved so that stone formation can be retarded, if not eliminated. The formation of a calculus in the urinary tract is insidious and subtle, giving few symptoms until the patient passes blood due to irritation by the calculus, or passes the calculus with the excruciating pain that is so characteristic of such passage. Final diagnosis: Staghorn calculus.

Case US-3

The radiographs presented here are from the same individual. This is a 55-year-old woman with recurrent infections and hematuria. The initial radiograph (US-3a) demonstrates several phlebolith-like densities in the pelvis that could be urinary stones, but are actually outside the urinary tract. There is faint calcification seen in the right renal area (solid arrows). The calcification assumes a configuration similar to staghorn calculi, but appear to be numerous small stones clumped together. Note that there are no calculi in the left kidney. A subsequent radiograph (US-3b) made during an intravenous urogram demonstrates a normal left collecting system and ureter, except

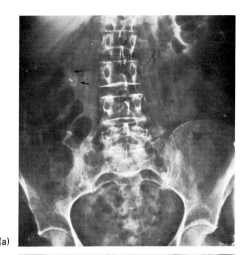
(a)

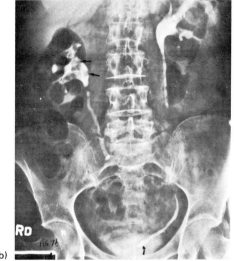
(b)

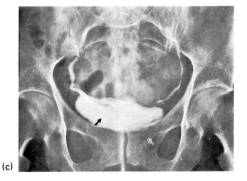
(c)

Case US-3

for a bulbous tip to the distal left ureter (curved solid arrow). The configuration of the distal ureter is classical for a uretero-cele.

A ureterocele is formed by a stenosis or narrowing at the most distal aspect of the ureter, with redundant mucosa and dila-tation of the ureter proximal to the area of narrowing. This assumes a "cobrahead" configuration, which is shown in this case, and can be of various sizes. It is a congenital abnormality. Because of the stenosis, there is stasis in the urine in the left collecting system that can lead to re-current infection and stone formation.

This individual actually has ureteroceles bilaterally, but the one on the right is not shown because of the small amount of contrast seen in the distal right ureter. The right ureterocele has, however, caused stasis of urine in the right collect-ing system so that there is formation of calculi in the right caliceal system and renal pelvis. Note that while the faint calcifications are seen on the preliminary film of the abdomen as positive or opaque densities, they are seen as negative or lucent defects in the contrast-filled right collecting system. The reason for this is that the calculi are not as dense as the iodinated contrast material that surrounds them, thereby giving a relative lucency to the stones. This lucency would be similar to a radiolucent calculus not seen on the preliminary film of the abdomen, yet causing a defect in the contrast-filled col-lecting system. Occasionally a nonradio-paque stone in the distal ureter will not be seen but would be suspected when obstructive changes are present. The final radiograph (US-3c) demonstrates the right ureterocele (solid arrow), which is two to three times larger than the left. Note that the entire right ureter is filled, suggesting

that urine and contrast material cannot be freely emptied from the right collecting system, leading to urinary stasis and cal-culi formation. Final diagnosis: Right ren-al stones in a patient with bilateral ure-teroceles.

Case US-4

The next three radiographs demonstrate the secondary signs of the passage of a urinary calculus, whether or not the cal-culus is opaque. The first radiograph (US-4a) demonstrates a persistent blush of the right kidney. This can be seen by exam-ining the lower poles of the kidneys (ar-rows), the right being more dense than the left. This means that there is pressure in the right collecting sytem, causing pres-sure in the renal tubular system as well, which causes stasis of contrast material in the renal parenchyma. When the pressure is relieved, the contrast material normally will pass freely into the collecting system. Because of this increase in pressure, there will be delayed visualization of the right collecting system when compared to the normal side. This is manifested by lack of opacification of the collecting system on one side when there is contrast material in the calices and renal pelvis on the normal side. Note that there is slight dil-atation of the right renal pelvis (3) and the proximal right ureter (2). If one would measure the length of the kidneys, the kidney with the obstructive changes would be larger than the nonobstructive kidney due to edema and swelling.

The second radiograph (US-4b) dem-onstrates a marked difference in the size of the collecting systems. The left collect-ing system shows moderate dilatation of the major and minor calices. There is also dilation of the renal pelvis (3) and the proximal left ureter (2) when compared to

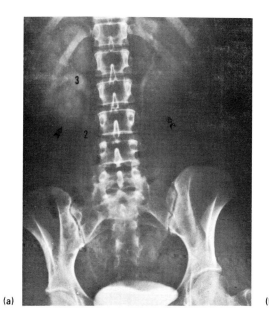

(a)

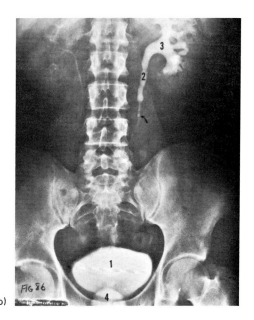

(b)

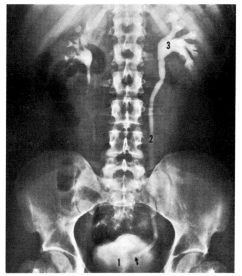

Case US-4   (c)

the nonobstructed right side. The site of obstruction is at the level of the left transverse process of L4 (solid curved arrow). This stone is in the proximal ureter, causing partial obstruction of the left collecting system leading to dilatation as shown.

Note that the distal left ureter is not dilated. The bladder (1) appears normal, but there is a soft-tissue density beneath the bladder (4), which is commonly seen in excretory urography representing the soft tissues of the penis overlapping the lower

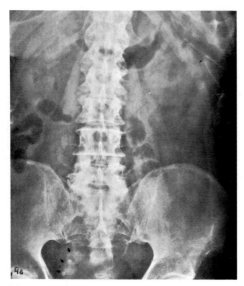

(a)

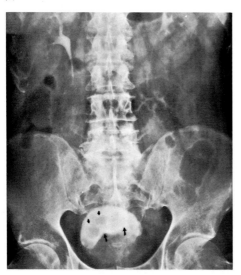

(b)   Case US-5

pelvis. The third radiograph (US-4c) shows a distal left ureterovesicle stone (solid arrow) causing proximal dilatation of the left renal pelvis (3) and left ureter (2). The bladder (1) is normal. Final diagnosis: Obstructive hydronephrosis due to stones.

Case US-5

This is a 70-year-old man with symptoms of prostatism, i.e., frequency of urination, reduced urinary stream, and hesitancy. Because of these symptoms an IVP was obtained to exclude upper urinary system abnormalities associated with prostatic problems. An IVP would also make it possible to evaluate the bladder and the prostatic area.

A radiograph of the abdomen (US-5a) shows slight to moderate degenerative spurring in the lower dorsal, upper lumbar spine area. There are phlebolithlike densities in the right aspect of the pelvis. There are three or four faint circular opacities, 1 to 2 cm in diameter, in the right aspect of the soft tissues of the pelvis (curved solid arrows). Some of them overlie the bony aspect of the sacrum. The remainder of the radiograph is unremarkable. A subsequent film during an intravenous urogram (US-5b) demonstrates contrast material in the normal upper collecting systems. However, in the bladder there are several intraluminal negative or lucent defects (curved solid arrows) in the contrast material. These densities represent the previously seen faint opacities in the right aspect of the pelvis. Also note that the bladder contour is not round and smooth as in the previous case. The floor or inferior aspect of the bladder has been uplifted by a nodular indentation (short solid arrows). This indentation is most likely due to prostatic enlargement, which by lifting the outlet of the bladder and the trigone is causing urinary stasis. Because of chronic stasis, bladder calculi have developed. Through a pathogenesis similar to that mentioned previously for upper urinary stones, the stasis in the bladder leads to the accumulation of biproducts in the urine, infection, and inflammatory change, which in turn favors the development of calculi.

Bladder stones may not be found on radiographs of the abdomen, since these stones are faintly opacified and overlie the bony structure of the pelvis. They can be of various sizes and shapes. Fifty percent have enough calcium to be seen radiographically. They are usually laminated. These types of stones are best seen during excretory urography or endoscopy of the bladder. Final diagnosis: Bladder calculi in a patient with prostatic enlargement.

Cases US-6 and US-7

The accompanying radiographs are of two different patients with similar pathological processes. Each demonstrates obstruction of the collecting system in different stages, but due to the same diagnostic entity. In the first case (US-6), note the size and shape of the renal pelves. They are dilated and somewhat rectangular in shape. The calices attached to the renal pelves are also dilated. At the inferior aspect of the renal pelves, where the outlet should be, there is a narrow ureteropelvic junction (solid curved arrows). A ureter of normal size is seen beyond this narrowing. The renal parenchyma (markedly curved solid arrows) is maintained in both of these patients despite the apparent obstruction. When obstruction is prolonged, the kidney will undergo obstructive atrophy; and the parenchyma will shrink. The left kidney shows no intraluminal filling defects in the renal pelvis. However, the right kidney shows multiple lucent or negative defects (short solid arrows) throughout the calices and renal pelvis, which are compatible with several etiologies. Any time a negative defect is seen in the contrast material in the urinary system, it

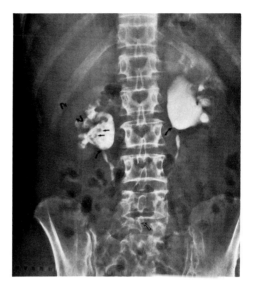

Case US-6

could represent a stone, blood clot, or tumor and cannot be differentiated without pertinent history and laboratory findings. In this individual, since there is obvious obstruction, the most likely diagnosis is calculi. Note that in the right kidney the caliceal structures are rounded and blunted, rather than the sharp cup design of normal individuals. This is due to obstruction and inflammatory change.

Renal pelvic junction obstruction is a common form of obstruction of the urinary system. It is congenital in origin, thought to be due to crossing vessels or adhesive bands, which narrow the ureteropelvic junction. Although some patients never have to undergo surgery for correction of this deformity, frequently surgery is indicated to prevent atrophy, scarring, and destruction of the kidney parenchyma. During surgery the redundancy of the renal pelvis is trimmed away, and the ureter is reinserted into the renal pelvis in the location best suited for fluid drainage.

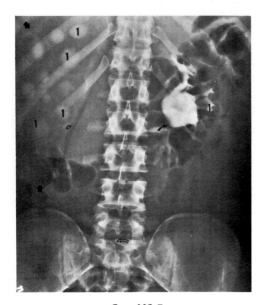

Case US-7

The second case (US-7) shows similar findings of ureteropelvic junction obstruction in the left kidney. Note here, though, that the calices (1) are sharp and cup-shaped, showing no changes of inflammation or obstruction despite the apparent narrowing at the ureteropelvic junction (curved solid arrow). The right kidney is markedly enlarged, and its edges are only faintly identified (solid fat arrows). The renal pelvis is not seen with contrast material, but is represented by a grey shadow overlying the proximal portion of the right iliopsoas muscle shadow. The calices (1) show marked dilatation with pooling of contrast material in the dependent portions of the collecting system when the patient is lying on his back. There is a halo of lucency about the puddles of contrast material in the collecting system, which is due to urine not containing contrast material lying in the periphery of these dilated calices. As the calices dilate in this pathological sequence, they

compress the renal parenchyma causing atrophy. A parenchymal stain is seen as crescents and rims at the edge of the dilated calices (straight open arrow). Note the marked renal parenchymal atrophy lying between the largest dilated contrast-filled calix in the upper lateral aspect of the right kidney and the solid fat arrow along the right lateral edge of the right kidney. Delayed films will show more complete filling of the collecting system. It is interesting that both of these patients demonstrate congenital failure to unite the spinous processes of S1 (curved open arrows). This lack of bony fusion is spina bifida occulta, which is a normal congenital variant. Final diagnosis: Stone formation and hydronephrotic change in congenital ureteropelvic junction (UPJ) obstruction.

Cases US-8 and US-9

The patients here demonstrate the same disease entity, but at different stages. The initial radiograph (US-8) demonstrates normal upper collecting systems. The ureters are of normal caliber, and empty into the bladder in a normal fashion with one exception. The interureteric ridge is horizontal rather than having the normal shallow U-shaped configuration. The distal ureters, as they enter the bladder, can be seen to be abnormally horizontal (solid arrows) rather than to make a normal slanted or oblique entrance into the posterior lateral aspects of the bladder. The most inferior aspect of the bladder is not completely filled with contrast material, giving a negative or lucent nodular defect in the lower aspect of the bladder. All of these findings are consistent with prostatic enlargement or any other condition that would uplift the bladder floor.

The second individual (US-9) also has

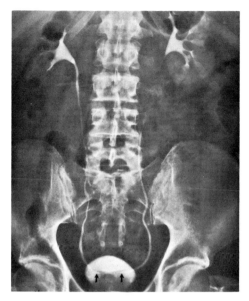

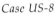

Case US-8

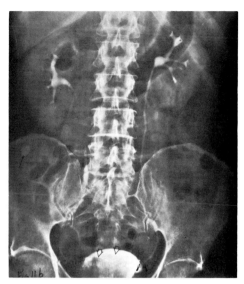

Case US-9

normal upper collecting systems, although in severe degrees of prostatic enlargement or bladder outlet obstruction, bilateral hydronephrotic changes can be present. Prostatic enlargement with outlet obstruction is the most common cause of bilateral hydronephrosis in men. Note the grossly misshapen bladder with nodular indentations (open arrows) uplifting the floor of the bladder. The distal ureters are hooked or have undertaken a J-shaped configuration (solid arrows) best seen on the patient's left side. The interureteric ridge has actually been inverted, but is not well seen on this film. Note that the inferior aspect of the bladder is irregular in outline and does not show the usual smooth surface. This individual demonstrates a more severe degree of prostatic enlargement and bladder deformity than the last patient, yet the upper collecting systems have yet to be affected by the disease process. Incidentally, there is a 1 cm scler-

otic density (long small arrow), irregular in outline, in the superior aspect of the right ilium. This represents a commonly seen normal variant, a bone island. It is of no clinical significance other than it can simulate sclerotic or osteoblastic bony metastasis.

Many of the phlebolithlike calcifications seen in these excretory urograms lie outside the urinary system and are obviously phleboliths. Calcifications over the course of the ureters that disappear when contrast material surrounds them are stones, not phleboliths.

Benign prostatic hypertrophy is frequently demonstrated on the excretory urogram. However, clinical history and physical examination may show significant disease without radiographic findings. Furthermore, as in this second individual's case, the physical findings showed minimal prostatic enlargement, but a marked degree of bladder deformity is seen by x-ray. Prostatic enlargement can be due to prostatic carcinoma, but is more commonly due to benign hyperplasia—a frequent disorder of men after 50. Since the prostate surrounds the urethra, it will narrow and obstruct the posterior urethra or bladder outlet. The bladder being muscular will become trabeculated, and even form diverticuli due to the chronic increase in tension or pressure in the bladder. Transurethral resection (TUR) of the prostate will alleviate the obstruction and narrowing, with both clinical and radiographic improvement. This reaming-out type of defect can frequently be seen on postoperative excretory urography as a triangular-shaped density at the inferior aspect of the bladder. Final diagnosis: Prostatic enlargement from benign prostatic hypertrophy (BPH).

INFLAMMATORY DISORDERS

Case Presentations

Case I-1

There are several radiographs included in case I-1. The initial radiograph (I-1a) demonstrates a normal right collecting system and bladder. A normal left ureter is visualized. Note the indistinct outline of the left renal pelvis (solid arrow) and the lack of good distention. The calices are not well seen on the right, but are normal in their contour. The kidneys are approximately of equal size. Usually, acute pyelonephritis causes no radiographic change. However, as in this case, edema of the collecting system mucosa will create linear lucencies and indistinct edges in the renal pelvis of the in-

volved kidney. The only other associated finding in acute pyelonephritis is swelling of the kidney, causing overall increase in size as compared with the opposite normal kidney.

Acute pyelonephritis occurs by several mechanisms. Hematogenous infection from distant sites is a known pathway for infection to get to the kidney. A more common route is urinary reflux from the bladder into the ureter and up into the caliceal system. Normally, urine travels in one direction down the ureter with the entry of the distal ureter into the wall of the bladder in such a fashion that a sphincter is created. When this mechanism is not present, reflux will occur, and any infection in the bladder would then spread to the ureters and kidneys in an ascending fashion.

The next pair of radiographs (I-1b and c) demonstrate a more chronic form of the disease, as this patient has had recurrent infection. This patient actually had bilateral ureteral reflux with recurrent pyelonephritis. The collecting systems are blunted (I-1b, solid arrows) or clubbed. There is atrophy of the renal parenchyma, best demonstrated on the accompanying tomogram (I-1c) of the renal areas. When the inflammatory process does take place, it involves the calyx and renal papilla. Following the inflammatory reaction and edema, scarring along with atrophy, takes place, which leads to thinning of the cortex in the area of the calyx (I-1c, solid arrow) and distortion of the caliceal structure. The parenchyma between each adjacent calyx is less affected. The pyelonephritic changes are more apt to be polar, occuring at the poles of the kidney, rather than along the lateral edge, unless the disease is extensive. While reflux is com-

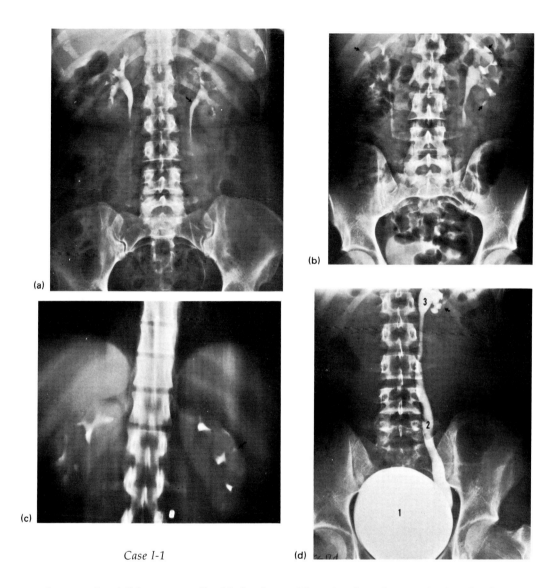

(a)

(b)

(c)

(d)

Case I-1

monly seen in children, not all of it leads to inflammatory atrophy and scarring of the collecting systems. It does occur more frequently in women than in men, due to the higher incidence of bladder infections in women. Patients may outgrow reflux, especially if infection is controlled.

The final radiograph (I-1d) demonstrates even further atrophy and distortion of a kidney involved with recurrent urinary tract infections due to reflux. This radiograph is a cystogram that was done in surgery. Contrast material was instilled into the bladder (1), and it is obvious that a large amount of contrast material refluxes up the ureter (2) into the left renal collecting system (3). Note the marked atrophy (solid arrow) and shrinkage of the kidney. Another method of demonstrating reflux is by instilling contrast material into the bladder via a urethral catheter inserted during the examination. If reflux is present, it may be seen as the bladder is filling or emptying during voiding. This is called a voiding cystourethrogram. Final diagnosis: Acute and chronic pyelonephritis due to vesicoureteral reflux.

Cases I-2 and I-3

The two radiographs presented are of two different female patients with the same disease process. Each of the patients demonstrated blood in the urine; and therefore, an excretory urogram was obtained to evaluate the urinary system. The radiographs demonstrate similar findings.

The first radiograph (I-2) demonstrates distortion, irregularity, and destruction of the minor calices. The normal cup-shaped calyx is no longer visualized. Several lucent round densities (solid arrow) are seen within the caliceal structure. Several collections of contrast material are seen in

the renal pyramid areas in the parenchyma adjacent to the minor calices (open arrow). The second radiograph (I-3) shows similar findings with clubbing and distortion of the caliceal systems. There are prominent accumulations of contrast material in areas outside the caliceal structures (solid arrows). These take many forms including linear streaks, amorphous accumulations, and circular collections (solid arrows). Both of these patients demonstrate renal papillary necrosis.

The etiology of papillary necrosis is not completely understood. It is known to have to do with ischemic changes in the renal pyramids and an associated inflammatory reaction. The renal pyramid tips or papillae undergo necrosis, and are sloughed into the caliceal system creating the lucent round densities as seen in the first patient. The place where the papilla is necrotic, but has not completely separated from the pyramid, may be surrounded by contrast material in the collecting

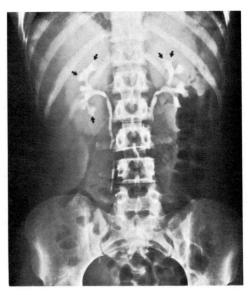

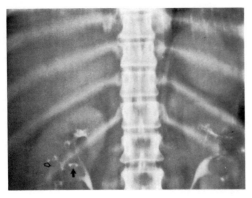

Case I-2   Case I-3

system, creating rings and streaks of contrast. There are multiple known etiologies that create ischemic changes, associated with this condition. This pathological process occurs in diabetics, aspirin and phenacetin abusers, sickle cell anemia patients, and patients with vasculitis. Occasionally, as part of the disease process, the necrotic debris will simulate the colicky pain of renal stones; and this is when the study is requested and the findings of papillary necrosis detected. Final diagnosis: Renal papillary necrosis.

Cases I-4 and I-5

When a clump of bacteria in the bloodstream is filtered out by the capillary system of the kidney, it most likely will be destroyed by the patient's defense mechanisms. When this does not occur spontaneously and the bacteria settle in the kidney, an inflammatory response will be created causing acute pyelonephritis. Normally, this is diagnosed and treated; but occasionally these small areas of infection are walled off by the body and escape detection. When this inflammatory process forms a focal area of necrosis and pus forms, there is an abscess. Luckily, renal abscesses are infrequent, but are seen in persons whose defense mechanisms are hampered.

Initially, as a renal carbuncle is being produced, little change is observed in the excretory urogram. Subsequently, loss of the renal edge and swelling in the area of the abscess may be noted with minimal distortion of the collecting system. As the abscess grows in size, more distortion of the collecting system is seen with bulging of the margin of the kidney. Liquefaction of the abscess or necrotic material has slightly less density than the surrounding contrast-containing renal parenchyma,

therefore giving a relative lucency to the abscess cavity. Medical treatment is usually the therapy of choice; but when these abscesses do not respond to aggressive antibiotic regimen, surgical incision and drainage must be done. Occasionally, spontaneous drainage will occur via a calyx. This is seen later as a diverticulum-like structure with a narrow neck representing a sinus tract that connects to the calyx.

The first radiograph in this group (I-4a) demonstrates a renal parenchymal abscess in the upper lateral aspect of the right kidney. A focal area of lucency (1) is seen with its edge (curved arrow) identified

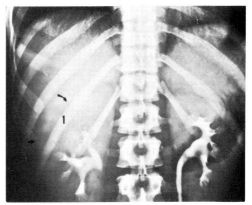

(a)

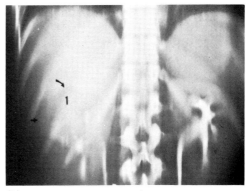

(b)

Case I-4

best superiorly. The adjacent parenchyma and the renal edge are not well demarcated because of the inflammatory reaction and edema in the adjacent tissues. This locally obliterates the normal fat stripe that is better seen inferiorly along the lateral edge of the kidney (solid straight arrow). There is distortion of the collecting system with incomplete filling of the caliceal structures in the area of the abscess. The kidneys otherwise remain normal, although the right kidney appears slightly larger than the left. The second radiograph (I-4b) shows the loss of the renal margin on a tomogram that was done as part of the excretory urogram. The markings on this film are the same as those in I-4a.

The second patient (I-5) shows a more extensive abscess of the left kidney. As a matter of fact, it involves the entire kidney. Gas produced by bacteria, usually gram negative bacteria, is seen as a lucency outlining the renal bed (solid fat ar-

rows). Linear lucencies are seen radiating from the central portion of the kidney, which is compatible with gas production by bacteria, actually in the tubules and parenchyma of the kidney tissue. This is an extensive and necrotizing infection, which will destroy the kidney, and is most frequently seen in diabetics. Final diagnosis: Renal abscess and suppuration.

Case I-6

This is a 70-year-old male patient with a 30-year history of hypertension, which could not be easily controlled. An excretory urogram was obtained for evaluation of his hypertension. Preliminary film of the renal area shows a dramatic appearance of the right kidney. The right kidney is completely calcified (solid curved arrows), deformed in its contour, and slightly shrunken. The calcification is in the form of globules with a consistency resembling putty. There are not many things that will calcify a kidney like this. While hemorrhage, tumors, cysts, and abscesses can cause calcifications, they usually are not this extensive. Tuberculosis is the most likely cause of calcification of an entire kidney. This is confirmed when

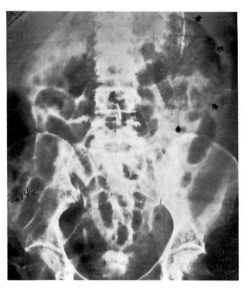

Case I-5

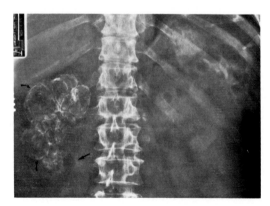

Case I-6

calcification is seen in the proximal right ureter, which overlies the right transverse process of L-3 (straight solid arrow). Tuberculosis is one of the two disorders that calcify a ureter, the other being schistosomiasis.

A chest x-ray film taken of persons with urinary tuberculosis may show the presence of active tuberculosis or previous tuberculous infection (50%). When the tuberculous bacteria invade the renal tissue (spreading to the kidney from the lung via the bloodstream), they cause a form of pyelonephritis that often causes changes similar to papillary necrosis with distortion of the caliceal structures As the disease progresses, the extensive, but indolent infection totally engulfs the kidney ultimately causing necrosis and calcification, the so-called autonephrectomy. This is what is presented in this case. Final diagnosis: Renal tuberculosis.

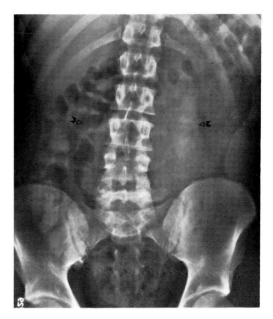

(a)

Case I-7

This patient is a 20-year-old man with left flank pain. Because of symptoms similar to renal and ureteric pain, an excretory urogram was obtained. The preliminary radiograph (I-7a) of the abdomen shows a single phlebolithlike density in the left aspect of the pelvis, just above the soft-tissue shadow of the penis. No other calcifications are noted. The spine is tilted slightly toward the left, consistent with the patient's symptoms of pain on the left. This scoliosis is due to spasm of the iliopsoas on that side similar to the changes that accompany abdominal pain as previously presented in appendicitis. Note, the right iliopsoas shadow (left arrowhead) is well seen and of normal size and configuration. The left iliopsoas shadow (right arrowhead) is large and not well defined. From the plain film alone, a di-

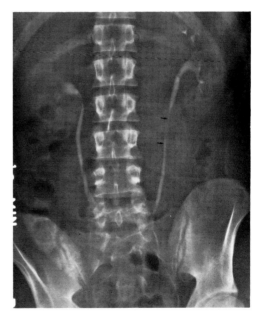

(b)

Case I-7

agnosis of a retroperitoneal abnormality, such as hemorrhage, infection, or tumor, can be suggested.

The 13-minute radiograph from an excretory urogram (I-7b) demonstrates a normal right caliceal system, ureter, and bladder. The left collecting system, while it appears normal in size, configuration,

and sharpness, is displaced to the left. The kidney is slightly further away from the spine than the right kidney, as is the ureter. Note that the proximal left ureter is slightly thinned (arrows) as it goes over the iliopsoas indicating a soft-tissue mass in that area. Since the patient has fever, has had no trauma, and is in an unlikely age group for a retroperitoneal tumor, the most likely diagnosis is a psoas abscess. This can be seen as a complication of pyelonephritis, and may even be seen in tuberculous infections.

If the patient had no fever, but a history of being injured, the diagnosis would have been retroperitoneal hemorrhage from blunt trauma to the left flank or back, with possible rupture of the kidney. An IVP would be done to see that the urinary system was intact. If there were no history of fever or trauma, a neoplastic growth

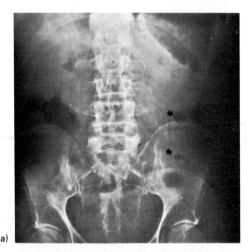

(a)

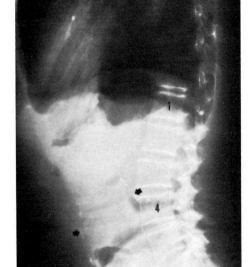

(b)

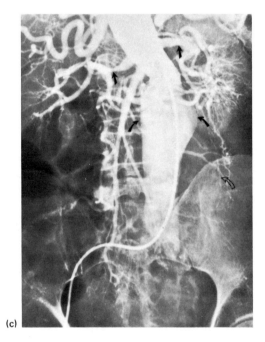

(c)

Case VD-1

must be considered. In this age group, lymphoma, retroperitoneal sarcoma, or spread of a testicular tumor would be likely possibilities. All could occur with similar findings. Final diagnosis: Left psoas abscess.

VASCULAR DISORDERS

CASE PRESENTATIONS

Case VD-1

This patient is a 76-year-old man with abdominal pain. A preliminary radiograph of the abdomen (VD-1a) demonstrates a curvilinear calcification (solid straight arrows) to the left of the lower lumbar spine. Other amorphous calcification is seen between the edge of the calcification and the spine. A lateral radiograph (VD-1b) of the abdomen demonstrates an elliptical calcification in front of the lower lumbar spine at L4 (solid straight arrows). Very fine irregular calcification is seen just anterior to the L5-S1 disc interspace on the lateral film and inferior to the sacroiliac joints in the soft tissues of the pelvis. This type of curvilinear calcification in the abdomen represents calcification in the abdominal aorta and branching vessels. The elliptical soft-tissue mass represents a moderately large, lower abdominal aortic aneurysm.

A subsequent abdominal aortogram (VD-1c) demonstrates a widened segment or bulge (curved solid arrows) below the renal arteries (solid straight arrows). Incidentally note that there is narrowing of the right renal artery where the arrow projects. While the intraluminal contrast material does show an aneurysm, it does not show an aneurysm that was as large

as the calcification seen to the left of the spine (curved open arrow) in the preliminary film. This means that while the lumen is still patent, allowing flow of blood, the wall of the aneurysm or the inner surface of the aneurysm contains a large clot. The clot, therefore, would be as thick as the distance between the contrast-opacified lumen, and the calcified linear densities seen on the original radiographs.

Abdominal aortic aneurysms are due to the process of arteriosclerotic disease. The degenerative changes in the abdominal aortic wall cause areas of weakening, which allows expansion of the lumen through these weaknesses creating bulges or aneurysms. Most aneurysms are small in caliber, causing no symptoms. Some larger aneurysms are easily palpable as pulsating masses near the midline of the lower abdomen. These aneurysms may create several complications. The aneurysm may leak or rupture causing a radiograph similar in appearance to the previously seen left psoas abscess. The formation of a clot in the aneurysm can lead to emboli thrown distally in the vessels of the lower extremities. This includes the blood flow to the kidneys and gut that are vitally important to the individual. It is therefore important not only to recognize the aneurysm itself, but to be aware of its location in respect to the vital vessels. This aneurysm would be an infrarenal lower abdominal aortic aneurysm.

The size of the aneurysm is also important. The surgeon will use the diameter of the aneurysm as a criterion for whether the patient needs surgery or not. Usually both walls of the aneurysm cannot be seen on the AP radiograph of the abdomen. Therefore, the most helpful radiograph, if the aorta is calcified, is the

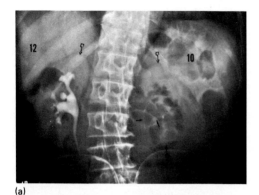

(a)

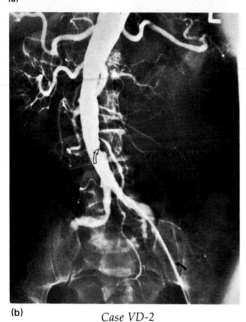

(b)

Case VD-2

cases. Final diagnosis: Abdominal aortic aneurysm.

Case VD-2

This patient is a 72-year-old man with hypertension. In evaluation of acute onset hypertension, hypertension in young adults, or hypertension that is suddenly uncontrollable, an IVP is an essential part of the patient's workup. There are many causes for hypertension in an individual. Ninety percent of hypertension cases are classified as essential hypertension, of which the cause is unknown. Along with this are other less common causes of hypertension, including pyelonephritis and congenital and obstructive changes of the kidneys, as well as neoplasm. However, 5% of the population has hypertension that has a specific etiology that may be amenable to surgery. This patient is such a case.

The 5-minute radiograph of the excretory urogram (VD-2a) shows a right kidney, which measures from pole to pole (boxed arrows) 12 cm in length. Its outline, although not well seen, is smooth with a normal-appearing nondilated collecting system that is not distorted. The left kidney is only faintly seen, measuring 10 cm from pole to pole (boxed arrows). Minimal contrast material is seen in the renal pelvis, which has a duplicated or bifid collecting system (solid arrows). The difference in the size of the kidneys and the obvious delay in excretion are two criteria for diagnosing renal artery stenosis leading to hypertension.

Arteriosclerotic disease is a diffuse process that may selectively stenose or occlude vital arteries. When this involves the renal artery, blood flow to the kidney is reduced, setting off a mechanism in

lateral. Here calcification, if present, can usually be seen in both the anterior and the posterior walls, allowing measurements that can be helpful to the surgeon. Recently we have been using for this purpose ultrasound, which can accurately determine the diameter of an aneurysm without the use of x-rays and does not depend upon calcification. Aneurysms above 6 to 10 cm in diameter are surgical that affected kidney to elevate the blood pressure. This mechanism involves the renin-angiotensin system. The stenosis usually occurs within the first centimeter of the renal artery, as it originates in the abdominal aorta. The remaining blood vessels to the kidney may be entirely normal, but the blood flow is such that the reduced pressure is sensed by a complicated mechanism near the glomerulus and tubules of the renal parenchyma. This sets in motion a sequence of hormonal changes in the body, climaxing in the constriction of peripheral vessels—leading to high blood pressure. Fibromuscular hyperplasia of the renal artery is a less common entity causing similar but more diffuse changes in the artery with the same effects.

In correlating the stenosis of the renal artery with the IVP, it is obvious that the reduction in blood flow to the affected kidney will make the kidney not only smaller in size, but also delay and decrease excretion of contrast in comparison with the normal kidney. Normally, kidneys should be within 1½ to 2 cm of each other in size, with the larger one usually on the left. In this case the left kidney is 2 cm smaller than the right. This individual shows minimal contrast in the left collecting system, while there is obviously good excretion or concentration of contrast material in the collecting system of the right kidney. This is due to a reduced blood flow and filtration rate. A third criterion for diagnosing renal artery stenosis on the excretory urogram is late hyperconcentration of the contrast material in the collecting system of the affected kidney. Since the pressure in the renal arterial system is reduced, flow through the kidney and flow into the renal tubules

is slowed. This slowing allows the contrast material to stay in the tubules for longer periods of time, increasing water absorption and concentrating the contrast material. This causes more opacity of the renal pelvis on a delayed (20 min.) film. This same phenomenon will be reflected by reduced flow down the involved ureter—so low volume runoff is another sign of renal vascular disease. These changes can be confirmed through the use of nuclear medicine techniques (Hippuran studies).

Final diagnosis of this disorder can be done by placing a catheter (VD-2b, solid curved arrow) into a femoral artery, using the Seldinger technique and guiding the tip of the catheter into the lower abdominal aorta. Contrast material can then be injected into the abdominal aorta outlining the abdominal vessels and their distribution. The accompanying radiograph demonstrates such an arteriogram. The lower abdominal aorta, before it divides into the iliac arteries, is slightly narrowed and irregular in outline (open curved arrow). This is due to arteriosclerotic changes in the wall and surface of the abdominal aorta. Note also that the abdominal aorta is somewhat tortuous in configuration rather than straight, as one would expect in a younger patient. The renal arteries are denoted by the solid straight arrows. The patient's left renal artery was occluded near the abdominal aorta, and the distal renal artery was opacified by collateral circulation, which is a common mechanism by the body to preserve organs. A stenosis of the renal artery can be observed in the angiogram of the patient with the abdominal aortic aneurysm (VD-1c). Final diagnosis: Renal vascular hypertension.

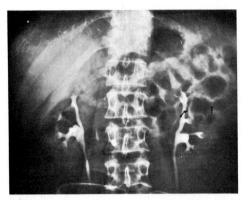

(a)

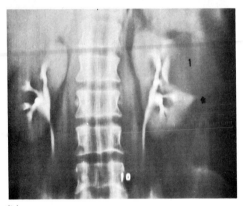

(b)

Case UM-1

URINARY MASSES &
NEOPLASMS

CASE PRESENTATIONS

Cases UM-1 and UM-2

There are three radiographs for discussion here. The initial radiograph (UM-1a) is a 5-minute radiograph from an excretory urogram. It demonstrates a normal right collecting system. In converse, the left collecting system is entirely normal, except for one calyx that is distorted, splayed, and elongated (curved solid arrow) in the mid portion of the left kidney. This is due to a large soft-tissue mass in the mid portion of the left kidney, extending laterally with the inferior edge of the renal mass (1) noted by the open arrow.

The second radiograph (UM-1b) is a tomogram taken during the excretory urogram showing a normal outline to the right kidney. The left kidney, however, shows a lucent 6 cm round density (1) that protrudes or extends from the lateral aspect of the mid portion of the left kidney. The deformed calyx is again identified more medially. At the junction of the mass and the renal parenchyma, inferiorly, one can see a triangular or beak-shaped opacity, which is in continuity with the renal parenchyma extending around the inferior margin of the lucent mass (solid arrow). This extension of the parenchyma, which is pulled out as the mass protrudes from the kidney, is a criterion that is most helpful in the diagnosis of benign simple renal cysts. The fact that the mass is lucent rather than solid (containing soft tissues) is also helpful in determining that this is a cystic structure. Note also that the margin of the lucency is smooth and thin-walled, rather than being irregular in outline and thick-walled, which is a manifestation of malignant change.

The third radiograph (UM-2) represents a different patient, a person with multiple simple cysts. The left kidney shows a 6 cm lucent smooth-walled density (1) in the same location as the previously seen simple cyst in the left kidney. The lower pole of the left kidney (open arrow) is irregular in outline and is not sharp and distinct like the lower pole of the right kidney. There is an even larger mass or cyst extending from this aspect of the kidney, but it is not in focus during the tomogram. This mass is noted to deviate the left ureter medially, near the number 12, which is a metallic marker for the depth of the tomographic section. The

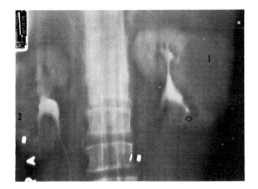

Case UM-2

right kidney shows a 2 to 3 cm, smooth-walled lucency (2) in the lower aspect of the kidney.

The origin of simple renal cysts is not known. When cysts extend from the lateral margins or poles of the kidney, they are easily diagnosed by the previously mentioned criteria. However, when the cyst appears near the center of the kidney or parapelvic region, it will distort the collecting system and retain its lucency, but no beak will be present. Patients can have one or multiple simple cysts of varying sizes. These cysts are not specifically associated with any particular clinical problems, but are frequently seen in older patients with obstructive uropathy. The problem with these masses is that they must be differentiated from malignant or neoplastic tumors. Definitive diagnosis of these cysts can be obtained by renal cyst puncture, ultrasound, arteriography, or computerized tomography of the abdomen. If a lucent mass is found by IVP, confirmation can be obtained by ultrasound and the mass can be definitely diagnosed by renal cyst puncture. If the ultrasound suggests a solid component, arteriography should be done next. If the IVP suggests a solid mass, arteriography should be next in line. Computerized tomography can confirm ultrasound and

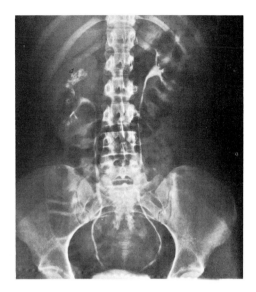

Case UM-3

arteriography findings. Final diagnosis: Simple renal cysts.

Case UM-3

This patient is a 19-year-old woman with hematuria. The excretory urogram demonstrates a normal left collecting system, as well as a normal right ureter. The right collecting system shows an unusual flowery appearance of the minor calices (open arrow). This is similar to the distorted caliceal pattern seen in papillary necrosis. Close observation, however, reveals that the minor calices are actually preserved, showing their normal discrete, sharp, cuplike appearance. This is best seen in the inferior aspect of the kidney. The flowery appearance is due to the accumulation of contrast material in the renal papillae. The appearance is of a tubular or linear variety that radiates towards the papilla and minor calyx. The contrast material is actually in the collecting tubules, which are abnormally dilated, or ectatic in the renal pyramid. This patient has a medullary sponge kidney.

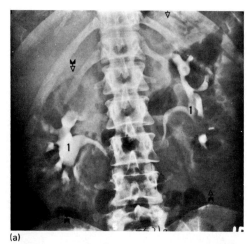

(a)

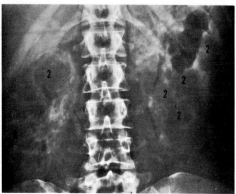

(b)

Case UM-4

Medullary sponge kidney is felt to be a congenital disease that can affect both kidneys, one kidney, or parts of one kidney focally. This patient has unilateral renal disease showing the classical changes of tubular ectasia. The distal aspects of the collecting tubules of the nephrons are congenitally dilated. As contrast material flows through the nephron, it accumulates in these dilated distal collecting tubules as urine would. The ectatic segments lead to stasis of urine, which as previously mentioned, may lead to chronic inflammatory processes and stone formation.

These patients frequently present with renal stones. While this disease entity can have serious complications, most of these patients will have a relatively normal life expectancy if appropriate precautions are taken to prevent infection and stone formation. Final diagnosis: Medullary sponge kidney.

Case UM-4

This patient is a 37-year-old woman with right upper quadrant pain. Physical examination of the abdomen revealed bilateral abdominal masses. In her radiographic evaluation, an excretory urogram showed not only what the abdominal masses were, but also the probable reason for abdominal pain.

The first radiograph (UM-4a) demonstrates markedly enlarged kidneys. The length of the kidneys or the distance between the upper and lower poles is well visualized (arrowheads). Not only are the kidneys large in size, but the collecting systems (1) are also large. There is slight dilatation of the collecting system, and several of the caliceal structures are distorted and flattened. It is as though something is pressing on the contrast-filled collecting system. In actuality, this patient has multiple cysts of varying size in both her kidneys. The cysts are of such a number as to enlarge the kidneys and distort the architecture of the kidneys. The lateral aspect of the right kidney is well seen. The renal parenchyma beneath this edge is not the normal uniform renal tissue, but is somewhat spotty or lucent in appearance. This lucency, as well as the poorly defined renal outlines, is due to the multiple cysts that are distributed throughout the renal parenchyma.

Multiple lucencies create a ''Swiss cheese'' appearance to the renal parenchyma, which is best seen on the 30-second blush film (UM-4b). This radiograph is presented out of sequence since the outline of the kidneys is not well seen. However, after knowing how large the kidneys are, and knowing that there are multiple lucent cysts (2) within the kidneys, one can see the renal shadows to better advantage. While only six cysts are delineated on the radiograph, there are hundreds of cysts of multiple sizes creating this abnormality. This abnormality is different from the multiple simple cysts seen previously, and this case represents polycystic disease of the kidneys.

Polycystic disease of the kidney is an inherited disorder. There are many theories as to its development. Most theories state that there is apparent obstruction of the tubules of the kidneys, either by malformation of the renal tubule, or a failure to unite the proximal and distal portions of the tubules in a normal manner. This defect usually appears in individuals as young adults and is often manifested by blood in the urine or hematuria. Some of the patients will not develop as many cysts or as large cysts as family members. Some will remain free of renal failure, the usual ultimate outcome of this condition. Final diagnosis: Polycystic renal disease.

Case UM-5

This patient is a 53-year-old man with hematuria. During his workup for hematuria, an excretory urogram and cystoscopy were done. A radiograph taken during cystoscopy shows a cystoscope in the bladder (UM-5, solid curved arrow). Apparently when direct visualization of the bladder showed no mucosal abnormality that would cause hematuria, contrast material was injected into the collecting systems by a ureteral catheter placed at the

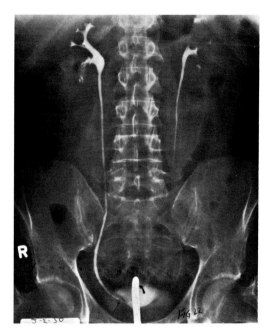

Case UM-5

ureterovesical orifice (long solid arrow). This retrograde pyelogram shows the left collecting system and ureter to be normal. There is irregularity and deformity of the calices (open arrow) of the lower pole of the right kidney, with the remaining calices appearing unremarkable. These findings are compatible with transitional cell carcinoma involving the lower pole of the right kidney.

Transitional cell carcinoma of the urinary system can occur at any site from the kidney to the bladder. That is why it is so important to see that the upper collecting system is well distended during an excretory urogram and special efforts made to distend these structures during the examination. This type of tumor is recurrent, and continuous follow-up must be obtained. If the carcinoma occurs in the renal pelvis or calices, it will seed the lower urinary system on the ipsilateral side. Since seeding of neoplastic growths can occur along the ureter and bladder area on that same side, when resection of the renal tumor is undertaken, that ureter and the part of the bladder containing that ureter is also resected.

The radiographic appearance of transitional cell carcinoma can be variable. It may appear as a polypoid or filling-defect type structure within the lumen of the collecting system, which cannot be differentiated from a stone or clot. It may present as a deformed calyx, or the calyx may show a moth-eaten appearance. The tu-

mor may also infiltrate the kidney diffusely, showing gross distortion of the kidney and collecting system without mucosal irregularity. These tumors are typically nonvascular; and, therefore, arteriography shows no vascular tumor "blush." Final diagnosis: Transitional cell carcinoma, renal collecting system.

Case UM-6

This patient is a 61-year-old man with back pain. The excretory urogram (UM-6a) demonstrates a normal left collecting system. The patient's right collecting system is distorted by a smooth lobular-type

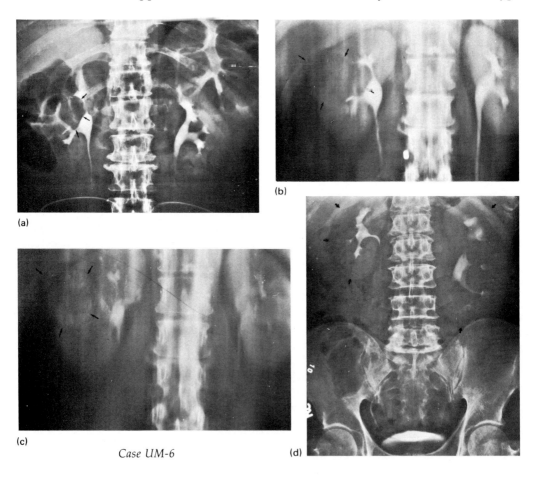

(a)

(b)

(c)

(d)

Case UM-6

mass, which indents the mid portion of the renal pelvis and calices (short solid arrows). A tomogram (UM-6b) through this kidney shows a 6 cm elliptical soft-tissue mass (short solid arrows), which lies in the mid portion of the right kidney, extending beyond the lateral confines of the kidney and to the renal pelvis. No characteristic beak to indicate a cyst is identified. The mass is not lucent, nor has it the smooth discrete wall characteristic of a benign lesion. Therefore, the mass is assumed malignant until proven otherwise.

The next step in evaluating renal masses that are assumed to be malignant is arteriography. At one point in the development of a protocol for mass lesions of the kidney, a bolus nephrotomogram was obtained. This is an injection of three times the amount of contrast material normally used for an IVP. The injection is timed so that tomograms through the kidneys would be taken at the optimum time for visualization of the mass. A single radiograph (UM-6c) from that sequence of films shows a vascular soft-tissue mass in the area of the previously seen mass. Its edges (solid arrows) are separate from the kidney, but ill-defined. This mass appears lobular, with a rim of soft tissue and lucent stellate-type center. This is characteristic of a malignancy, most likely renal cell carcinoma of the kidney. An angiogram would show similar findings.

Renal cell carcinoma is a second variety of carcinoma that occurs in the kidney. This carcinoma usually appears on the radiograph as a mass lesion protruding from the kidney and distorting the collecting system. At times this carcinoma is difficult to distinguish from a cyst, and it may even contain calcification and be lucent. A renal cell carcinoma typically metastasizes to the regional lymph nodes, and then may seed the entire body, including bones, liver, and lungs. It may also directly invade the surrounding renal bed, parasitizing vessels as it grows. Another form of renal cell carcinoma is the diffuse infiltrative renal cell carcinoma, which is seen on the fourth radiograph in this set (UM-6d). Note the normal right kidney (solid arrows on patient's right) and the diffusely enlarged left kidney (straight solid arrows on patient's left). Since the tumor is diffuse throughout the kidney, there is minimal distortion of the collecting system, except that the collecting system is large. It has an appearance similar to polycystic renal disease, but is unilateral. Polycystic renal disease is almost always bilateral. Final diagnosis: Renal cell carcinoma of the kidney.

Case UM-7

This patient is a 74-year-old man with hematuria. Again, an excretory urogram (UM-7) was obtained, which shows normal upper collecting systems. The bladder is slightly irregular in outline, which can be due to trabeculation of the bladder. Trabeculation of the bladder is usually seen with increase in bladder muscle tone, as a part of bladder outlet obstruction and prostatic enlargement. A stellate density (curved solid arrow) at the base of the bladder is indicative of a previous transurethral resection (TUR).

Also in the bladder (1) is a lucent, irregular, nodular soft-tissue density (arrowhead) measuring 2 to 3 cm located in the right upper lateral aspect of the structure. This represents the typical appearance of a transitional cell carcinoma occurring in the bladder. Most of the transitional cell carcinomas of the bladder are so small that they are not visualized on an IVP.

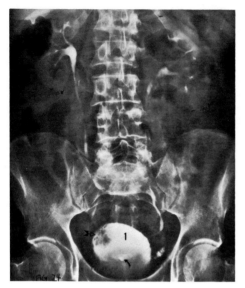

Case UM-7

These are seen endoscopically through the cystoscope and are usually removed at that time. However, when they are asymptomatic, they may attain sizes that can be seen on an IVP showing this characteristic deformity. Although this tumor appears large, its cell type may not be aggressive and it may be easily excised.

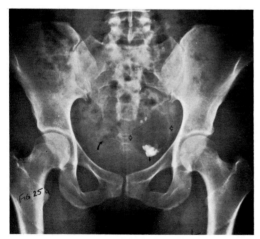

Case GD-1

In another case a small tumor, only a few mm. in size, may be so aggressive that it will require complete bladder excision. The usual symptom for these tumors is painless gross hematuria. They tend to recur, and frequent regular endoscopy is necessary. Final diagnosis: Transitional cell carcinoma of the bladder.

GENITAL DISORDERS

CASE PRESENTATIONS

Cases GD-1 and GD-2

The female patients shown here are both approximately 30 years of age. They have the same findings, that of a pelvic mass. A preliminary radiograph (GD-1) of the pelvis in the first patient demonstrates a lucent, smooth, somewhat egg-shaped soft-tissue density (open arrows) in the left aspect of the pelvis. At the inferior aspect of this soft tissue density is a densely calcified, irregular-in-outline structure (solid straight arrow). Just above the lucent mass are several half centimeter calcifications similar to phleboliths.

The only large lucent structure in the pelvis should be the gas or stool-filled rectosigmoid colon. The rectum sits low in the pelvis near the midline. In this individual the rectum contains waste material (solid curved arrow). Stool is represented by a granular-appearing lucency, and is also seen in the cecum and right colon. The rectum may be slightly to the right of the midline suggesting a soft-tissue mass on the left. The only other large gas-containing structure that may lie in the pelvis is the cecum, but this is normally on the right usually above the pelvis. These findings are therefore compatible with a mass in the left pelvis that has an unusual but specific density within it. The lucent structure in the mass represents fat, which is less dense than the surrounding soft tissues. The dense calcification in the inferior aspect of the mass are shadows of teeth and particles of bone, which grow in this particular type of tumor. This tumor is a dermoid or teratoma of the left ovary.

The second patient (GD-2) also shows a left-sided pelvic mass containing fat compatible with a small dermoid cyst (open arrows). However, there is also a large soft-tissue mass coming out of the pelvis, extending into the lower abdomen. Normally, gas shadows are seen in the pelvis, but in this individual there is a round haziness (solid arrows) that is compatible with a pelvic mass. There is minimal indentation on the bladder (1). This patient had a hemorrhagic infarction of the right ovary; and the large mass represents the ovary, which is expanded with blood and clots.

Pelvic masses are unusual in men. Usually this will represent a distended bladder. However, in women multiple pelvic masses can occur that create soft-tissue densities that sometimes indent the bladder, distort the ureters, and raise the colon and small bowel out of the pelvis. Also in women, enlargement of the uterus can occur with pregnancy, fibroids, and carcinoma. Similarly, ovaries can undergo both benign and malignant cystic change.

A dermoid cyst can appear like any other mass, but it is distinguished from the other masses by its contents of fat, bone, and teeth. Also, hair and other segments of the body can occur in this tumor, as this tumor develops from multiple embryological germ layers and, therefore, has the ability to produce many

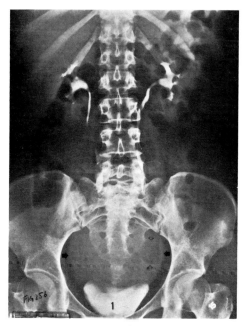

Case GD-2

types of tissues. Final diagnosis: Pelvic mass with (1) dermoid cyst of the ovary and (2) hemorrhagic infarction of the ovary.

Case GD-3

This patient is an 89-year-old woman with complaints of an abdominal mass. Like the previously presented patients, there is a haziness in the lower abdomen and pelvis with absence of gas shadows. All of the gas shadows lie across the upper abdomen. There is fine, irregular calcification in the right aspect of the upper pelvis, but in the left aspect of the pelvis this calcification is a large, dense mass (1). This calcification is rather characteristic, being nodular and lobular. A soft-tissue mass in the pelvis with this type of calcification is characteristic of a uterine leiomyoma or fibroid. The uterus in this patient probably contains multiple fibroids,

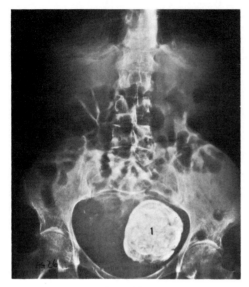

Case GD-3

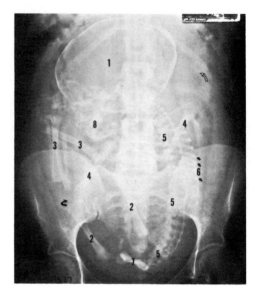

Case GD-4

only one of which is densely calcified. The remainder of the soft-tissue mass in the right aspect of the pelvis represents at least one or more uterine fibroids of various sizes, one of which has faint calcification (right upper aspect).

Uterine fibroids are benign tumors arising from the smooth muscle of the uterus. They can be asymptomatic or can cause extensive bleeding. The tumors undergo calcification as they degenerate. Fibroids can be of any size and position in the pelvis. They are usually near the midline sitting just above the bladder, and can be easily recognized when they contain the irregular popcorn-type calcification seen in this case. Final diagnosis: Calcified uterine fibroid.

Case GD-4

This patient is a 28-year-old woman who was near term in her pregnancy. An x-ray film (GD-4) was obtained because the fetal head was not felt in the normal position in the pelvis. The x-ray film confirms that the fetus lies in a breech presentation with both lower extremities extending into the right upper quadrant of the abdomen. Today, fewer radiographs of pregnant women are done because ultrasound can diagnose many abnormalities.

Note the displacement of the maternal gut, most of which lies in the upper quadrants. The colon remains in the periphery of the abdomen, but is not filled with gas. Many fetal parts can be identified. The fetal head (1) lies in the upper aspect of the maternal abdomen with a U-shaped mandible (8) along the base of the skull. The fetal spine (5) is noted along the left aspect of the maternal abdomen. Multiple ribs (6, curved arrows) are identified. The bony pelvis (7) is the most inferior aspect of the fetus with the attached femora (2) extending towards the right. The fetal tibiae and fibulae (3) are seen extending towards the right mid abdomen, whereas the humeri (4) are seen on either side of the abdomen. Although the placenta is usually not discretely seen on radiographs, there is a homogeneous soft-tissue density along the left aspect of the maternal abdomen, which suggests the placenta (open curved arrows).

There are restricted indications for x-ray use during pregnancy. Indications include acute abdominal disorders and multiple or abnormal fetuses. Also in some cases, diagnosing the position of the fetus is important as the obstetrician may elect to do a cesarean section. A special technique can actually measure the birth can-

al, maternal pelvis, and fetal head to determine if there is disproportion between the head and the birth canal. Fetal age can be ascertained by noting the epiphyses of the knee (if they have developed). This fetus is at 36 weeks (at least) gestation as the distal femoral epiphyses are identified (sharply curved solid arrow). Incidentally, one should note that the pubic symphysis is slightly separated, which is a normal finding in late pregnancy, as the ligaments become lax in preparation for the passage of the fetus through the birth canal. Final diagnosis: Near-term fetus in the breech presentation.

6

Skull and Spine

NORMAL SKULL AND FACIAL BONES

It would be beyond the scope of this book to completely review the anatomy of the skull and facial bones. Therefore, only certain important structures will be delineated. In the examination of the skull, four routine views are obtained. They include the AP, PA, lateral, and Towne's views. These views will ordinarily show all the pathological conditions affecting the skull, but there are a few specialized views needed to show difficult areas—including the base of the skull and the facial bones.

Figure 6-1 is an AP view of the skull. The frontal (1) and ethmoid (2) sinuses are well delineated. The orbits (3) are well outlined, showing adjacent overlying structures. The lesser wing (curved open arrow) and greater wing (solid straight arrow) of the sphenoid bone are discrete structures overlying each orbit. The supraorbital ridge (curved solid arrow) forms the superior margin of the orbit.

The PA film of the skull (Fig. 6-2) demonstrates other normal findings. The sagittal (curved open arrow) and lambdoid (open straight arrow) sutures are well outlined as irregular wavy lines of the skull

tables. The petrous bone demonstrates various structures of its anatomy, including the internal auditory canal (solid small straight arrows) and one of the semicircular canals (curved solid arrow). The mastoid tip and air cells (fat solid arrow)

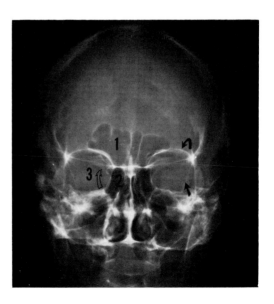

Figure 6-1

are also clearly shown. The Towne's view
(Fig. 6-3) shows similar findings with the
petrous bone and the mastoid area (7),
also showing the internal auditory canal
(small straight arrows). Both petrous tips
should be symmetrical. The lambdoid suture (larger solid arrow) is again noted
between the parietal and occipital areas.
Projecting into the foramen magnum is
the dorsum sellae with its posterior clinoids (open arrow).

The lateral view (Fig. 6-4) again shows
the frontal (1), the ethmoid (2), and the

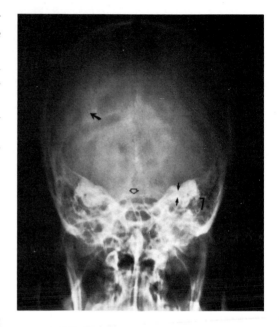

Figure 6-3

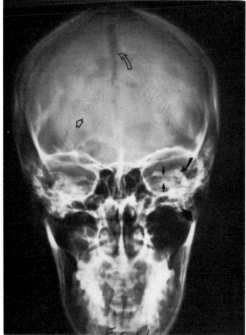

Figure 6-2

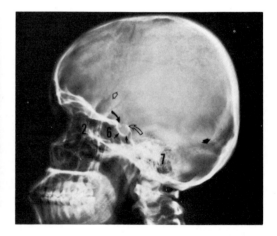

Figure 6-4

mastoid (7) sinuses, including the sphenoid sinus (6). Sitting above the sphenoid sinus, which lies in the body of the sphenoid bone, is the sella turcica. The anterior clinoids (solid curved arrow) and posterior clinoids (curved open arrow) are well shown. It is important to observe the floor of the sella turcica (small solid straight arrows) as a solid white sheet of cortical bone, the lamina dura. The height of the sella turcica should be 11 to 12 mm in depth, and its anterior-posterior diameter should be no longer than 16 mm. Also noted in the lateral view are the meningeal artery grooves (straight open arrow) along the inner tables of the lateral cranial bones. The coronal suture is also in this area, but is not well delineated on this radiograph. The lambdoid suture (fat solid arrow) is again identified posteriorly.

The facial bones require special views. Most of the facial bones can be interpreted from a Waters view (Fig. 6-5) of the skull. The zygoma or malar bone (5) is well outlined, showing its many processes that fuse with the many bones of the face and cranium. Note that the superior and inferior margins of the orbits, as well as the nasal arch (solid arrows), are well outlined. Cone-down lateral views of the nasal area (Fig. 6-6) will better demonstrate the nasal bone (solid straight thin arrow) and the inferior nasal spine (solid fat straight arrow). The mandible requires further specialized views, but can be observed on all the views so far outlined. Note that the Waters view shows excellent visualization of the sinuses, especially the frontal, ethmoid, and maxillary areas.

Before discussing the pathological conditions occurring in the skull, several normal variations should be pointed out. The

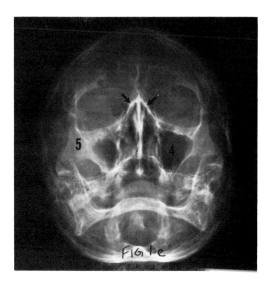

Figure 6-5

pineal gland, which lies in the mid portion of the brain, is calcified in adults in approximately 50% of the cases. A calcified pineal (open straight arrow) can be identified on the lateral and PA views of the skull in Figures 6-7 and 6-8. Note that the pineal gland lies in the midline, slight-

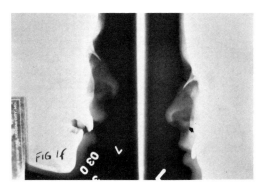

Figure 6-6

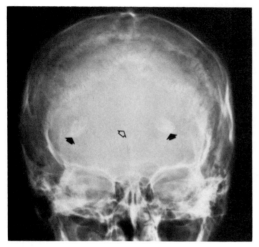

Figure 6-7

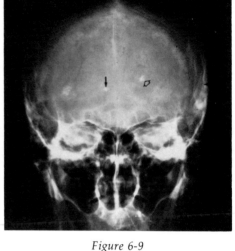

Figure 6-9

ly posterior and superior to the sella and the petrous pyramids. This gland should be within 3 mm of either side of the midline on the AP and the PA views. The choroid plexi (solid straight arrows) are frequently calcified and lie in the atria of the lateral ventricles. They can be seen overlying each other on the lateral radiograph and on either side of the pineal gland on the PA radiograph.

Figure 6-9 represents a 75-year-old man

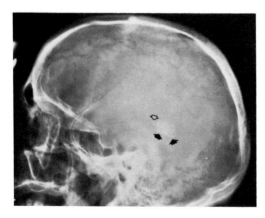

Figure 6-8

with a subdural hematoma. Note that the pineal gland (solid straight arrow) is deviated to the right of the midline, more than the allowed 3 mm. The patient's left choroid plexus is deviated towards the midline. Both of these signs of deviation represent a mass (subdural hematoma) occupying the surface of the left hemisphere and displacing the structures to the right. These signs are useful in localizing masses within the cranium. Small arrows point to the inner tables of the skull.

Frequently, additional bone, called hyperostosis frontalis interna, is deposited along the inner aspect of the frontal bone of the skull. This formation is a benign process having no clinical significance, but it does have a characteristic appearance. The increased density seen on the PA film (Fig. 6-10) never crosses the midline. The lateral film (Fig. 6-11) demonstrates this flowery, flocculent density (solid straight arrow) beneath the inner table of the frontal bone.

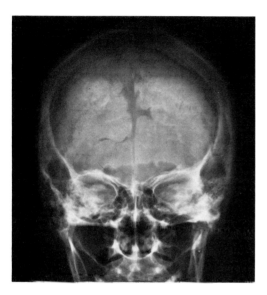

Figure 6-10

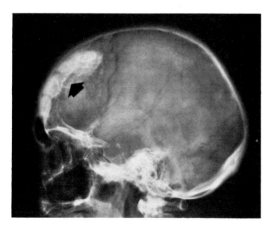

Figure 6-11

CASE PRESENTATIONS

Cases B-1 and B-2

The two skull radiographs presented here represent two different individuals with the same pathological entity, but the entity is secondary to two different mechanisms.

Osteomyelitis of the skull is most commonly due to the direct extension of a suppurative process from the scalp or paranasal sinuses. Direct contamination, such as from trauma or postoperative procedures, is another common cause. Hematogenous spread from distant infection is less common. As they do elsewhere in the skeleton, the radiographic changes often lag behind the clinical symptoms and signs by one to two weeks. Isotopic bone scans can be positive much earlier.

The first patient (B-1) demonstrates postoperative changes, including burr holes, metallic sutures, and metallic clips. This patient has undergone a craniotomy, but during the convalescent or healing stages has developed an infection in the bone flap. Multiple lucencies (small solid arrows), which are not seen in the adjacent skull, are seen scattered throughout the bone fragment. These areas of rarefaction are due to bone reabsorption from infection. As the process continues, the small areas of destruction will coalesce, forming larger areas of lucency. As the process becomes more chronic, sclerotic bone will be deposited around the areas of rarefaction in repair attempts. Frequently, significant edema will overlie this area of infection. If the focus of infection had been one specific area rather than the diffuse bone flap, a spreading lucency, rather than this diffuse process, would be seen radiating from a central area.

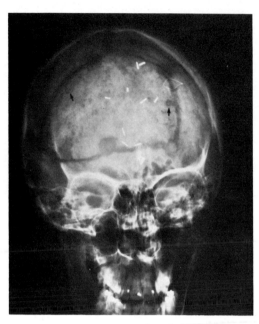

Case B-1

The second patient (B-2) shows no frontal sinus. This patient has had chronic frontal sinusitis with infection of the surrounding bone. The frontal sinus is completely opacified except for a small air bubble (small solid arrows) in the central portion of the sinus area. Note that the surrounding bone is increased in density due to the slow, chronic osteomyelitis that is common with infection spreading from adjacent sinuses. Final diagnosis: Osteomyelitis secondary to postoperative intervention and frontal sinusitis.

Cases B-3 through B-7

These are cases of individuals with the same pathological processes, but with varying degrees of involvement. Inflammation of the mucosal membranes of the paranasal sinuses causes inflammatory and edematous changes that can be seen radiographically. The first radiograph (B-3) in the series demonstrates a Waters view in a patient with minimal changes

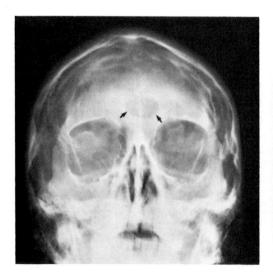

Case B-2

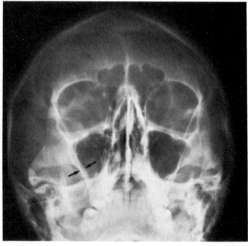

Case B-3

of sinusitis. The maxillary sinuses are lucent structures, triangular in shape, sitting in the body of maxillary bones. The superior and lateral wall of these sinuses shows a fine sclerotic margin that is well defined. There is a ½ cm mucosal membrane thickening (solid arrows) demonstrated best along the lateral wall of the right maxillary antrum. This mucosal membrane thickening can be due to inflammation secondary to either infectious (bacteria or virus) or allergic causes. The next individual (B-4) demonstrates further mucosal membrane thickening (solid arrows) of the maxillary antra. Also noted is an air/fluid level (open arrow) in the left maxillary antrum. This represents blood, fluid, mucus, or pus gravitating to the inferior aspects of the maxillary antrum in a patient who was positioned upright. When edema and inflammatory changes cause thickening of the mucosal membranes of a sinus, it also involves the mucosal membranes of the ostia or openings of the sinuses into the nasal cavity. Such swelling obstructs the opening allowing poor drainage, thereby creating fluid accumulation in the affected sinus.

A third radiograph (B-5) in the sequence demonstrates further opacification of both maxillary antra with bilateral air/fluid levels (open arrows) and probable involvement of the frontal and ethmoid sinuses, as there is clouding of those areas as well. Note that, despite the intense inflammatory changes that are present, the thin, delicate, white line of the maxillary antra remains intact (curved solid arrow). As the process becomes chronic, this mucoperiosteal line becomes obscured, indicating that this is a chronic process. The next stage would be osteomyelitis involving the adjacent bone as previously seen.

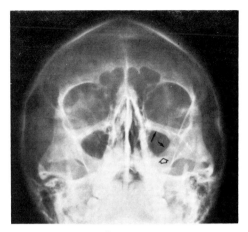

Case B-4

The next radiograph (B-6) demonstrates mucosal membrane thickening (solid arrows) of the sphenoid sinus. This sinus is not as frequently involved as the maxillary and the frontal sinuses and is seen only on the lateral radiograph. It too can cause

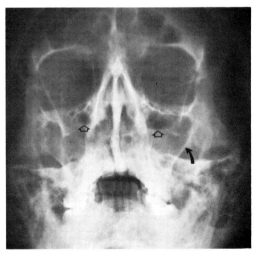

Case B-5

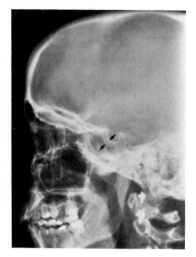

Case B-6

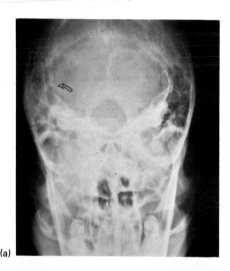

(a)

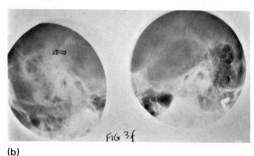

FIG 3f

(b)

Case B-7

the common symptoms of nasal discharge, sinus fullness, and headaches.

The final pair of radiographs (B-7a and b) demonstrate a specific variety of sinusitis that does not involve the paranasal sinuses. The sinus air cells in the temporal bones of the skull do not drain into the nose. They are, however, closely associated with the structures of the ear. Infection in the ear can, therefore, spread to adjacent structures through the thin bony septa, leading to a sinusitis of the mastoid sinus air cells. Note in the Towne's view (B-7a) that there is opacification of the patient's right mastoid air cells (curved open arrow). Discrete sinus air cells are not identifiable due to the accumulation of edema, inflammatory cells, and exudate from the infection. Cone-down views of the right and left mastoid sinuses (B-7b) show the opacification of the right mastoid sinus (curved open arrow) with loss of the fine septa (small solid straight arrow) that separate normal left sinus air cells. A further extension of this inflammatory process through the thin bony structures of the skull can lead to meningitis, a frequent complication of this disorder. Final diagnois: Sinusitis with mastoiditis.

Cases B-8 and B9

Case B-8 is a 69-year-old woman with fatigue and confusion. Her entire skull series was normal except for the lateral view (B-8). Note that the posterior aspect of the lamina dura or floor of the sella turcica has been reabsorbed and is no longer visible (solid arrow). This is an early sign of increased intracranial pressure. The entire sella turcica may be demineralized, but the earliest finding in increased intracranial pressure is the loss of this lamina dura of the anterior aspect of the dorsum sellae and the posterior aspect of the sellar floor. As the intracranial pressure increases, further demineralization of the sella turcica is produced—including erosions of the dorsum sellae. In the adult, no other signs are radiographically visible for this condition.

However, in the child several signs of increased intracranial pressure can be seen. The most frequent sign up to the age of 12 to 14 years is the separation of the sutures. The lambdoid, sagittal, and particularly the coronal sutures are most frequently involved. As the sutures increase in width, there is prominence of the suture interdigitations (B 9, solid straight arrows). As the child reaches adulthood, the sutures become rigid, and this sign is not seen. A less reliable sign of increased intracranial pressure is the increased digital markings seen on the skull tables. This apprears as a "beatenbrass" appearance of the inner table of the skull, supposedly due to transmitted pulsations of the convolutions of the brain. However, between the ages of five and ten this scalloping of the skull can be a normal variation. The demineralization of the sella turcica seen in adults is less frequently seen in children. The pressure is decompressed by the spreading of the sutures, thereby reducing the pressure before erosion of the sella occurs. Final diagnosis: Increased intracranial pressure.

Cases B-10 through B-16

This series of patients show manifestations of intracranial masses. Radiographic changes from intracranial neoplasms or tumors are the exception rather than the rule. The skull series infrequently demonstrates pathological changes that are secondary to a growing mass within the skull. Besides the shift of the pineal gland

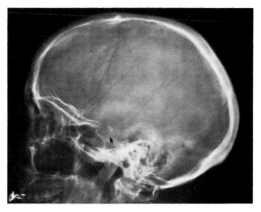

Case B-8

or other usually calcified structures, calcification in the tumor or adjacent to the tumor can be demonstrated. Calcification occurs in 10% to 15% of all brain tumors. Oligodendrogliomas are the most frequently calcified tumors. However, these are rare tumors. Therefore, the most frequently calcified tumor is the meningioma, and second is the fast-growing, necrotic, highly malignant glioma. Bone destruction or alteration of the normal symmetry of the skull may also be seen.

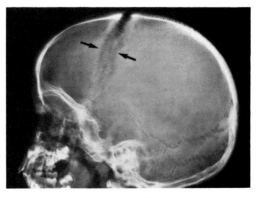

Case B-9

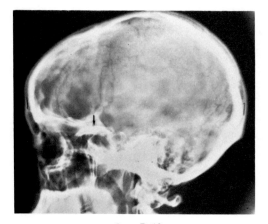

Case B-10

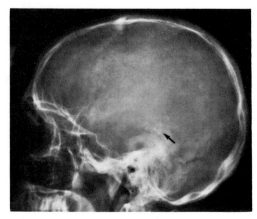

Case B-12

The first patient (B-10) demonstrates a densely sclerotic planum sphenoidale (solid arrow), which is the posterior aspect of the floor of the anterior cranial fossa, sitting just superior and anterior to the sella turcica. This is a common location for meningiomas. These tumors cause bone reaction and hyperostosis in the adjacent bony structures. It is not infrequent for meningiomas to appear like this.

The second individual (B-11) shows a similar production of bone in the parasagittal area (solid arrows). This also represents a meningioma in a common location.

The third patient is a 62-year-old man. His intracranial calcification is a focal area of irregular densities (B-12, solid arrow)

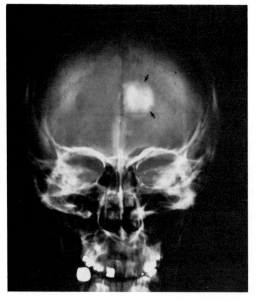

Case B-11

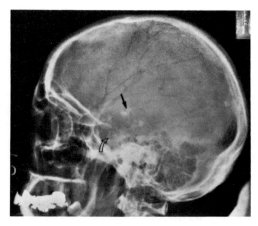

Case B-13

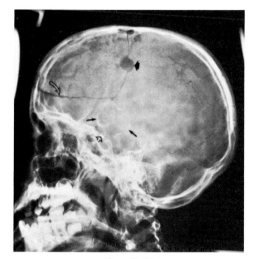

Case B-14

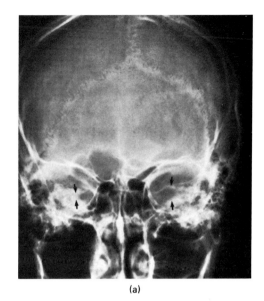

(a)

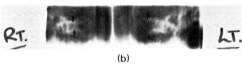

RT. LT.

(b)

Case B-15

just above the petrous pyramid. The film in B-13 shows a similar focal area of irregular calcifications (solid straight arrow) in the perisellar area. However, in this patient the sella turcica has been destroyed (curved open arrow). This combination of abnormalities help to identify the cell type of this tumor. While a craniopharyngioma would cause a similar pattern, this individual had a chordoma involving the sella turcica.

The next individual's radiograph (B-14) demonstrates postoperative changes in the frontal area, manifested by a burr hole (solid straight arrow) and saw line (curved open arrow). There is also curvilinear calcification above the sellar area (solid straight arrows). A metallic ½ cm × 1 mm density is seen just above the sella turcica beneath the calcification, representing a surgical metallic vascular clip (open straight arrow). This individual has an intracranial aneurysm. This could just as well be a calcified arteriovenous malformation, as these two entities are the only vascular tumors that calcify in the skull.

The next three radiographs (B-15 a and b; B-16) represent two individuals with an acoustic neuroma. These tumors characteristically grow in the internal auditory canal or its opening (meatus). Before changes in the radiograph are apparent, clinical symptoms may be present including hearing loss, tinnitus, dizziness, or loss of balance. As the tumor grows, bony changes will occur in the petrous tips. The film in case B-15a demonstrates asymmetry in the petrous tips with widening of the patient's left internal auditory canal (solid arrows), as compared to his right. This is best delineated on a tomogram through the petrous pyramids in Case B-15b. The film of the second individual (B-16) does not demonstrate well-defined internal auditory canals, but does demonstrate asymmetry in the tips of the

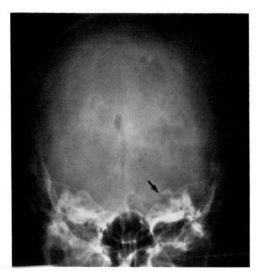

Case B-16

petrous bones. Note the bony erosion (solid arrow) of the patient's left petrous tip, due to a growing acoustic neuroma. A meningioma or other cerebellar pontine-angle tumor could give similar changes.

In the past, isotopic brain scanning has been a good study to evaluate intracranial symptoms. Since the advent of CT scan-

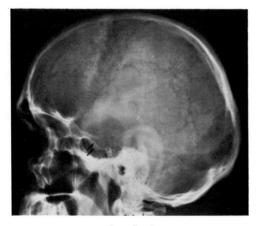

Case B-17

ning, it is used only as a screening device or for evaluation of gross vascular asymmetries in the neck and head. CT head scanning has revolutionized neuroradiology by precisely defining intracranial abnormalities. It is beyond the scope of this book to thoroughly discuss this topic. Final diagnosis: Intracranial tumors manifesting tumor calcification and bone erosion.

Cases B-17 through B-19

These three cases are individuals with the same disease process.

The pituitary lies in the sella turcica. Neoplastic growth of the pituitary can lead to changes in the sella turcica that are easily recognized. The first radiograph (B-17) demonstrates a double-floor sella turcica (solid arrows). This is due to asymmetrical enlargement of the sella. The side of the sella not affected by the neoplasm is relatively normal in configuration. However, as the sellar tumor enlarges, it pushes the floor of the sella anterior and inferior—creating this so-called "double floor." When the tumor enlarges symmetrically only one floor will be identified. This is seen in case B-18. Note that the sella turcica is enlarged beyond the normal limits for size. The clinoids are thinned, but the sellar floor (solid straight arrows) remains intact. The floor is slightly ballooned inferiorly due to this enlarging mass. As the neoplasm continues to grow, there will be destruction of the sella turcica, which on plain radiographs may be extensive.

The film in case B-19a is of an individual with this kind of destruction. Note that the sellar floor is no longer identified and that there is marked thinning of the dorsum sellae and posterior clinoids. The sphenoid sinus is totally opacified because neoplasm is in that confined space. However, a tomogram (B-19b) through this area demonstrates thinned anterior and posterior clinoid processes and dorsum sellae (solid arrows). While the floor is not visible on the plain film, the tomogram demonstrates a thin, irregular sellar floor, which has ballooned even further and more extensively than the previous sella.

Pituitary tumors comprise from 9% to 18% of all intracranial tumors, with by far the greatest majority being chromophobe adenomas. Basophilic adenomas do not enlarge the sella turcica, while eosinophilic adenomas commonly produce growth hormone, creating acromegaly in the adult and gigantism in the child. In the acromegalic adult, there is enlargement of the paranasal sinuses, overgrowth of the mandible, and thickening of the calvarium. None of these changes are seen in the cases presented. Final diagnosis: Pituitary tumors with sellar changes.

Cases B-20 through B-23

The next series of radiographs demonstrate neoplasms of the sinuses. The initial radiograph (B-20) is of a 19-year-old woman with dizziness and headaches. Because of these symptoms a sinus series was included in the skull workup. The Waters view demonstrates a large, round soft-tissue opacification of the left maxillary antrum. There is a large polypoid mass filling the entire sinus with its edge (solid arrows) seen just below the infraorbital ridge.

This mass most likely represents a large retention cyst of the maxillary antrum— retention cysts are the most common type of mass in a sinus and are frequently asymptomatic. This cyst is due to an overenlargement of an occluded glandular

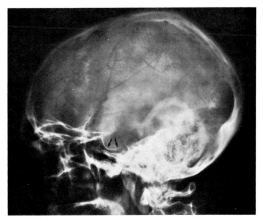

Case B-18

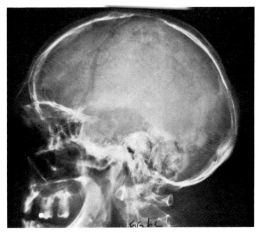

(a)

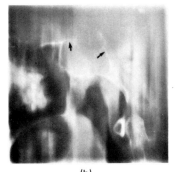

(b)

Case B-19

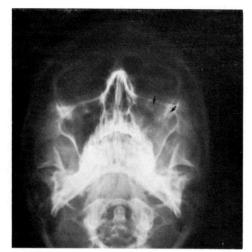

Case B-20

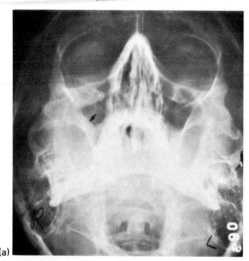

(a)

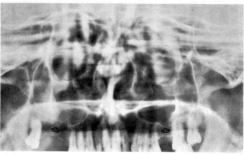

(b)

Case B-21

structure. Such masses usually occur in the inferior aspect of the maxillary antrum and can be of various sizes. Other benign masses occurring in the sinuses include adenomas and mucoceles. Characteristically, a mucocele, when enlarged, will expand the affected sinus, causing bone destruction from the inside out. This type of destruction is not commonly seen in the maxillary sinus areas, and therefore would not be a likely consideration in this individual.

Malignant tumors of the paranasal sinuses manifest themselves initially as inflammatory-like changes. The film in Case B-21a is a 45-year-old woman with markedly thickened mucosal membrane density in the right maxillary antrum (solid arrow). No obvious bone destruction is seen, and the mucoperiosteal line appears intact. However, a subsequent panorex view (B-21b) of the maxillary bones demonstrates asymmetry in the floor of the maxillary antra. The right maxillary antrum shows irregular bone destruction (open arrow) as compared to the normal mucoperiosteal line on the left (right side of radiograph). Chronic maxillary infection would obliterate the entire mucoperiosteal line. In this individual only a focal area of bone destruction is seen, therefore indicating a neoplastic process. Biopsy is mandatory for definitive diagnosis.

The next two radiographs demonstrate advanced stages in neoplasms of the sinus. The first individual (B-22) shows extensive destruction of the sella turcica (solid arrow) with opacification of the sphenoid sinus. The anterior aspect of the sphenoid sinus is bulging anteriorly as seen by the solid curved arrow. A mucocele could similarly expand the sphenoid sinus, but the extensive bone destruction points toward a neoplasm. The last indi-

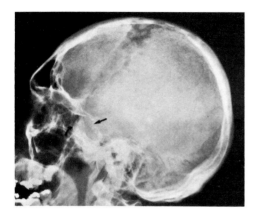

Case B-22

vidual (B-23) demonstrates extensive destruction without expansion of the left maxillary bone and zygoma (curved arrows). Only an aggressive neoplastic process could destroy the face in this way. Final diagnosis: Tumors of the paranasal sinuses.

Cases B-24 and B-25

These cases are two individuals with a dense homogenous structure overlying the calvarium. The first individual (B-24) shows a 2 cm density in the inferior aspect of the frontal-parietal area (solid arrows). The second individual (B-25a) shows a larger 4 to 5 cm density overlying the posterior-inferior aspect of the left parietal area (solid arrows). The third radiograph (B-25b) shows a tangential view of the second individual showing that these structures actually are sclerotic densities adjacent to the outer table of the skull and protruding externally. A soft tissue mass is clinically palpable. Both of these individuals have osteomas of the cranial vault.

Osteomas of the skull are benign neoplasms that occur both on the inner and outer table of the skull. They consist of

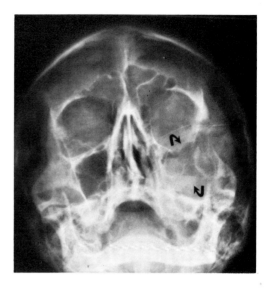

Case B-23

dense sclerotic bone, which is smooth in contour, having no signs of invasion. The hyperostosis must not be confused with that which occurs with a meningioma. When the tangential view is obtained and the protrusion is identified, the diagnosis is clinched.

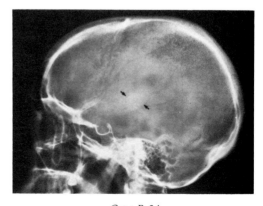

Case B-24

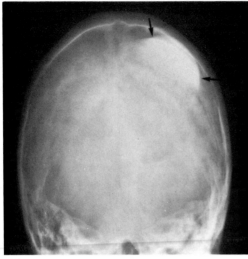

(a)

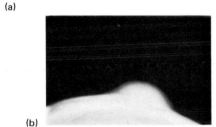

(b)

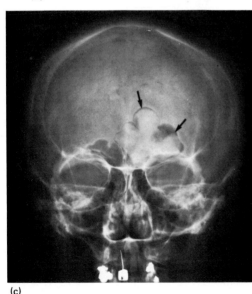

(c)

Case B-25

There is a variety of osteoma that occurs in the sinuses, commonly the frontal sinus. It starts as a small, homogeneous calcification gradually expanding until it conforms to the inner outline of the sinus, as demonstrated in B-25c (straight solid arrows). While these masses may be incidental findings, they occasionally will create problems leading to symptoms that require surgical intervention. Final diagnosis: Skull osteomas.

Case B-26

The next patient is a 45-year-old woman with headaches and accompanying nausea, vomiting, and incontinence. Skull radiographs were obtained because of her symptoms. There is a discrete lucency (curved open arrow) in the left frontal area of the skull (B-26a). Its margins are well defined without a sclerotic rim. Small white septa can be seen radiating towards the innermost aspects of this lucent skull lesion. This represents a hemangioma of the calvarium.

These lesions typically occur in the diploë between the skull tables. They are asymptomatic, frequently seen as incidental findings on radiographic workups. If these lesions are inadvertently biopsied because they are not recognized, they bleed considerably.

There are two other lucencies of the skull tables that need consideration here. One is a discrete lucency with a sclerotic rim, without the bony septa seen in hemangiomas. This lesion is also an incidental finding representing an epidermoid tumor or cholesteatoma of the skull. It apparently represents a congenital inclusion of epithelial tissue as the clavarium develops. Most of these lesions are round and well circumscribed with a sclerotic rim because they have been there for a period of years. A curved open arrow demonstrates this lesion in case B-26b.

The third lucency of the skull table is that which occurs with eosinophilic granuloma. This lesion typically shows an irregular lucency, which is well demarcated, without a sclerotic rim or central calcification. Its edges are beveled, giving a geographic outline to its rim. Obviously a single metastasis from a distant site could have a similar appearance. This disease is one of three disorders occurring in the Histocytosis X Complex. Final diagnosis: Hemangioma and epidermoid of the skull.

Cases B-27 and B-28

The next two radiographs represent the same disorder. Both lateral skull views demonstrate multiple small lucencies in the skull tables.

The first individual (B-27) shows less than a dozen obvious lucencies, but as closer examination is done, small less discrete lucencies are identified. Note that the lucencies are well demarcated, but with irregular, ill-defined edges. No sclerotic margin is seen, nor central calcification noted.

The second individual (B-28) shows a similar process, but there are many more lucencies involving the entire skull and cervical spine. Note that the lucencies involve the diploë (solid arrow) of the skull table. Metastases, when they do occur, usually involve the marrow spaces of which the diploë is one.

Multiple lucent or osteolytic densities of the skull table are compatible with metastatic tumors from many sources. Commonly, these originate in the breast, lung, and prostate. Both of these patients had primary carcinomas in the lung. Osteolytic metastases are usually numerous, ill-

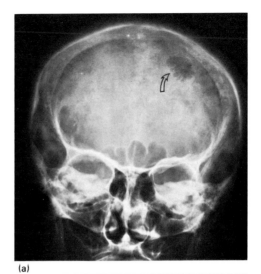

(a)

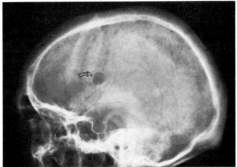

(b)

Case B-26

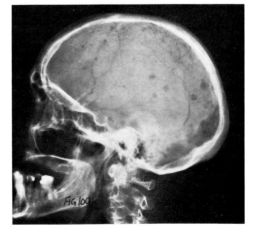

Case B-27

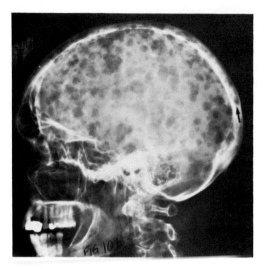

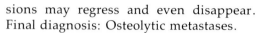

Case B-28

sions may regress and even disappear. Final diagnosis: Osteolytic metastases.

Cases B-29 through B-35

These cases are a series of patients with trauma to the skull. The films in cases B-29 through B-34 represent linear skull fractures involving the cranium. A simple nondepressed linear fracture is manifested by a sharp, discrete lucent line as though someone cut the radiograph with a knife. It has no branching or undulation, and its edges are nonsclerotic. Case B-29 shows a fracture involving the inferior aspect of the frontal-parietal area (curved solid arrow). Case B-30 shows a fracture through the inferior aspect of the parietal-temporal area (curved open arrow). Case B-31 shows a linear fracture in the occipital area (curved solid arrow).

defined radiolucent areas of various sizes. This is in contrast to multiple myeloma, which gives a similar appearance but whose multiple radiolucencies are usually uniform in size from 5 to 10 mm in diameter. Osteoblastic or bone-producing metastases can be seen in metastatic carcinoma of the lung, breast, prostate, and GI malignancy. With treatment, these le-

In evaluation of a patient with head trauma, the neurological physical examination is most important whether or not the patient exhibits a skull fracture. Patients may have considerable intracranial damage without an obvious skull fracture, and on the other hand, can have an exten-

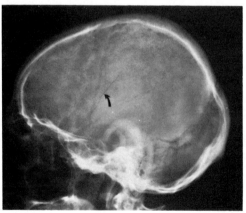

Case B-29

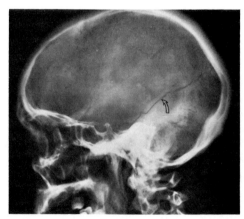

Case B-30

sive fracture without underlying brain injury.

There are certain other characteristics of skull fractures which are important. The fourth radiograph (B-32) demonstrates an air/fluid level in the sphenoid sinus (solid arrow). In a patient with trauma, this would be indicative of blood in the sphenoid sinus from fracture into that structure. These fractures are not routinely seen on standard skull x-rays, and views of the base of the skull or tomograms would be needed to definitely identify the fracture. A fracture line that crosses the middle meningeal artery groove should arouse some interest. A fracture in this area could tear the middle meningeal artery, causing an epidural hematoma that can rapidly lead to the patient's death. Fracturing of this area is clincally important for the radiologist and clinician to note.

Skull x-rays following trauma may exhibit air intracranially when a fracture has transected an air containing space such as

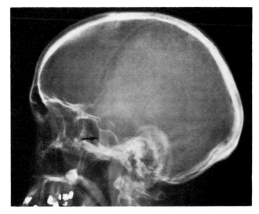

Case B-32

a paranasal sinus. The accompanying radiograph in case B-33 shows a lucent structure just inside the inner table, low in the frontal region of the anterior fossa. There is an air/fluid level (solid curved arrow) present demonstrating that fluid is also present. With a history of trauma, and without an obvious fracture located, fracture to the frontal or ethmoid sinus is suspected. The importance of this observation is that there is a communication between the sterile environment of the central nervous system and the non-sterile

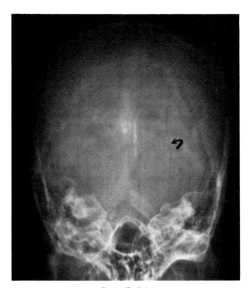

Case B-31

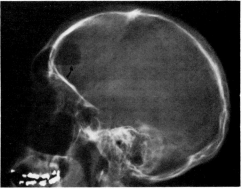

Case B-33

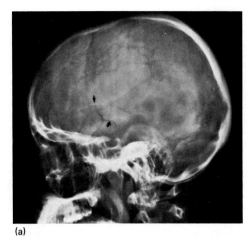

(a)

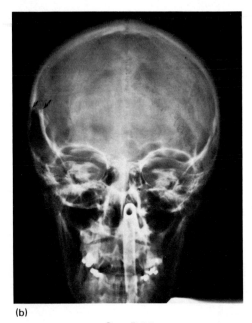

(b)

Case B-34

The next individual (B-34a and b) demonstrates a depressed skull fracture. In this type of fracture, the fragment is depressed intracranially beneath the inner table of the skull. On the AP radiograph (B-34a) the fragment is at least 1 cm closer to the midline than the inner table of the intact skull (arrows). Unless the fracture is seen tangentially, it is often difficult to diagnose this. However, there are characteristics on the lateral skull film (B-34b) that can make that diagnosis without the accompanying AP film. When a fracture occurs, there is a linear lucent line (small curved solid arrow) indicating a fracture. However, slightly anterior and superior to this line is a white curvilinear density (straight solid arrow), which is created by an overlap of bone fragment edges. This then tells the observer that the fragments are not side by side, but one on top of the other, creating increased thickness for the x-ray beam to travel through. This results therefore in an increase in opacity. Depressed skull fractures are surgically corrected when there is underlying neurological damage. If no underlying injury is present, surgery would only be indicated for cosmetic reasons.

Two other types of skull fractures should be mentioned. A fracture which involves the suture, such as demonstrated in case B-35 is called a diastatic fracture. This fracture line (curved open arrow) is seen involving the posterior aspects of the skull, but extending into the lambdoid suture. A fracture that continues to enlarge following the usual time for healing is called a growing fracture. This is due to tearing of the underlying dura, with protrusion of meninges and cerebral spinal fluid into the fracture line. Pulsations from blood flow continously widen the fracture line creating the enlarging defect.

environment of the mucosal membrane of the nasal cavity. Not only is meningitis a possible complication to this type of fracture, but also continous leakage of cerebral spinal fluid is possible through the tear in the meninges and break in the skull base.

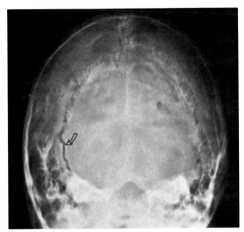

Case B-35

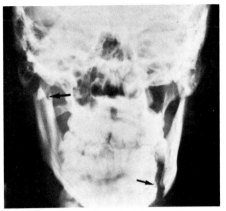

Case B-36

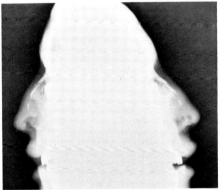

(a)

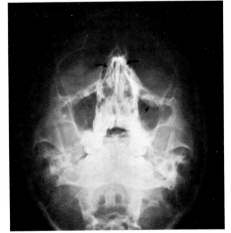

(b)

Case B-37

This is the so-called leptomeningeal cyst. Final diagnosis: Skull fractures.

Cases B-36 through B-40

The next series of radiographs represents examples of facial trauma. The first case is the typical mandibular fracture (B-36). There is a discontinuity of the patient's right mandibular ramus just below the condylar neck (left solid arrow). There is also discontinuity of the patient's left mandibular body (right solid arrow), with slight separation or diastasis of fracture fragments. In fractures of the mandible, the bony structure is considered a continuous ring, much like the pelvis. When one fracture line is present, a second one should be looked for, as is demonstrated in this patient.

The next patient (B-37a) demonstrates a comminuted depressed fracture of the nasal bone. The inferior nasal spine is intact. Normally, there are multiple small lucent lines in the nasal bones due to vascular and neural grooves. These lines usually run parallel to the long axis of the nasal bone. Lines at right angles to the long axis of the nasal bone should be considered fracture lines, even if no other evidence of fracture is seen. Note that the most distal aspect of the nasal bone is depressed and completely separated from a middle fragment, which is also depressed in relationship to the proximal nasal bone.

A Waters view of the same individual (B-37b) demonstrates a discontinuity of the nasal arch (solid curved arrows). Although the lateral view may show a normal nasal bone, there should be a continuous nasal arch on the Waters view. Discontinuity of the nasal arch, in itself, is a manifestation of a nasal fracture.

This same individual in case B-37b shows a second commonly seen fracture. This patient had a blow to the nose and orbit, with resultant fracturing of the nose and increase in the intraorbital pressure. The soft-tissue contents of the orbits under pressure can protrude into the weakest bony structure—the medial aspect and the floor of the orbit. When the floor is fractured, the soft-tissue contents of the orbit will protrude into the superior aspect of the maxillary sinus, creating a soft-tissue defect (small solid straight arrow). This is a so-called blow-out fracture of the orbit. While no discrete bone fragments of the floor are identified, the lateral aspect of the superior maxillary roof appears slightly disorganized, suggesting bony injury.

A second individual (B-38) with the same abnormality shows not only the soft-tissue protrusion (solid straight arrow) of the orbital contents into the maxillary sinus, but also disruption of the bony floor of the orbit (curved open arrow). Note that the inferior orbital rim is intact; it is not necessarily involved with blow-out fractures. These patients may exhibit ab-

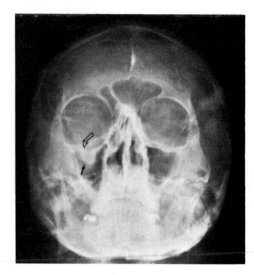

Case B-38

normal or restricted eye movement when orbital muscles are snared in the fracture fragments.

Cases B-39 and B-40 represent other commonly seen facial fractures. These are fractures involving the malar or zygoma bone seen in blunt trauma to the cheek. Case B-39 demonstrates multiple fracture sites (solid arrows). There is a fracture of the inferior orbital rim, lateral wall of the maxillary sinus, zygomatic process of the malar bone, and diastatic fracture of the zygomatic frontal suture. This type of fracture is commonly called a tripod fracture. Case B-40 also demonstrates comminuted fracture of the malar bone body with a fracturing of the zygomatic process and lateral maxillary sinus wall (solid arrows). It is important to note whether this fragment is depressed and is best seen in submental vertex views of the skull. Final diagnosis: Facial fractures.

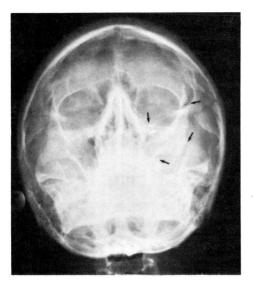

Case B-39

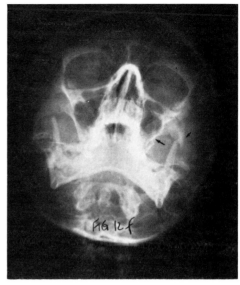

Case B-40

Cases B-41 and B-42

These are the cases of a 56-year-old man and a 76-year-old woman, both of whom entered the hospital with clinical problems of cerebral vascular accident. Each had a skull series during evaluation. The first patient (B-41) shows lucency of the skull table which is fairly well demarcated in the frontal parietal area by normal adjacent bone (curved open arrows). The stage of this disease process represents a destructive or lytic process with no attempt at healing. This is osteoporosis circumscripta, a phase of Paget's disease of the skull. As this process progresses, an attempt to heal creates a different radiographic pattern. While lytic destruction is occurring, there is also bone production occurring simultaneously—giving a skull that shows multiple irregular, dense, sclerotic nodules with small areas of rarefaction producing a "cotton-wooly" ap-

pearance. At the same time the skull table appears thick as seen in B-42a.

Paget's disease of bone can occur in all parts of the skeletal system including the skull and facial bones. Involvement of the base of the skull by this soft, abnormal bone often leads to CNS problems. A

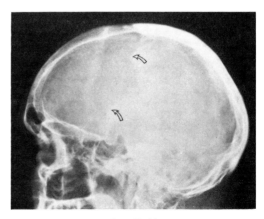

Case B-41

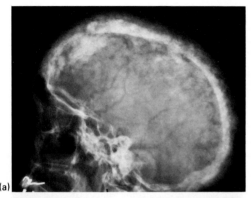

(a)

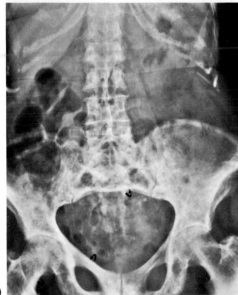

(b)

Case B-42

radiograph of the pelvis (B-42b) from the second individual demonstrates extensive Pagetoid change of the hips, pelvis, and sacrum. This is manifested by coarse, dense trabecular margins with thickened cortices (curved arrows). A hallmark of the disease is enlargement of the bone size. This enlargement differentiates this process from osteoblastic metastasis. Final diagnosis: Paget's disease.

Case B-43

The next pair of radiographs belong to a 33-year-old man being treated for renal failure. Skull and hand radiographs were obtained for evaluation of his clinical status. The film B-43a demonstrates a lateral view of the skull. Note that the skull bones are demineralized, with a spotty irregularity of the calvarium. This represents the so-called "salt-and-pepper" manifestation of hyperparathyroidism. The accompanying film of the hands (B-43b) demonstrates the reabsorption of bone involving the shafts of the distal phalanges (curved open arrow) and the shafts of the intermediate phalanges (solid straight arrow). The bony reabsorption of the phalanges characteristically occurs most noticably along the radial aspect of the shafts of the intermediate phalanges of the fingers. There are other areas in the skeletal system where reabsorption of calcium from bone occurs—distal ends of the clavicles, medial proximal tibial metaphysis, cortical bone surrounding teeth, and end-plates of vertebral bodies. Renal osteodystrophy or hyperparathyroidism seen in renal failure occurs because of elevated levels of parathormone. Calcium is depleted from its bony warehouse, which causes a generalized bony demineralization and the previously mentioned changes. Osteosclerosis can occur concomitantly with the deposition of calcium in periarticular tissues and blood vessels secondary to metastatic calcification. Brown tumors may also be found in the skeletal system, but all of these changes may regress when transplantation has corrected the metabolic problem. Final diagnosis: Secondary hyperparathyroidism due to chronic renal failure.

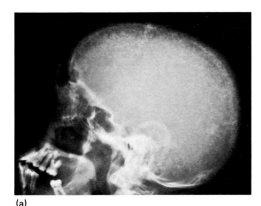

(a)

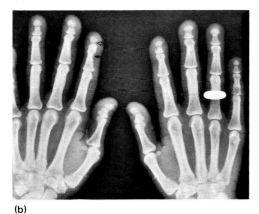

(b)

Case B-43

THE SPINE

Normal Spine Radiographs

In the radiographic examination of the spine, usually only AP and lateral radiographs are obtained. There are special views, however, for specific areas in the spine, which will be discussed. In the evaluation of abnormalities of the spine, the normal anatomic structures, as well as their interrelationships with adjacent structures, must be known. It is beyond the scope of this book to completely describe normal anatomy, but several important anatomical areas will be discussed.

The AP radiograph of the neck (NS-1a) demonstrates the lower two thirds of the cervical spine. The vertebral body of C7 is outlined with dotted lines, and adjacent vertebral bodies can then be seen, both in the cervical and dorsal spine. The spinous processes are tear-drop structures, which overlie the midline of the spine and can be seen by the dotted oval. A line drawn through the spinous processes of each cervical vertebra should be straight, signifying no malalignment. The upper one third of the cervical spine is seen with a specialized odontoid view. A cone-down view with the x-ray beam perpendicular to the C1–C2 area is utilized for best detail. C2 is well visualized with the odontoid process (solid arrows) between the lateral aspects of the C1 ring (dotted line).

The lateral view of the cervical spine (NS-1c) is probably the most important view obtained. It shows alignment of all the vertebral bodies, lateral masses, and spinous processes. If the entire vertebra of C7 is not on the film, the examination is incomplete. A line drawn through the anterior and posterior edges of the vertebral bodies and the base of the spinous processes (dotted line) should be a continuous uninterrupted line. This ensures no malalignment or dislocation. The intervertebral disc spaces (curved solid arrow) should be relatively equal in height. The anterior aspects of the odontoid process (open arrow) of C2 should be within 2½ mm of the posterior edge of the anterior ring (solid arrow) of C1 in the adult and up to 5 mm in children. A true lateral view should show each lateral mass (dotted trapezoid) of the same vertebra over-

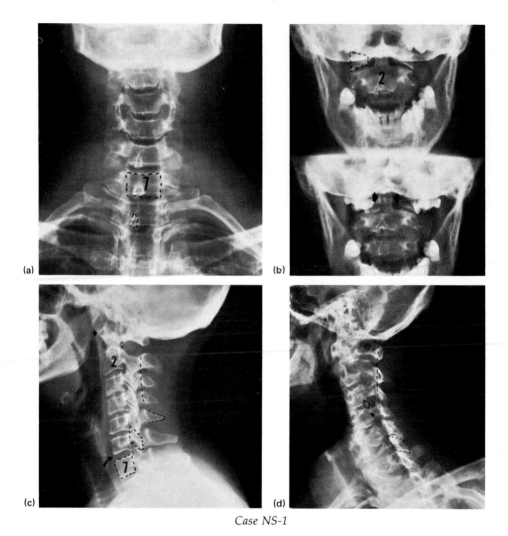

Case NS-1

lying each other perfectly. Alteration in this relationship suggests unilateral sub-luxation. The spinous processes of the cervical spine are shown by the dotted angle, with the spinous process of C7 being the largest. The soft-tissue shadow between the curved open arrow, the posterior wall of the hypopharynx, and the anterior surface of the cervical vertebral

bodies represents the prevertebral soft tissues. There are various measurements for this thickness, but this should never exceed one third the AP diameter of the C4 vertebral body. If this is thickened, it usually represents soft-tissue edema or hemorrhage from trauma.

An oblique view (NS-1d) of the spine demonstrates the neuroforamina (open ar-

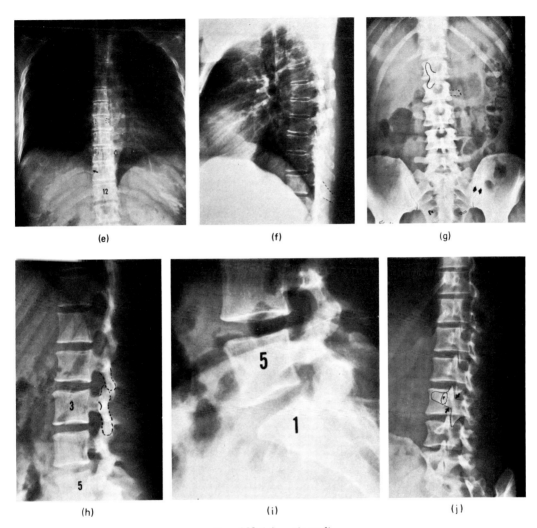

(e) (f) (g)

(h) (i) (j)

Case NS-1 (continued)

row) where the spinal nerves exit. Again, line continuums can be drawn, as is demonstrated by the dotted line. The lateral masses (dotted trapezoid), including the pedicle (solid arrow) of each cervical vertebra, can be easily seen.

Similar anatomical parts can be seen in the dorsal spine. The AP radiograph (NS-1e) demonstrates a square vertebral body with concave edges, becoming only slightly larger as progression goes from T1 to T12. The pedicles are well outlined, as a pair of circles on either side of the midline (dotted circles). The spinous processes are pointing markedly inferior, and therefore are not readily identified in the view. The transverse processes (solid arrow) are obscured by adjoining ribs. The proximal part of each rib articulates, not only with the transverse process, but with the edge of the vertebral body. There is a thin soft-tissue line (open arrow) that can be seen on either side of the spine. This should be uniformly straight; otherwise it is abnormal. The lateral view (NS-1f) demonstrates square-shaped vertebral bodies with thick cortical end-plates. The intervertebral disc spaces are uniform in height. Each paired pedicle is identified in profile (dotted line) as are the spinous processes seen as a dotted line more posteriorly.

Examination of the lumbar spine is a common radiological procedure for backache. An AP film (NS-1g) shows the vertebrae more discretely. There are five lumbar vertebral bodies, which increase in size slightly as the sacrum is approached. The transverse processes (dotted line) overlying the iliopsoas muscles are easily seen. The L1 lamina is divided into halves by a continuous black line. The lamina gives rise to not only the spinous process, but also the superior and inferior articulating facets. In this view the sacrum is also seen to good advantage showing its multiple neuroforamina (curved open arrow). The sacrum's articulation with the pelvis is at the sacroiliac joints (solid straight arrows). In this patient an intra-uterine device (IUD) is seen in the pelvis (curved solid arrow). The lateral radiograph (NS-1h) shows to good advantage the vertebral bodies and disc spaces. The L4–L5 intervertebral disc space should be the largest, with a highly variable L5–S1 disc interspace. Normally, L5–S1 disc interspace will be approximately half of the L4–L5 disc interspace area. The laminae of the vertebrae are noted by dotted lines with the inferior aspect of the lamina of the L2 articulating with the superior aspect of the lamina of L3. The transverse process is represented by a curved solid

line. A spot-lateral film (NS-1i) shows to good advantage the relationship of the L5 vertebra to the sacrum.

An oblique film of the lumbar spine (NS-1j) was obtained to show the relationships of the articulating facets and the pars interarticularis area (solid arrows). A solid line is drawn around the edge of half of a lamina and its transverse process as well as around the pedicle which lies en face. With a little imagination, a "Scottie dog" is visualized. This configuration is looked for on the oblique films when looking for congenital or traumatic injuries of the posterior elements and pars interarticularis area.

CASE PRESENTATIONS

Cases SP-1 and SP-2

These films represent two common congenital variations of the cervical spine. The first radiograph (SP-1) demonstrates a bony projection (solid arrow) from the transverse process of C7. Normally, cervical vertebrae do not have ribs, but occasionally anomalous cervical ribs will develop at the C7 level. Normally, there are only 12 pairs of ribs attached in pairs to each dorsal vertebra. Cervical ribs are seen as incidental findings on the chest radiograph. However, they can be associated with clinical symptoms when they interfere with the nervous or the vascular supply to the upper extremities. These patients will complain of numbness of their upper extremities in certain positions, and surgery may be needed to correct this abnormality.

Similarly, the second radiograph (SP-2) was obtained for trauma. It shows fusion of the vertebral bodies of C4 and C5, as

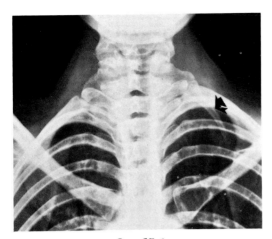

Case SP 1

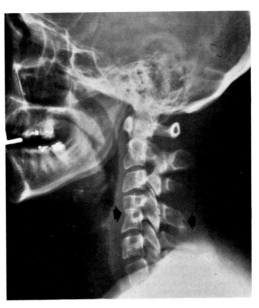

Case SP-2

well as fusion of the lateral masses and spinous processes (solid arrows). This is a coincidental finding in a patient without limitation of motion in the neck as long as only three or fewer vertebrae are involved. This defect is due to failure of the vertebrae to segment during development. This type of deformity can be associated with symptoms when changes are extensive or associated with spinal cord abnormalities. Final diagnosis: (1) Cervical rib. (2) Congenital block vertebra.

Case SP-3

Case SP-3 is a 52-year-old man with low back pain. Radiographic evaluation of the lumbar-sacral spine area reveals an abnormality at the L5–S1 area. Note that the posterior margin of L5 vertebral body (curved solid arrow) is 1 to 2 cm forward of the posterior aspect of S1 (curved open arrow). This represents forward subluxation of L5 on S1. Commonly this is due to a defect in the pars interarticularis area (solid straight arrow) of L5. There is a controversy at the present time concern-

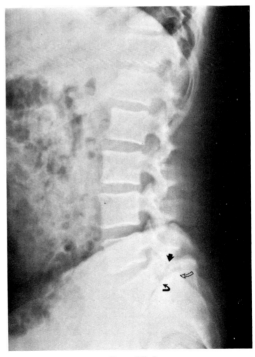

Case SP-3

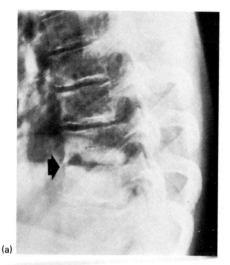

(a)

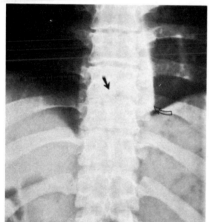

(b)

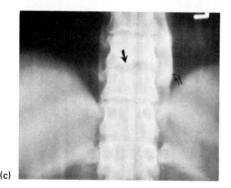

(c)

Case SP-4

ing whether this defect is congenital or traumatic in origin. In any event, this defect allows the superior aspect of the lamina of L5 and the rest of the lumbar spine to slip forward on the inferior aspect of the posterior elements of L5 and the sacrum. This subluxation is called spondylolisthesis and is a grade II variety. A grade I slippage would be represented by the forward subluxation of the L5 vertebral body only one fourth the distance of the AP width of S1. A grade III variety of course, would be forward subluxation of L5 over three fourths the AP dimension of S1. The break in the pars interarticularis area of L5 is called a spondylolysis. This defect can occur without subluxation and is best seen on oblique radiographs of the lumbar-sacral spine (neck fracture of the Scottie dog).

This is a common problem seen today. It may be asymptomatic and seen only as an incidental finding on examination of the lumbar-sacral spine. However, it can be the source of chronic recurrent low back pain, but is infrequently operated upon. Final diagnosis: Spondylolisthesis L5–S1.

Case SP-4

This patient is a 28-year-old woman with back pain. Routine views of the dorsal and lumbar-sacral spine show an abnormality, and therefore cone-down views were obtained in the AP and the lateral dimension. The lateral radiograph (SP-4a) demonstrates loss of the intervertebral disc space height (solid arrow). The vertebral body surfaces of the adjoining vertebrae show ill-defined margins. This is especially true of the more superior vertebra which also shows lucencies in the inferior anterior surface. The AP radiograph (SP-4b) shows similar findings, but they are less well defined. There is irregularity of the vertebral body surfaces (solid arrow). There is thickening of the paraspinal soft tissues stripe (curved open arrow) bilaterally more on the patient's left than on the right. A tomogram (SP-4c) done in the AP dimension better defines the changes in the adjoining vertebral body surfaces, showing the bone destruction (solid arrow), the loss of intervertebral disc space height, and the paraspinal soft tissue thickening (curved open arrow).

Infections of the spine are usually due to the hematogenous spread of bacteria, most notably by staphylococci or gram-negative bacteria. Less commonly, tuberculous bacteria can give similar changes. The earliest x-ray finding in osteomyelitis of the intervertebral disc space and the adjacent vertebra is the destruction of the disc. This is manifested by a loss in the height of the disc. As the infection involves the end-plates of the adjacent vertebra, there is bone destruction noted along the vertebral body surfaces. This is manifested by a lucency and irregularity of its vertebral surfaces. As the disease becomes chronic, sclerosis becomes prominent. Healing of this process finally results in fusion of the vertebral bodies, occasionally with increase in angulation of alignment. The inflammatory process spreads to adjacent soft tissues, causing edema and pus formation that leads to a thickened paraspinal stripe. In tuberculosis, this inflammatory soft-tissue response may calcify, giving the characteristic appearance of Pott's disease. Treatment is with antibiotics, and surgery is rarely necessary except for sampling the bacteria for specific antibiotic treatment. Final diagnosis: Disc space infection with adjacent osteomyelitis of vertebral bodies.

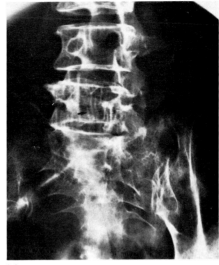

(a)

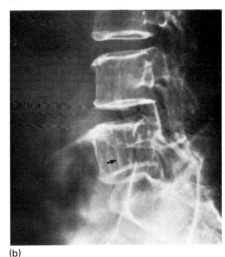

(b)

Case SP-5

Case SP-5

The pair of radiographs (SP-5a and b) demonstrate an abnormal trabecular pattern of the vertebral body of L5. Note that there are vertically oriented striations due to coarse trabeculations (solid arrow). The adjacent vertebral bodies show uniformly calcified vertebra. This pathological appearance is compatible with a hemangioma of the L5 vertebral body.

This is one of the most common benign tumors of the spine. The vast majority are asymptomatic, seen only incidentally on radiographs of the spine. The coarse trabecular bony structures of the vertebral bodies are surrounded by and produced by the dilated vascular spaces of the hemangioma. Occasionally, this pattern can be seen to extend into the posterior element. Because of the weakness that is created in the vertebral body, a compression fracture may occur with adjacent hemorrhage. Note that the course lines are vertically oriented, which is typical for this abnormality. Final diagnosis: Hemangioma at L5.

Cases SP-6 through SP-8

The next series of radiographs represents three individuals with the same pathological process. The first radiograph

(SP-6) demonstrates compression of the C7 vertebral body (solid arrow). However, close examination of this vertebral body shows lucency, suggesting that this is a pathological fracture or fracture due to a pathological process softening the vertebral body. No other changes characteristic of a neoplastic process are noted in the spine. There are slight degenerative spurs present. This patient was a 58-year-old man with carcinoma of the lung and metastatic bony destruction of the spine.

The next radiograph (SP-7) is an AP radiograph of the dorsal-lumbar spine. Note that there is almost total opacification of the right chest due to postoperative and carcinomatous change. However, pay particular attention to the pedicle and the lateral aspect of the T12 vertebral body. The pedicle is not a discrete circular structure as seen in other vertebral bodies. The lateral aspect of the vertebral body (solid arrow) appears moth-eaten and does not contain the normal amount of calcium. This represents metastatic destruction of this vertebral body from carcinoma of the

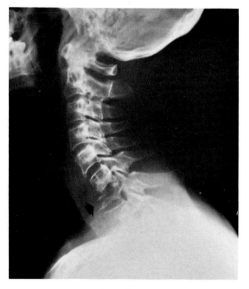

Case SP-6

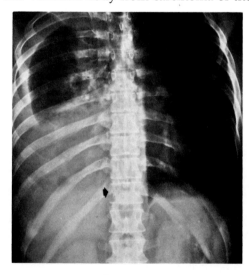

Case SP-7

lung. No other metastatic disease is seen, although there is a fracture deformity of the right 11th rib.

The AP and lateral films in case SP-8a and b are from the same individual. This individual is a 61-year-old man with cancer of the prostate, which has spread throughout his entire body, giving multiple metastatic lesions. Metastatic changes in this individual are of two varieties. The first variety is a sclerosis or osteoblastic change best seen in the vertebral bodies (open straight arrows). Bone destruction or osteolytic metastasis is seen in the vertebral bodies (solid straight arrows) as well. Several of the pedicles are missing on the AP film, best demonstrated at the level of the solid straight arrows. Note that there is a degenerative spur seen in the lower dorsal spine (solid curved arrow).

Metastatic tumors involving the spine are the most common form of malignant tumors of the spine. As seen in these individuals, both bone production (osteoblastic change) and bone destruction (osteolytic change) can occur. The most common primary malignancies leading to osteolytic metastasis are carcinomas of the lung, breast, kidney, or prostate. Similar osteolytic bone destruction can be seen in multiple myeloma. It is not infrequent for multiple myeloma to appear as a diffuse demineralization of the skeletal system without specific discrete lytic densities. Both multiple myeloma and metastatic carcinoma, producing osteolytic metastasis, lead to pathological fractures commonly seen in ribs and vertebral bodies and eventually to compression deformity. Expansile lytic defects can occur with certain types of tumors such as multiple myeloma, or renal cell, and thyroid carcinoma.

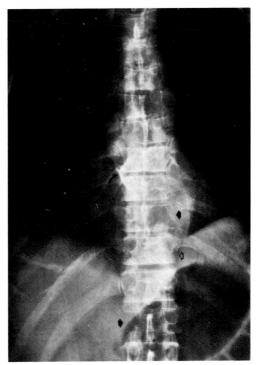

(a)

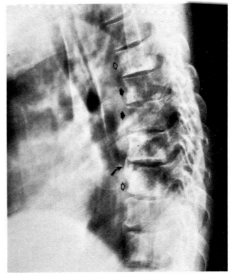

(b)

Case SP-8

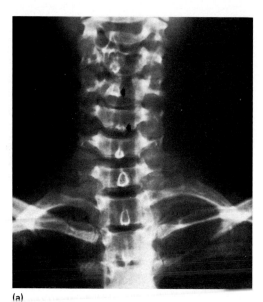

(a)

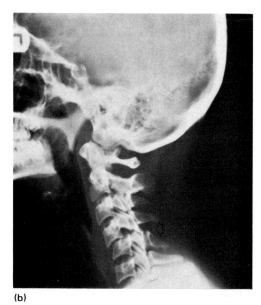

(b)

Case SP-9

Bone production or osteoblastic change is commonly seen in breast carcinoma, prostatic carcinoma and GI malignancies and infrequently in lung carcinoma. While the sclerosis suggests reinforcement of the structure, the bones are actually weakened by the metastatic process as the bone production is of a pathological nature.

Several types of malignancy can give both osteolytic and osteoblastic metastasis. Breast carcinoma can do both, with osteoblastic changes seen when the patient is being treated. Prostatic carcinoma is another common imitator of both types of changes. Ninety percent of the lung metastases are lytic. Lymphomatous tumors may give mixed changes as well. Knowing the patient's age and sex and the type and location of the metastasis can frequently yield the specific cell type or origin of the primary tumor. In contradistinction to inflammatory lesions of the spine, malignant tumors of the vertebral column rarely involve the intervertebral disc space. Final diagnosis: Osteolytic and osteoblastic metastasis.

Cases SP-9 through SP-16

The next series of radiographs demonstrates multiple fractures of the spine due to trauma in different areas. Varieties or different types of fractures are also demonstrated.

The first pair of radiographs (SP-9a and b) demonstrate AP and lateral films from a 19-year-old woman. The AP radiograph shows malalignment of the spinous processes. Note that the spinous process of C4 and C5 (solid arrows) are offset and not in a straight line. This suggests dislocation at the C4–C5 level. A lateral view demonstrates obvious forward subluxation of C4 on C5 of approximately 1 cm. Note that no obvious fracture is seen, nor is there an increase in the prevertebral soft tissues, which would suggest edema. There is, however, widening of the space between the spinous processes (straight open arrow) and narrowing of the intervertebral disc space. This is compatible with disruption of the ligaments and the disc at this level. The radiographic appearance of the subluxation and soft-tissue injury suggests that the spinal cord is compressed, but this patient was relatively asymptomatic. Case SP-10 demonstrates a similar subluxation of C2 on C3 (curved solid arrow). However, in this individual there is thickening of the prevertebral soft tissues (solid straight arrow) indicative of hemorrhage and soft-tissue edema, as well as compression of C3, C4, and possibly of C5. Both of these individuals had a flexion injury of the cervical spine.

The next radiograph (SP-11) demonstrates fracture of the pedicles of C2 (solid arrow). Note that there is angulation of C1 and C2 body angled forward, and there is an increase in the space between the posterior aspects of C1 and C2. This means that the posterior ligaments between C1 and C2 are torn also, and, therefore, C1 and the body of C2 are free to slip forward on the rest of the spine with flexion, which can lead to cord injury.

The patient in case SP-12 represents a relatively stable fracture of the spinous process of C7 (solid arrow). This is created by sudden stopping of an extension motion, the so-called "clay shovelers fracture." Ligamentous injury is also present.

The next pair of radiographs (SP-13a and b) demonstrate yet another variety of fracture-subluxation. In the AP view, (SP-13a) there is a vertical fracture line

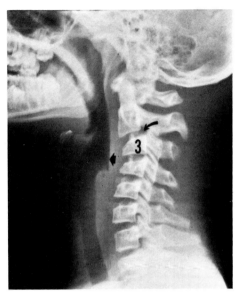

Case SP-10

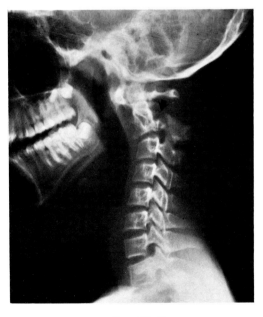

Case SP-11

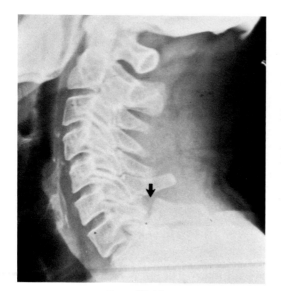

Case SP-12

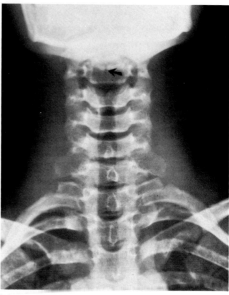

(a)

through the body of C3 (solid arrow) and probably of C4. Other routine views were unremarkable. However, one oblique radiograph (SP-13b) demonstrates interruption of the continuous straight line at C4–C5 (curved solid arrow) connecting the anterior aspects of the lateral masses. Therefore, there is subluxation of the lateral masses.

Injuries to the dorsal-lumbar spine are similar. Compression of the spine by extensive flexion causes a common fracture—a compression fracture. This is demonstrated in the film in case SP-14, involving the L1 vertebral body. There is anterior wedging of L1 with the other vertebral body heights remaining normal. The posterior aspect of L1 is also unchanged. A similar, but more extensive, type of injury is seen in case SP-15. Again, there is compression and anterior wedging of L1. However, this fracture is of a burst variety with multiple fragments pro-

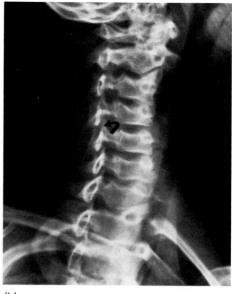

(b)

Case SP-13

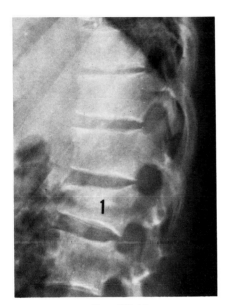

Case SP-14

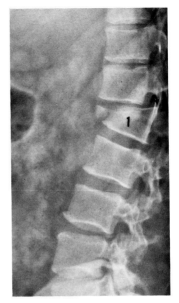

Case SP-15

duced when the vertebral body exploded. There is also soft-tissue injury as T12 has slipped forward on L1 (solid curved arrow). This is due to an acute extensive flexion injury of the lumbar spine. Subluxation of this vertebral body could then lead to cord or nerve root compression. Keep in mind that the spinal cord ends at about L1, with the remaining spinal canal filled inferiorly by the multiple lumbar and sacral nerve roots.

A less frequent fracture is demonstrated in case SP-16. There is a fracture through the pars interarticularis area (solid straight arrow) of the lamina of L3. This type of injury may need surgical support as the upper lumbar spine could slide on the lower lumbar spine at the level of the fracture site if there is destruction of the ligamentous attachments.

It must be noted that minor trauma to the spine can cause severe nerve or spinal

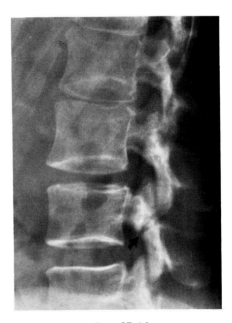

Case SP-16

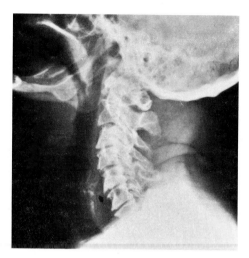

Case SP-17

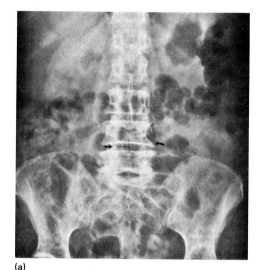

(a)

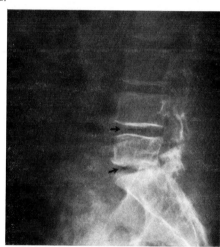

(b)   *Case SP-18*

cord injury with radiographs demonstrating minimal injury. On the other hand, extensive trauma seen radiographically may be associated with minimal nervous injury. The important thing in the management of these patients is to know whether the fracture is stable or unstable, and if there is the possibility of cord compression. Final diagnosis: Spinal fractures and dislocations.

Cases SP-17 and SP-18

The next set of radiographs are from individuals with similar radiographic problems. The first radiograph (SP-17) is a lateral cervical spine radiograph. Note that there is loss of the typical square shape of the vertebral bodies. Their edges are irregular in outline with small bony projections commonly called spurs (solid arrow). The intervertebral disc spaces are narrowed in several areas. There is sclerosis or increase in bone production about the intervertebral disc space areas. All of these changes are due to degenerative arthritic change in the cervical spine, with degenerative disc changes as well.

The next pair of films (SP-18a and b) are AP and lateral films of the lumbar spine from the same individual. While there is no loss of height of the disc space, there is a horizontal lucency seen in the L4–L5 and L5–S1 disc interspace areas (solid straight arrows). There are also small spurlike protrusions from the vertebral body edges best seen on the AP film (solid curved arrow). Sclerosis involving the vertebral bodies surfaces at the L5–S1 level is seen, but it is not as marked as that seen in the cervical spine. These changes also reflect degenerative arthritic changes.

As a person grows older, bony spurs are often visualized along the margins of vertebral bodies. These spurs can occur in the physiological process of aging. They also can be exaggerated by recurrent trauma or as a reparative process secondary to degenerative change in the intervertebral disc. Frequently, these changes are asymptomatic. Occasionally, these spurs may project into the neuroforamina or posteriorly into the spinal canal, producing neurological changes and symptoms.

As a disc undergoes aging and degeneration, the space between the vertebral bodies becomes narrower. Gas may accumulate in the space left by the disappearing disc, manifested on a radiograph as a lucent horizontal line commonly referred to as vacuum phenomenon. The adjacent vertebrae will try to repair or stabilize this defect by causing bony overgrowth or spurs and adjacent bony changes known as osteosclerosis. When this process is extensive, spurring and bone bridging can narrow the spinal canal (AP dimension) below 12 mm, which is the lowest limit allowable before spinal compression occurs. Surgery to remove the spurs from a neuroforamen or to decompress the spinal cord may be warranted.

It must be mentioned here that there are few changes on plain films of the spine that are indicative of herniated disc disease. Only a myelogram can show this abnormality, but there are frequently as-

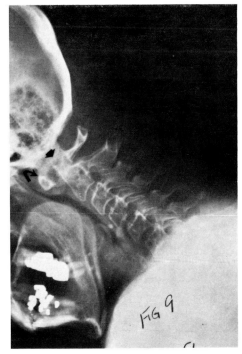

Case SP-19

sociated hypertrophic degenerative changes in the spine. Final diagnosis: Hypertrophic degenerative arthritis.

Case SP-19

The next radiograph represents a 60-year-old woman with rheumatoid arthritis. There are extensive changes of rheumatoid arthritis seen in the extremities, with very few changes seen in the spine. The only synovial joints in the spine are the articular facet joints and a small synovial sac in the C1–C2 area. Changes in the articular facets are similar to those seen in the extremity joints. There is narrowing of the joints with bony demineralization and articular erosions. As the disease progresses, fusion of this area may develop.

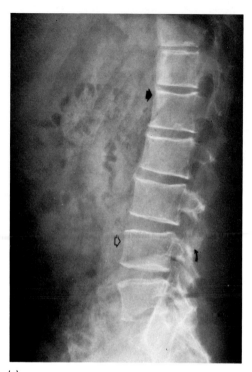

(a)

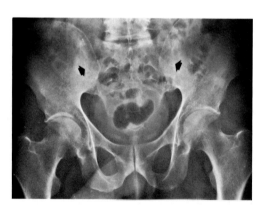

(b)

Case SP-20

There is, however, one synovial joint in the cervical spine that is important. A small synovial sac occurs between the posterior aspect of the odontoid process and a ligament running transversely from one side of C1 to the other, holding the odontoid process anterior in the spinal canal of the C1 region. If rheumatoid changes occur in this sac, erosion involving the transverse ligament may occur, causing the ligament to rupture. When this occurs the odontoid process is free to move in the spinal canal, compressing the spinal cord.

A single view of the cervical spine in the lateral projection (SP-19) shows this patient in flexion. Note that the odontoid process (solid straight arrow) is posterior in relationship to the anterior C1 ring (solid curved arrow). This is due to disruption of the transverse ligament. This subluxation is best seen with the head in flexion and may not be demonstrated in extension or neutral positions. Final diagnosis: Rheumatoid arthritis, rupturing the transverse ligament allowing subluxation of C1 on C2.

Cases SP-20 through SP-22

The next series of radiographs represents three young adults with the same disease process and similar radiographic manifestations. The first pair of radiographs (SP-20a and b) are from the same individual. The lateral lumbar-sacral spine (SP-20a) demonstrates characteristic squaring of the upper lumbar and the lower dorsal vertebral bodies. This squaring is due to erosions of the anterior-superior aspect of the vertebral bodies (solid straight arrow). The normal smooth corners and the concave anterior surface (straight open arrow) of normal vertebrae

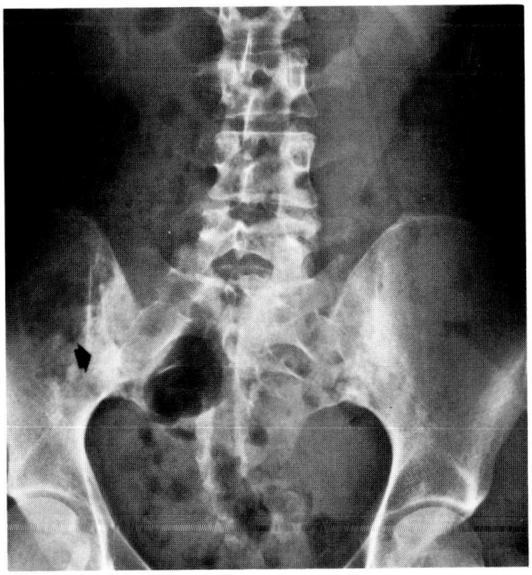

Case SP-21

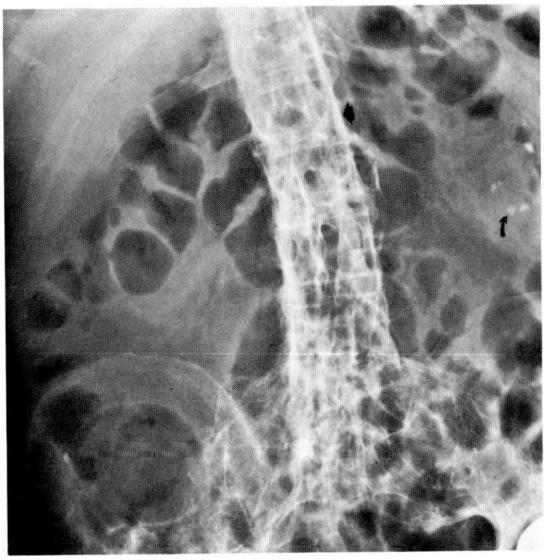

(a)

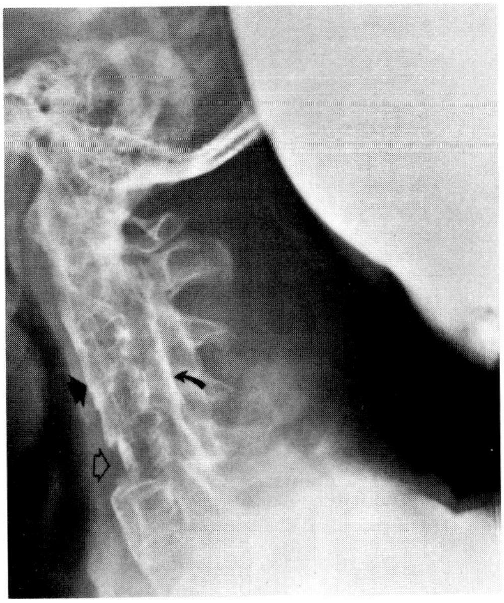

(b)

Case SP-22

are not seen. Note that the articular facet joints are ill defined, suggesting arthritic change (curved solid arrow).

The same individual, in a film of the pelvis (SP-20b) shows ill-defined sacroiliac joints (solid straight arrows). This is due to an involvement of the arthritic process in the sacroiliac joints. Only the lower two thirds of the sacroiliac joints are synovial joints. Case SP-21, from a different individual, shows even further change in the sacroiliac joints with loss of the joints and adjacent sclerosis along the iliac aspect of the joint (solid straight arrow). Similar changes are seen in the pubic symphysis (open straight arrow). As the disease progresses there is obliteration of the sacroiliac joint with fusion. A similar process takes place in the facet joints of the spine. This leads to ankylosis or fusion of the facet joints and costal vertebral joints.

Ligamentous calcification and fusion (SP-22a, solid straight arrow) is common and gives a "bamboo" appearance to the spine. Note in this patient that there are numerous renal calculi (curved solid arrow) as well as cup arthroplasties bilaterally. The entire process of ankylosing spondylitis or Marie-Strumpell's disease begins in the sacroiliac joints spreading cephalad into the cervical spine. Similar changes are seen in the cervical spine with fusion of the posterior elements and calcification of spinous ligaments (SP-22b, solid straight and curved arrows). Not infrequently this rigid spine is complicated by fractures with subluxation (open straight arrow).

This variety of arthritis involving the spine and pelvis is still considered by some to be a variant of rheumatoid arthritis. However, many people have separated this into a distinct entity. Its previous name, rheumatoid spondylitis, is no longer correct, and it should now be referred to as ankylosing spondylitis. Final diagnosis: Ankylosing spondylitis.

7

The Upper Extremity

Since the thrust of this text is frequent radiographic diagnosis, it is only proper that we allocate considerable space to the upper extremity. Normal anatomical structures in the upper extremity may be altered by many pathological processes. Smashed fingers, falls with injuries to the wrist, elbow, and shoulder result in nearly half of the radiographic studies done on outpatients.

Trauma is not the only pathological process involving the extremities. The hand is an excellent area for evaluating metabolic disease. The shoulder in the upper extremity, and the pelvis and the hip in the lower extremity are frequent sites of metastatic lesions. Degenerative joint disease is a major area of concern in virtually all the joint areas, particularly the knees and hips. In the upper extremity, degenerative joint disease is common, but rheumatoid processes tend to be more crippling. Primary bone tumors are relatively infrequent in their overall occurrence, but their greatest incidence is in the lower extremity.

Our discussions in reference to each film will be relatively brief. It is hoped that our examples will serve as guides in the development of your learning to evaluate radiographic findings. As we enter a new anatomical area for evaluation, normal films will be presented as a standard.

To start our studies of the shoulder, two normal films of the right shoulder are presented.

SHOULDER

CASE PRESENTATIONS

Case UX-1

Two films are presented, for we routinely make all extremity radiographs at least in two different projections. We prefer to take films at right angles to each other, but a lateral film taken through the chest has only limited value. The lateral film is used to evaluate fractures in the surgical neck of the humerus, but it has little other value. Therefore, films of the shoulder are made in internal and external rotations. If specialized views are required, oblique films will show the relationship of the head to the glenoid or an axillary view will be made to identify either anterior or posterior displacement of the head. Unfortunately, if a patient has a dislocated shoulder, axillary views are virtually impossible to obtain. Therefore, we will try to help you make the diagnosis without the use of difficult or complicated supplementary views.

Film UX-1a is made in internal rotation; Film UX-1b is in external rotation. Iden-

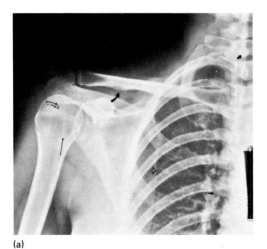

(a)

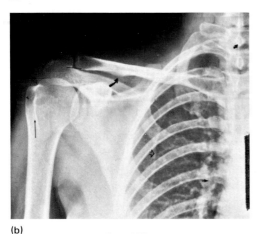

(b)

Case UX-1

tical style arrows are used to point out the same anatomical points on the two films. For example, the long, slender, delicate arrow over the humerus is directed toward the bicipital groove. As the humerus moves, the location of the groove changes considerably. The heavy curved arrow pointing cephalad has the base of the arrow on the coracoid process of the scapula. The point of the arrow is directed toward the attachment of the coracoclavicular ligament on the clavicle at the junc-

tion of the distal and middle third. The large open arrow is directed toward the supraspinous groove in each projection. The short open arrow is directed toward the edge of the scapula as it superimposes on the lung fields. The small dark arrow toward the medial side of the film identifies a dorsal transverse process. In this case it is the transverse process of the seventh dorsal body. The delicate black line seen along the inferior margin of the distal clavicle points out the parallel alignment between the inferior margin of the acromion process and the inferior lateral end of the clavicle. A short solid arrow with a slight curve is directed toward an annular density in the superior medial portion of the radiograph. This is the spinous process of the first dorsal body. The configuration of the spinous processes changes as the level changes. For example, the second and third spinous processes are elongated. The third and fourth spinous processes appear as virtually vertical lines rather than circles.

A number of other anatomical areas are not indicated by arrows. The transverse process of D1 is very prominent. The first rib, of course, arises from the first dorsal body and extends anteriorly. The cortex of the humeral shaft is relatively dense, but tapers to a fine line as the metaphyseal end of the humerus is reached. Over the head of the humerus, only the fine trabecular pattern of the bone is identified—the cortex here being very thin and sharp.

Shoulder films frequently give an excellent view of the apical lung fields. Here there is no significant pathology. We use shoulder films to evaluate patients with Pancoast's tumor or with metastatic disease that may involve the upper ribs or dorsal spine.

In virtually all films of the shoulder, the

head of the humerus appears to be super-imposed on the acromion. The acromion process is posterior to the humeral head and serves to protect this portion of the shoulder as a roof. Because of this roof posterior dislocations of the humeral head are relatively infrequent. Since the clavical and anterior portion of the acrom-ion tends to roof the humerus superiorly, dislocations tend to go forward and down into the axilla. This will be shown later. Keep in mind this normal set of films, we may be referring to them later.

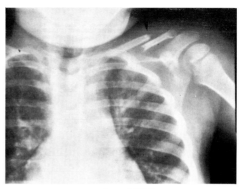

Case UX-2

Case UX-2

Case UX-2 is a two-year-old child who was brought to the emergency room com-plaining of pain in the shoulder following a fall.

This is the most frequent fracture of the upper extremity in children under the age of two. This is a transverse fracture through the clavicle at the junction of the middle and outer third. There is approx-imately 1 cm of override at the fracture site. This will result in some loss of length initially; however, as the bone repairs and models, this loss will be corrected. No joint-space involvement is present. Ribs and chest appear normal. Treatment of fractures of the clavicle in children is al-ways conservative. Some type of a yoke to pull shoulders back and maintain the length of the clavicle is attempted.

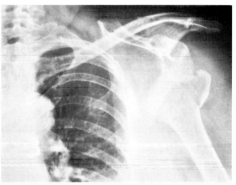

(a)

Case UX-3

Case UX-3 is a 63-year-old obese wom-an. Films were made following a fall. She came to the emergency room unable to move her left arm at the shoulder.

The humeral head is dislocated from the glenoid cavity—it sits inferior to the gle-noid. From the single AP projection (UX-3a) it is difficult to know if the humerus

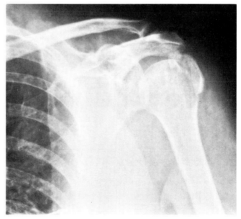

(b)

Case UX-3

is posterior or anterior to the glenoid. However, when the head is displaced downward, it is invariably in the subglenoid or subcoracoid area. This displacement represents anterior dislocation. Special views can be attempted to prove the point. Oblique views may be very helpful; stereoscopy is acceptable, axillary views are difficult to obtain and transthoracic views are of more value in injuries of the surgical neck of the humerus or below.

In addition to the obvious dislocation, there is a fracture through the tuberosity of the humerus. Even the mechanism of this fracture is demonstrable on the film since the fracture is produced by impaction of the inferior rim of the glenoid on the tuberosity. A vertical fracture in the tuberosity of the humerus is one of the most frequent fractures about the shoulder. It can occur with or without dislocation.

Film UX-3b was made following a reduction of the anterior dislocation. The tuberosity fragment has fallen into good

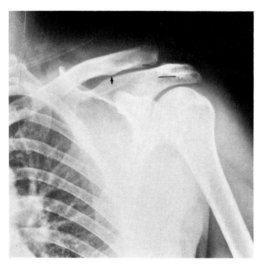

Case UX-4

position. In patients that do not have an associated anterior dislocation, the fracture of the tuberosity looks much as seen here, only the degree of displacement will vary. There are instances in which only a vertical fracture line is noted. In others, such as this, the tuberosity is slightly displaced from the head itself. Final diagnosis: Anterior dislocation of the shoulder with vertical fracture of the tuberosity. Successful reduction is demonstrated.

Case UX-4

Case UX-4 is a 32-year-old man who had fallen on the ice while playing hockey.

In the film, the humerus articulates with the glenoid normally. No fractures are identified. However, the level of the black line along the inferior margin of the distal clavicle and inferior margin of the acromion process respectively indicates that there is at least 1 cm superior displacement of the distal clavicle. This is the classical appearance of acromioclavicular separation. The distance between the coracoid process and the eminence of the lateral clavicle as evidenced by the small dark arrow is somewhat increased. A tear in the coracoclavicular ligament is an important part of acromioclavicular separation.

There are occasions when radiographs of the shoulder will not demonstrate the separation at the acromioclavicular joint. If initial studies show no fracture and this is the point of clinical suspicion, additional films should be taken with the patient supporting weight in the involved hand. The absence of fracture is important for the patient's safety and comfort. Weight-support radiographs will then exaggerate the separation of the clavicle from the acromion process. When weight-supporting films are obtained, it is helpful to show both shoulders together. This can be done with a 7 × 17 cassette placed crosswise. The first radiographs should be made without weight support and then a second film made with weight being supported in each hand. Final diagnosis: Acromioclavicular separation.

Case UX-5

Films UX-5a and b were taken of a 32-year-old man. The patient was a known epileptic, who had had seizures in the recent past. Following a seizure, the patient noted discomfort and poor utilization of the shoulder.

The radiograph of the shoulder in the AP projection shows a subtle but important abnormality. The humeral head in this circumstance has been described as having a "light bulb" appearance, or the term "pseudocyst" of the humeral head has been used. In any event, there is something different about the head of the humerus as one sees it in this projection. In the case we are presenting, the head is at the normal height; and in the single view one has the impression it may be adequately seated in the glenoid. If the head had been high in position so that it was superimposed on the acromion process, a diagnosis of posterior dislocation could be made from the anterior projection only. Since that is not the case here, additional films were required. The second film presented is a transthoracic view, which is always difficult to interpret when dislocations are in question. The small dark arrows point to the inferior margin of the glenoid. The upper solid arrow points to the superior portion of the glenoid. It is barely visible through the humeral head. Most of the head of the humerus is posterior to this point.

An oblique film would have been help-

ful here. An axillary view is virtually impossible with this type of dislocation. Stereoscopic studies in the AP projection would be of help.

Regardless of the views available, a high index of suspicion must always be maintained when there has been loss of shoulder function secondary to a traumatic event. The anterior dislocatons that we

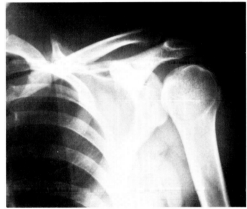

(a)

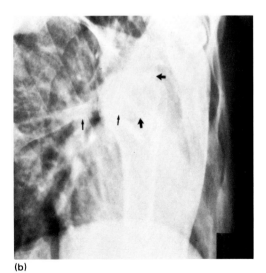

(b)

Case UX-5

have shown previously are relatively easy to diagnose. Posterior dislocations are missed on many occasions. In fact, one study has reported as many as 75% of patients with posterior dislocations of the shoulder have been radiographed at least twice before the diagnosis was established. The history of seizures is important, although other forms of trauma may produce the same type of dislocation. The AP view is helpful and may in some instances be diagnostic, but usually some other supportive view will be required. Final diagnosis: Posterior dislocation of the shoulder.

Cases UX-6 through UX-8

Three cases of fracture of the scapula are presented together. Each shows a different aspect of trauma. In addition to being an important stabilizing factor of the upper extremity, the scapula serves as a protective shield to the posterior rib cage and lung. In each of the cases we are

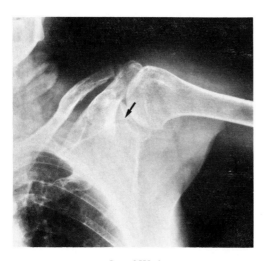

Case UX-6

presenting there are obvious fractures in the scapula, but in none of the cases is there a rib fracture or any evidence of lung contusion.

Case UX-6 is a 74-year-old woman who fell on a stairway, with most of the force being transmitted directly up the humerus. Note that there are degenerative changes at the acromioclavicular joint. The heavy dark arrow points to a split in the glenoid. There is little, if any, displacement of fragments, although the inferior lip of the glenoid may be slightly depressed. It is interesting that, at the same time this film was made, another film was made in a slightly different projection that did not show the glenoid fracture. This emphasizes the point that two views should be made of the shoulder, even though one of them cannot necessarily be a lateral view.

Fractures that enter an articular margin carry some increase significance for they tend to result in degenerative joint disease. This may be even more important to this elderly woman for she is already showing degenerative changes. Final diagnosis: Fracture through the glenoid of the scapula.

Case UX-7 is a 46-year-old woman who fell in such a way that the force of the fall transmitted through at least a part of the scapula, the humerus being spared. The heavy dark arrow points to a major split in the inferior portion of the scapula. There is some separation of the large lateral fragment. The open arrows are directed toward some linear areas of increased bone density. We normally think of fractures as radiolucent lines, such as the one outlined with the heavy dark arrow, but fractures can present as an area of increased density. This happens when two fragments of bone become superimposed upon each other. In this instance the flat bone was fractured and fragments displaced in such a way that a margin of the fracture slid under the other fragment; and a line of increase density resulted. Apparently, articular margins are not involved here. Final diagnosis: Comminuted fracture of the scapula.

Case UX-8 is a 16-year-old youth, also the victim of a fall. Two radiographs are presented here for the changes are considerably more subtle than that seen in the previous cases. The heavy arrow points cephalad to an irregular line just below the glenoid in the AP projection (UX-8a). Since this is heavier than the usual vascular line, and no epiphyseal line occurs here, fracture becomes the diagnosis of first choice. However, a film made in an oblique projection (UX-8b) is even more convincing, since the irregular line can be identified and apparently both the superior and inferior cortex are involved. There is no displacement of fragments, and the fracture line probably stops below the articular margin. The open arrow in the AP view of the shoulder is directed toward a radiolucent line across the proximal humerus. It looks amazingly like the fracture line in the scapula, but it represents an unclosed epiphysis. Since the patient is 16 years of age, the epiphysis cannot be expected to close for another one to two years. This epiphyseal line traverses the proximal humerus, and is seen in a more conventional manner beneath the small dark arrow. With the arm tilted slightly, the superior and inferior portions of the same epiphyseal line do not superimpose. Final diagnosis: Undisplaced fracture of the scapula. It does not involve the articular margin, and other than relief of pain will require little in the way of special management.

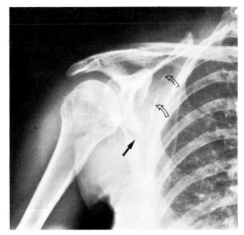

Case UX-7

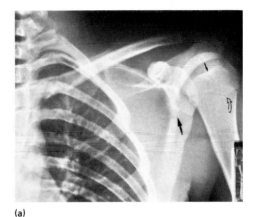

(a)

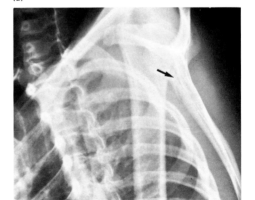

(b)

Case UX-8

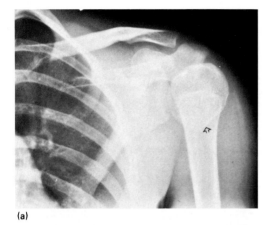

(a)

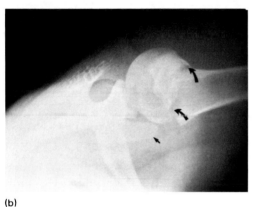

(b)

Case UX-9

Cases UX-9 and UX-10

The next two cases represent fractures of the proximal humerus. The two patients have not fused their epiphyses. The fracture in the younger child is far from subtle, even if epiphyses are closed, fractures occur high in the humeral neck, or as we showed in the case of anterior dislocation, the tuberosity may split vertically.

Case UX-9 is a 17-year-old youth who was injured playing football. In the AP view of the shoulder (UX-9a) one gets the impression that there is an additional line lower in the humerus. This is indicated by the open-faced arrow. The epiphyseal lines seen superior to this point are evident and do not appear unusual.

The axillary view (UX-9b) is helpful in defining the nature of the injury. A small dark arrow points to the coracoid process of the scapula which is anterior. The curved dark arrows point to the fracture line, which is continuous with the epiphyseal line. However, a portion of the metaphysis of the humeral shaft has been displaced with the head of the humerus posteriorly. This fracture, then, interrupts the epiphyseal line anteriorly and extends across the metaphysis to the posterior portion of the upper shaft of the humerus. The Salter classification of epiphyseal injuries is useful diagnostically, but is even more important in prognosis. See Table 1, page 221. This is a Salter type 2 injury in which the epiphyseal line is fractured and a corner of the metaphysis is attached. It is a combination of epiphyseal slip and fracture. Simple epiphyseal slips without fracture of the metaphysis are Salter type 1. Type 2 epiphyseal injuries of the proximal humerus are unusual due to the V-shape of the epiphysis, which tends to lock the epiphysis in place.

Involvement of the epiphysis and epiphyseal line is always important to note, for it can result in growth disturbances. These fractures occur frequently, and have the potential for growth arrest. Final diagnosis: Fracture of the proximal humerus, Salter type 2.

The second proximal humeral fracture (Case UX-10) is not presented as a subtle diagnostic problem. It is simply a transverse fracture through the proximal humerus. This area will constrict with further growth and development, and this

SALTER'S

CLASSIFICATION OF EPIPHYSEAL INJURY

TYPES
SALTER

I

EPIPHYSEAL SEPARATION IN THE LONG AXIS.
NO FRACTURE.
EASILY REDUCED.
GOOD PROGNOSIS.

II

EPIPHYSEAL SEPARATION ALONG THE PLATE
LINE TO A LONG AXIS FRACTURE LINE
THROUGH THE METAPHYSIS.
DIFFICULT REDUCTION.
GOOD PROGNOSIS USUALLY.

III
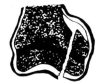
EPIPHYSEAL FRACTURE SEPARATION, INTO
JOINT SPACE.
ACCURATE REDUCTION IS NECESSARY.
PROGNOSIS DEPENDS ON REDUCTION.

IV

EPIPHYSEAL FRACTURE ACROSS THE PLATE
AND THROUGH THE METAPHYSIS IN THE
LONG AXIS.
PERFECT REDUCTION MAY REQUIRE
OPEN PROCEDURE.

V
COMPRESSION INJURY.
PROGNOSIS GUARDED.
SHORTENING DEFORMITIES.

Chart 1

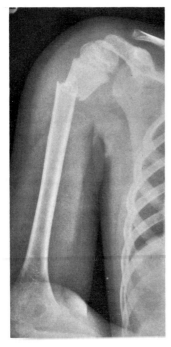

Case UX-10

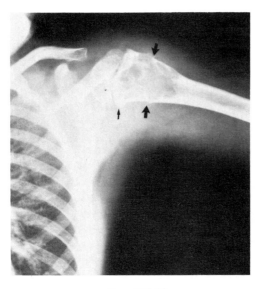

Case UX-11

will probably represent the surgical neck of the humerus. Fractures of the humerus can be transverse as is obvious here, or they can be spiral and comminuted depending upon the degree and mechanics of the trauma. No epiphyseal centers nor joint spaces are involved in this injury. Maintenance of length and general alignment is important. Final diagnosis: Transverse fracture of the proximal humerus.

Cases UX-11 through UX-19

Our next group of cases involves pathological processes in the shoulder and adjacent structures. These processes have both similar and dissimilar radiographic appearances. All are malignant, and all involve other portions of the body as well as the upper extremity. These lesions will appear again in differential diagnoses on films involving other anatomical locations.

Case UX-11 is a seven-year-old boy admitted with pain in his shoulder following relatively minor trauma. There was no history of discomfort prior to the injury.

The film of the shoulder is taken with the arm extended. Other views were also obtained, but this view showed the lesion best. There is an evident deformity of the proximal humerus. The deformity involves the metaphysis and extends nearly to the epiphyseal line. The small dark arrow points to the rather dense provisional zone of calcification on the metaphyseal side of the growth plate. The epiphyseal center that is forming the humeral head appears to be normal. The metaphysis is moderately expanded and fails to show the usual tubulation that occurs in a growing child. Multiple septations or fine bony bands are seen traversing the expanded and more radiolucent proximal humerus. The heavy dark arrows

This book belongs to Timothy J. Frohlick SSAN 553-86-7720
Give it back, you goddamned thief!

point to a break in the cortex on two sides of the humerus indicating that there has been a pathological fracture. The fracture is considered a pathological one since it involves an abnormal segment of bone.

Our final diagnosis is a pathological fracture through a humeral bone cyst. The cyst is considered benign and while it does appear to have multiple loculations, it would be classed as a simple cyst. It has been stated that a fracture through a cyst of this type will result in hemorrhage and healing of the cyst. Certainly this has been stated by many authors prior to us and is a generally accepted axiom, however, some authors have raised a question as to whether the fracture has a significant role in the healing of the bone lesion. Surgical procedures where bone chips or other foreign material are impacted in the area does seem to result in some healing of the cystic structure, and it is reasonable to assume that a fracture also speeds up the corrective process.

These cystic lesions are rather characteristic in their appearance. They invariably are at the metaphyseal end of the long bone. As the child grows, they appear to move more toward the diaphysis and eventually disappear.

Case UX-12 is a 65-year-old woman admitted with multiple sites of skeletal pain. A major area of discomfort was the right shoulder and the chest. The history was important in that the patient had had a breast removed for malignant disease four years earlier. She has been on chemotherapy including androgens.

The radiograph of the shoulder presents areas of bone destruction and bone production. Small dark arrows in the surgical neck of the humerus show poorly defined areas of bone loss. The one directed toward the cortex shows how the cortical

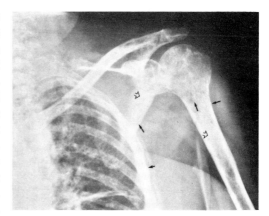

Case UX-12

bone is being destroyed. Note how much thinner the cortex is directly beneath the arrow than the cortex is on the opposite side of the humerus. Another solid arrow is directed toward a lytic lesion in the inferior portion of the lateral scapula. The fourth solid arrow is directed toward a pathological fracture in the fifth rib approximately in the mid axillary line. There is evidence of callus formation here. On close inspection, there are at least two or three other ribs involved above the level of this arrow.

The open-faced arrows are directed toward the areas of increased bone density. Sometimes it is difficult in the presence of osteolytic disease to know whether normal bone that remains is truly normal or if it is involved with an osteoblastic process. Here the arrows are directed toward a portion of the bone where the trabecular pattern is poorly defined and the margins of the increased density are fluffy and amorphous. No soft-tissue masses are identified here, except one identified as callus around healing rib fractures.

The final radiographic diagnosis is perfectly consistent with the clinical suspi-

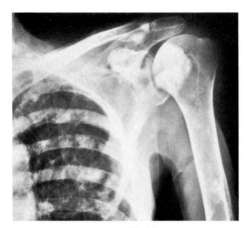

Case UX-13

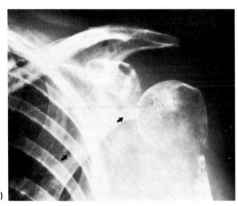

(a)

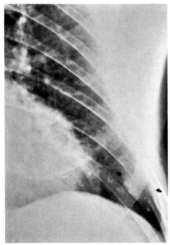

(b)

Case UX-14

cion of metastatic disease to bone, but the fact that there are osteolytic and osteoblastic changes present means that this is most likely a breast primary. Certainly when patients have been on androgens as part of their chemotherapeutic regime, osteoblastic lesions occur.

Case UX-13 is a 76-year-old man admitted to the hospital with generalized skeletal discomfort. He has known carcinoma of the prostate.

The radiograph of the shoulder girdle and ribs demonstrates classical osteoblastic metastatic disease. The humeral head shows dense bone formation along its articular margin. Other nodular areas of increased density are in the humerus. The third and fourth ribs are markedly dense in their curved regions, which are at approximately the posterior axillary line. The inferior margin of the scapula is also dense, as is the mid clavicle. No pathological fractures are noted. While we know that osteolytic changes usually precede or occur along with osteoblastic lesions, certainly here the osteoblastic process predominates.

Our final diagnosis here is osteoblastic metastasis. Odds are greatly in favor of this being from the prostate, although lung, breast, GI malignancy and occasionally Hodgkin's disease will produce osteoblastic lesions.

Case UX-14 is a 65-year-old man admitted to the hospital because of anemia and back pain. An initial chest radiograph (UX-14a) suggested probable shoulder pathology.

The radiographic changes in the shoulder are those of extensive bone destruction. The process appears to be entirely osteolytic. There is a break in the cortex seen in the surgical neck of the humerus. The small dark arrows are directed to changes in the scapula. One is just posterior to the glenoid where there is some destruction of bone. Another dark arrow between ribs points to a destructive lesion in the inferior margin of the scapula.

A second film (UX-14b) showing the lower rib cage is presented. This is the same patient and shows what is a very helpful sign in this case. The three dark arrows surround an area of rib destruction with what appears to be some increased density of a soft-tissue type surrounding the bony lesion. There is some expansion of the bone in the area of the lateral arrow.

The differential diagnosis from the shoulder film alone would include metastatic disease, such as might be encountered from the lung, breast, kidney, thyroid or multiple myeloma. The rib change described here is helpful in the differential diagnosis, but is far from pathognomonic. The expanding rib lesion with a low-density soft-tissue mass around it is very suggestive of multiple myeloma. This does not mean that osteolytic metastasis cannot produce this process. However, most cases are like that of the patient (UX-12) who had cancer of the breast; the destructive lesion produced a fracture and there was subsequent healing. In multiple myeloma pathological fractures occur, but there is considerable hemorrhage around them; this produces much of the soft-tissue density described.

Multiple myeloma involves those areas that are very rich in bone marrow, and tends to involve the cortex only by extension. A radiograph of the spine is helpful in the differential diagnosis since multiple myeloma tends to involve the vertebral bodies to a greater extent than it does the vertebral pedicle. Multiple myeloma tends to avoid the mandible, but does involve the cranial vault rather extensively. There-

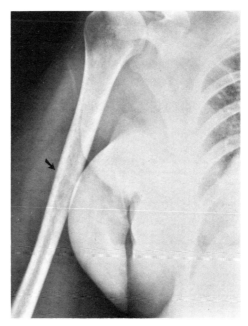

Case UX-15

fore, if one has multiple radiographs one can usually make a diagnosis of multiple myeloma with reasonable accuracy. Final diagnosis: Multiple myeloma involving scapula, humerus, and ribs.

Case UX-15 is that of a 53-year-old woman admitted because of a swollen arm. There was redness present, but little increase in temperature.

The radiograph of the humerus shows a very fine type of bone destruction associated with some periosteal elevation. The solid arrow points to some elevation of the periosteum. This is a minimal finding. The punctate areas of bone loss are scattered over a large area, and the soft-tissue density seen in the axilla is the patient's breast. On skeletal survey other parts of the bony skeleton were involved.

The differential diagnosis here must include osteomyelitis, as well as metastatic

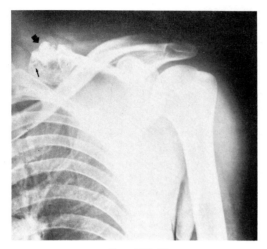

Case UX-16

disease. However, if it is metastatic disease, the process is certainly different than those seen previously. Most of the changes here are cortical with subperiosteal infiltration. It is a rule of thumb that if a bone lesion looks like osteomyelitis and clinically as well as radiographically there is some evidence for osteomyelitis, lymphoma must be considered the differential

diagnosis. In this case, the patient also had enlarged lymph nodes. These were biopsied and proved to be lymphosarcoma. Infrequently, lymphoma, usually Hodgkins disease, can produce osteoblastic changes. Final diagnosis here is lymphomatous involvement of bone. The case is presented primarily to make the point that it is difficult to differentiate a malignant process in bone from an infectious process.

Case UX-16 is that of a 35-year-old man who was admitted with an unusual asymptomatic bump on his back. Duration of the pathological process was unknown.

The shoulder radiograph shows an area of gross pathology involving the upper medial portion of the scapula. Here a large bony projection extends out from the ridge of the scapula. A dense sclerotic cap is seen at the superior portion, as evidenced by the heavy closed arrow. The small delicate closed arrow points to a small cystic area seen in the body of the mass. There is no appreciable deformity of the rib cage; and this mass while attached to and blending with the scapula, apparently does not alter the margin of the rib cage.

The pathology here is characteristic of an osteochondroma or cartilaginous exostosis. The radiolucent areas are cartilage arrests within the bony mass. The dense portion of the mass represents amorphous calcification and bone. These tumors are always larger than suspected radiographically, since there is usually a large cartilage component on the superior aspect (cap) of the lesion.

Final diagnosis is osteochondroma of the scapula. These tumors are generally considered to be benign. However, when they arise from a flat bone they have a 2%

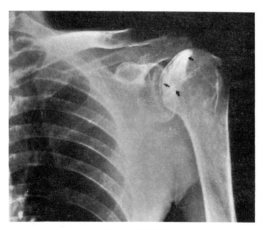

Case UX-17

to 6% incidence of malignant transformation. Certainly if there is evidence clinically of growth or pain, an excision biopsy is required. Lesions near the central axis of the body (spine) should be closely observed; a malignant transformation is more likely here than in those lesions that are peripheral in the extremities.

Case UX-17 is a 56-year-old man that was admitted to the orthopedic clinic with pain and discomfort in the shoulder. The patient was a known alcoholic.

The radiographs of the shoulder in the AP projection show an unusually dense humeral head. The curved dense arrows point to the margins of the chalky-appearing density within the humeral head. The trabeculations are still visible for the most part, but the bone appears to be very compact. The inferior curved arrow also demonstrates an irregular line that extends to the articular surface of the humerus. Here there appears to be a break in the cortex, suggesting a fracture line. The third arrow, a more slender solid arrow, points to the surface of the compact bone of the humeral head, which appears to be covered by a thin shell of bone with 1.0 mm of radiolucent space between the shell and the compact bone. The joint space is not altered. The scapula appears to be uninvolved. The chest and ribs are considered normal.

This is a classical radiographic picture of avascular necrosis of the humeral head. With the reduced blood supply the bone dies and tends to become chalky in appearance, and microscopic fractures occur. As a result of the fractures there is some actual impaction of the surface of the bone, and therefore we see not a shell over the top of the humerus, but a normal edge of the articular margin with the more central part of the humeral head impacted.

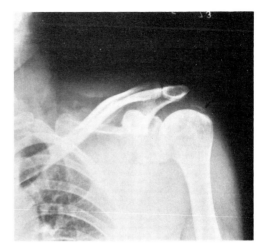

Case UX-18

This entity in adults is associated with alcoholism or with chronic use of steroids and other less frequent causes. With corrective therapy, some of these cases are reversible. Others require surgical intervention as they lead to degenerative arthritis.

Case UX-18 is a 40-year-old woman who was seen because of severe shoulder pain. The pain was of relatively short duration. It was much worse when elevating or rotating the arm such as might result from an attempt to brush or comb her hair.

The radiographic features are classical in their appearance. There are linear soft calcifications seen in the region of the supraspinatous groove. All other features of the shoulder are unremarkable. Final diagnosis: Calcific tendinitis of supraspinatus tendon.

Case UX-19 is a 67-year-old woman, who suffered from generalized rheumatoid arthritis. Changes were more marked in her hands and feet, but she did have considerable loss of function in her shoulder.

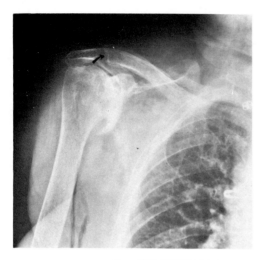

Case UX-19

The AP film of the shoulder reveals classical changes of rheumatoid arthritis. Rheumatoid arthritis characteristically destroys cartilage and produces bone erosions. The joint space between the glenoid and the humerus is virtually destroyed. As a result of the cartilage loss, there is considerable reactive change in the glenoid, and along the articular surface of the humerus. Cystic changes are not a striking feature here, but there is generalized demineralization of bone. The trabecular pattern, while it remains, is poorly defined in the area of the glenoid neck and inferior margin of the glenoid. The dark curved arrow is directed toward the end of the clavicle. There are a number of erosive changes that occur with rheumatoid arthritis. The inferior margin of the distal clavicle frequently is eroded to the point where it has a "sharpened stick" appearance. Such is not the case here where the joint space at the acromioclavicular joint is reasonably well preserved.

Rheumatoid arthritis is usually accompanied by some soft-tissue atrophy. This is not evident in this instance, but other joint areas tend to show this before the shoulder. The lung, in this instance, remains clear, showing little or no evidence of rheumatoid fibrosis. Final diagnosis: Rheumatoid arthritis of the shoulder, with generalized demineralization of bone and cartilage destruction.

Case UX-20

Case UX-20 is somewhat similar to case UX-19 in that there is generalized demineralization of bone. However, in this instance there is preservation of the cartilage joint space between the glenoid and humerus. There is also no evidence of narrowing at the acromioclavicular joint. In fact, the distal portion of the clavicle has a fluted appearance with some fine serration of bone. It gives the appearance of loss of the articular end of the clavicle.

Slight cortical bone absorption is noted at the inferior margin of the humeral neck, and in the region of the supraspinatous groove. The lungs remain clear and the ribs show nothing but demineralization.

The final diagnosis here is that of secondary hyperparathyroidism. The patient is known to have chronic renal failure. She has been undergoing dialysis for nearly four years.

The differential diagnosis between rheumatoid arthritis and hyperparathyroidism, primary or secondary, may present some difficulties. However, there are some fundamental differences that we have tried to point out here. The most important rule is that rheumatoid arthritis is a disease that produces local cartilage destruction and marginal bone erosion on both sides of the acromioclavicular joint. The demineralization that accompanies rheumatoid arthritis is the result of dis-

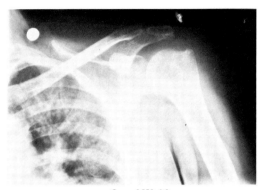

Case UX-20

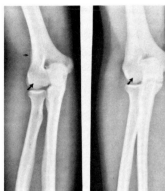

Case UXE-1

use. On the other hand, hyperparathyroidism is a systemic disease that results in loss of calcium from bone with much demineralization, but in general the cartilage is undamaged. The marginal bone changes that are seen in hyperparathyroidism are due to actual cortical reabsorption, but usually only the clavicular side of the acromioclavicular joint is involved.

ELBOW

Since rotation of the forearm and wrist (supination and pronation) is part of elbow function, the elbow joint is more complicated than a simple hinged joint. The standard hinged motion of the elbow takes place primarily between the ulna and the humerus, with pronation and supination occurring between the radius and its articulations with the ulna and humerus. The elbow actually consists of three functioning joints; the humerus and the ulna, the humerus and the radius, and the radius and the ulna.

CASE PRESENTATIONS

Case UXE-1

The normal adult elbow that is presented here will not be described in great detail, but it will be used as a reference from time to time. The sloping solid arrow is pointing toward the lateral condyle of the humerus. This is formed from the capitulum epiphysis and may also be referred to as the capitulum. Its importance lies in its relationship to the radial head. The radial head is always directed toward this prominence of the humerus regardless of the patient's position or projection of the radiograph.

The only other arrow used is to point out a variant in a normal elbow. This small solid arrow points to the lateral margin of the distal humerus. Here, attention is called to a very thin line that looks like a periosteal elevation. This is frequently a confusing finding in the AP or the oblique projection. It represents only a thin edge of the bone projected laterally. It is of no significance, except to be recognized as a

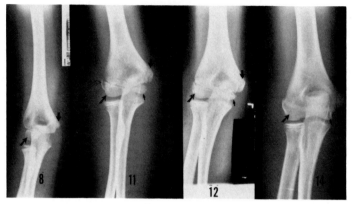

Case UXE-2

normal finding. As we encounter abnormal findings about the elbow, you will want to return to the film of the normal elbow for comparison.

In general, we prefer three views of the elbow; the AP, the lateral, and the oblique. A number of radiology offices, however, take only an AP and a lateral view—which in general constitutes an adequate study. The oblique view simply opens the radial head to better visualization and offers a slightly different perspective of the bone trabecular pattern in the intercondylar portion of the distal humerus.

Case UXE-2

The film is actually a composite of the AP radiographs of the elbow in four individuals of differing ages. This is presented to help clarify the development and the maturation of the structures about the elbow. During the period in life when the epiphyses are open, evaluation of the elbow probably produces more variability and more confusion to the part-time or learning radiologist than any other joint area.

The films presented here are AP projections of four boys aged 8, 11, 12, and 14. Similar types of arrows are used to direct your attention to the development process of a given area. The medial epicondylar epiphysis is designated by a short heavy solid arrow directed downward. Its position, growth, and maturation is seen over this 6-year interval.

The capitulum, which is the portion of the humerus that articulates with the radial head, is indicated by a solid dark arrow with a sloping base. It is clearly defined as a rounded structure in the initial film at age 8 and gradually changes to a smooth articular condyle, as seen in the adult.

The small solid arrow is directed toward the trochlea, which is the epiphysis of the medial condyle of the humerus. The epiphyseal center is seen first on the film of the 11-year-old. This center is roughly triangular in shape and presents many variable appearances. On the film of the 12-year-old, it is moderately fragmented. This is a feature that can be considerably more dramatic than is shown here and still be normal. By the time the child is

14, the trochlea and the capitulum have fused together and are being molded into very respectable articular condyles similar to that seen in the adult.

Arrows were not used to point to the radial head. Clearly its growth and maturation are evident and even at 14 the epiphyseal line is still open.

If the growth and the development of a bony area are understood, radiographs presented following trauma will be less confusing. There is a tendency to radiograph the opposite side for comparison when trauma occurs. This should not be necessary. Certainly the diagnostic yield in radiographing untraumatized extremities is zero, and if we are to keep the radiation exposure to a minimum, persons interpreting radiographs should be so familiar with the growth and development of areas that comparison views are unnecessary. Of course some confusing cases may require a single comparison view, but it should not be routine.

Another normal variant is indicated on the elbow of the 11-year-old by an open arrow. This is the epiphysis of the lateral epicondyle of the distal humerus. It appears as a vertical line and is frequently mistaken for an avulsion fracture. This epiphysis is relatively variable in its appearance and is usually present for approximately two years before it fuses to the capitulum.

Case UXE-3

Case UXE-3 is a 55-year-old woman who had fallen on her outstretched hand. She was complaining bitterly of pain in the elbow at the time of examination. There was modest restriction of motion.

The radiograph is presented for two reasons. First, it shows a relatively subtle vertical fracture line in the radial head.

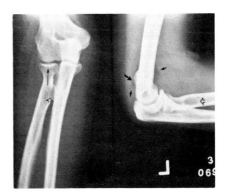

Case UXE-3

This vertical fracture line is indicated by the solid long slender dark arrow in the AP projection. There is no appreciable displacement of the fragments.

The second reason for presenting the film is to demonstrate the displacement of the fat pads about the elbow. The posterior fat pad evidenced by a heavy dark arrow posterior to the distal humerus and a small vertically directed black arrow just posterior to the elbow joint. This fat pad normally sits in the olecranon fossa and is not visible in either the AP or the lateral projection. However, when intracapsular hemorrhage or fluid develops, as occurs in virtually all fractures, blood occupies the joint space and the fat is displaced outward. Visualization of the posterior fat pad with trauma should be construed as indicating a fracture even if no fracture line is seen. We will frequently recommend that the elbow be supported and that the films be repeated in seven to ten days, for we know fractures may undergo some marginal bone absorption and the fracture line becomes more evident after a period.

The anterior fat pad is of similar significance. It is seen on a normal elbow, but is usually in a more vertical position than is seen here. Our rule of thumb is that if the anterior fat pad is displaced more than 30° from the humerus it is considered to represent edema or an intracapsular effusion. It has a triangular shape.

The open-faced arrows point to an area that is sometimes confusing in elbow films. In the lateral film of the elbow there appears to be a hole in the radius, just above the arrow. This, of course, is not a hole, but a relatively radiolucent portion of the radius as seen through the radial tuberosity. The open arrow in the AP projection points to the same area. The cortex of the radius is thinned as the tuberosity forms. Final diagnosis here is that of a vertical fracture line in the radial head with an intracapsular effusion, clearly demonstrating displacement of the posterior fat pad.

Case UXE-4

Case UXE-4 is a 5-year-old boy who was hit by an automobile. He sustained multiple skeletal injuries. A single radiograph is presented here. A film at right angles to this was obtained. However, it was not considered to be important for our usage here.

There is an obvious fracture of the proximal ulna. This fracture presents no diagnostic challenge and is not even identified

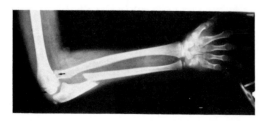

Case UXE-4

by arrows. A second injury, which is fully as important, probably more important in the long run, is the dislocation of the radial head. Recall that on all normal views of the elbow the radial head is directed toward the capitulum. This is true regardless of the radiographic projection or position of the patient. A small black solid arrow points to the posterior portion of the capitulum of the humerus. A second similar arrow is directed down the neck of the radius to indicate its directional plane. It is evident that there is at least a 2-cm dislocation of the radial head from its usual direction.

The mechanism of the force is not difficult to envision. It most likely was a direct blow to the proximal ulna with some pronation of the wrist resulting in a tear of the supporting structures about the elbow. Final diagnosis: Fracture of the ulna with associated dislocation of the proximal radius (Monteggia's fracture, dislocation).

Case UXE-5

Case UXE-5 is a 3-year-old girl who was brought to the emergency room following a fall. There was obvious swelling and refusal by the patient to move the elbow.

Radiographs of the elbow in the AP and the lateral projections show the fracture line running through the condyle of the distal humerus. A solid black arrow points to the rather indistinct fracture line in the olecranon fossa. A slight break in the cortex is seen on the medial side of the distal humerus. There is also considerable swelling on the medial side of the elbow.

The lateral view shows more clearly the bony fragment extending posteriorly. The solid dark arrow on the flexion side of the elbow is directed toward the fracture line. The second solid arrow directed toward the humerus from the posterior is identifying the displaced posterior olecranon fat pad, which lies nearly 5 mm posterior to the bony fragment.

Supracondylar or intracondylar fractures of the distal humerus are the most common fractures about the elbow in children. As a general rule a positive fat pad sign in a preadolescent child is a supracondylar or intracondylar fracture of the distal humerus until proven otherwise—just as a positive fat pad in an adult usually means a radial head fracture until proven otherwise.

There is very little alteration in alignment, although the distal fragment is displaced slightly posterior. The length of the humerus has not been significantly altered. It is evident that with flexion of the elbow the triceps tendon will improve the position of the distal fragment. Final diagnosis: Intracondylar fracture of the distal humerus.

Case UXE-6

Case UXE-6 is a 10-year-old boy who fell on his elbow while playing. He was admitted to the emergency room with a markedly swollen and painful elbow.

The radiographs of the elbow clearly show soft-tissue swelling over the medial side of the distal humerus. The medial epicondylar epiphysis has been displaced downward and laterally. The lateral film does not show this epiphyseal center; therefore, it has not been significantly displaced either forward or backward. The open-faced arrow is directed toward the epiphysis. A very tiny shell of bone is seen in the space between the epiphyseal center and the distal humerus. This represents a periosteal tear from the metaphysis. Other features of the elbow joint are not remarkable. The radial head is

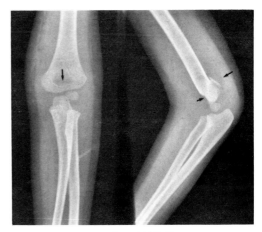

Case UXE-5

normally directed in each view. It is surprising that there is not a well-defined posterior fat pad, but one is not seen here.

Avulsion of the medial epicondylar epiphysis is a relatively frequent injury in children. It is an important one since it does involve a growth center. The displacement of the epiphyseal center varies considerably. The displacement here is minimal. It can be displaced to the point where the entire epiphyseal center is free in the joint space. If this occurs, it will act as a foreign body and produce locking of the elbow. Since a growth plate is in-

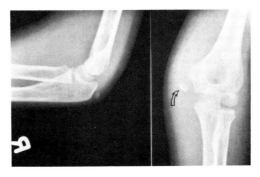

Case UXE-6

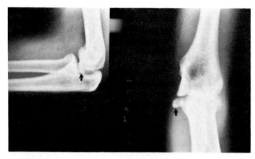

Case UXE-7

volved, surgical pinning is not usually done. However, if the epiphyseal center is free in the joint space, more aggressive therapy may be needed. Final diagnosis: Avulsion of the medial epicondylar epiphysis.

Case UXE-7

Case UXE-7 is a 16-year-old boy who had been injured a year before. He was now complaining of intermittent locking of the elbow.

This case is a follow-up or a sequel to Case UXE-6 in which there was a recent

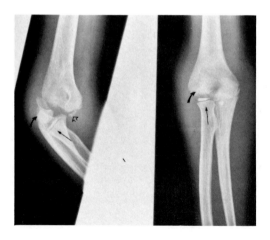

Case UXE-8

fracture dislocation of the medial epicondylar epiphysis.

The heavy dark arrow points toward the epiphysis in each projection. It is noted in the AP view and is loose in the joint space. In the lateral projection it is superimposed on the ulna and the radial head. The distal humerus is flattened on the medial side. This represents an alteration in the growth pattern of the distal humerus. It is amazing that the epiphysis has remained viable, even as a loose fragment in the joint space. This is frequently the situation. Final diagnosis: Old fracture dislocation of the medial epicondylar epiphysis with the epiphysis free in the joint space, acting as a loose body.

Case UXE-8

Case UXE-8 is a 10-year-old boy who had suffered a fall. The radiographs are rotated so that we have neither a true AP nor a true lateral view. This is frequently the case when a severe injury occurs about the elbow; however, landmarks are identifiable and the significant injury can be identified.

The dark long slender arrow follows the direction of the radius, with the point directed toward the radial head. This arrow is placed principally for direction. The curved arrows are directed toward the capitulum, which in the semi-AP projection is superimposed on the distal humerus. In the oblique projection, the capitulum is not aligned with the radial head, but is displaced posteriorly and is associated with an avulsion fracture of the distal humerus.

The open-faced arrow on the oblique projection points toward some bone fragments. The presence of these does not represent an additional injury, but is a developing trochlear epiphysis that is unusually fragmented. This is not part of the patient's injury. There is a rather marked soft-tissue swelling.

The final diagnosis is that of a fracture of the distal humerus, which involves the epiphysis or the capitulum. Since there is a fragmented metaphysis with it, it would be classed as a Salter type II epiphyseal fracture. (See chart #1, page 221.)

Case UXE-9

Case UXE-9 is a 60-year-old man complaining of stiffness and locking of the elbow.

The important pathology is obvious. There are multiple bony ossicles seen in the joint space. They are principally noted on the anterior side of the elbow, although at least one is superimposed on the olecranon when viewed in the lateral projection.

There is joint space narrowing between the radius and humerus, and there is minimal spurring on the medial articular process of the proximal ulna. These findings are considered degenerative in origin.

The final diagnosis is osteochondromatosis of the elbow. There is some associated osteoarthritis. There was no known history of trauma, which is one of the stimuli for the formation of osteochondroma. Others result from proliferations of the synovial lining of the joint space, and still others are unknown in their cause. The present film does show the limits of the elbow joint space. It extends farther up the distal humerus than we ordinarily expect. It also stops at the radial neck, and in the mid portion of the olecranon, as viewed laterally.

Cases UXE-10 through UXE-12

If we were to present the many radiographic manifestations of congenital anomalies here, we would soon lose sight of our goal to present only frequent radiographic diagnoses. However, we will demonstrate three such cases of congenital variations about the elbow.

Case UXE-10 is a 5-year-old girl admitted to the orthopedic clinic because of difficulty in pronation and supination of the hand.

A single lateral radiograph is presented here since this shows the important defect. In our discussion of the lateral elbow, we made the point that the radial head is

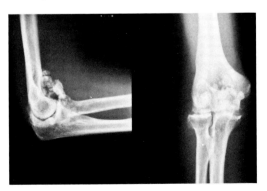

Case UXE-9

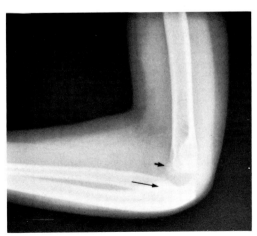

Case UXE-10

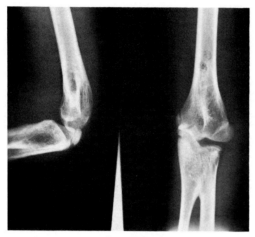

Case UXE-11

always directed toward the capitulum. This is true even in poorly positioned films. Here the long slender arrow is in mid portion of the shaft of the proximal radius, and the arrow points toward the head. The short dark arrow points to the

capitulum. There is nearly 2 cm misalignment, with the radial head directed posteriorly.

The final diagnosis is congenital posterior dislocation of the radial head. This may occur as a single anomaly or it may occur with multiple other anomalies such as the Nail-Patellar syndrome, Cornelia de Lange syndrome, or even multiple cartilaginous exostosis. When this anomaly is found, look for other pathological processes, particularly in the skeleton and kidneys.

Case UXE-11 is a 10-year-old boy who was also having difficulty with pronation and supination. The radiographs of the elbow clearly show the reason for the problem.

No arrows are needed on this study. There is complete fusion with bridging of the bone trabecular pattern between the radius and ulna. This may also be an isolated congenital anomaly, or it could be secondary to cross-healing fractures or even healing infectious disease. This finding is usually congenital and isolated. Repairing this anomaly has presented quite a challenge to orthopedic surgeons over the years. Unfortunately, results of treatment are frequently less than desirable, and if the deformity is established to be a congenital one, it is usually left alone.

Case UXE-12 is a young adult who was admitted to the emergency room because of trauma. The finding here is an incidental one. The large dark arrow is directed toward a bony process on the flexion side of the distal humerus.

This is a supracondyloid process. It is a vertical structure that appears on the anterior surface of the humeral shaft in approximately 1% of persons of European extraction. It is rarely associated with symptoms, but may be associated with

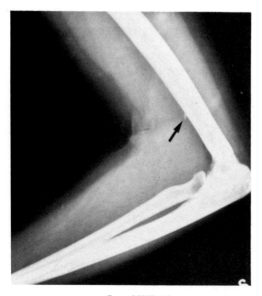

Case UXE-12

pressure on the median nerve. It is shown here only to be identified and is not to be confused with other entities.

HAND AND WRIST

CASE PRESENTATIONS

Case UXH-1

Case UXH-1 is the radiograph of a normal adult male. It is presented principally for review of anatomical detail about the wrist. It will also be of value in noting growth and development when compared to subsequent films of children and adolescents.

The following letters are used as labels for the carpal bones on each of the films presented:

GM--greater multangular

LM--lesser multangular

C--capitate

H--hamate

T--triquetrium

P--pisiform

L--lunate

N--navicular

These carpal bones are labeled in each projection to give the best possible idea of their position in that projection. In some instances, there is so much superimposition of bony structure that labeling seemed inappropriate.

Case UXH-2

Case UXH-2 is a male infant two and a half years of age. His film differs markedly from that of the adult. In addition to the distal radial epiphysis, there are only two carpal bones identified—the hamate and

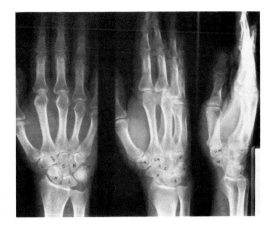

Case UXH-1

the capitate. The heads of the metacarpals are forming. The epiphysis at the base of the thumb metacarpal has not yet formed. There are small flat epiphyses at the base of the proximal phalanges.

The small dark arrow is directed toward the provisional zone of calcification. This occurs at all epiphyseal centers. It is directed toward the distal radius, where it is broad and rather indistinct. It is generally more dense than the adjacent metaphysis since it is here that the calcium

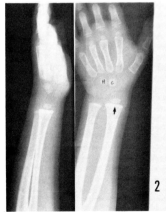
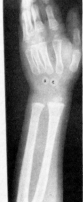

Case UXH-2

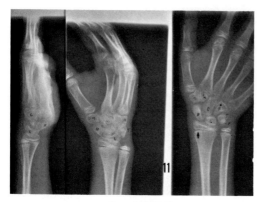

Case UXH-3

is being deposited. It is then converted to bone. This is the way bones grow in length. While there is no question as to the shape and identity of bony structures in the hand and the forearm, it is quite apparent that these structures are immature.

Case UXH-3

Case UXH-3 is an 11-year-old girl. Certainly there has been a great deal of maturation by age 11. Most of the adult carpal bones are easily identified, only their shapes are more immature and ovoid compared with the well-differentiated

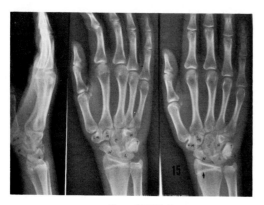

Case UXH-4

adult bony structure. The small dark arrow is again directed toward the provisional zone of calcification, which is now much sharper in its definition and more localized at the epiphyseal plate than was seen in the infant.

The lateral view shows the distal ulna to be dorsal in its position. This is not abnormal, but is a reflection of positioning at the time the radiograph was made.

Case UXH-4

Case UXH-4 is a 15-year-old girl. The epiphysis at the distal radius has not yet closed. The epiphyseal line is sharp and the provisional zone of calcification well defined. The distal radius and ulna are the only remaining epiphyseal centers still open in this patient. A sesamoid at the distal end of the thumb metacarpal is well developed. The sesamoid that will subsequently appear at the interphalangeal joint of the thumb has not yet appeared. Virtually all of the carpal bones have the mature contour, and from the appearance of the epiphyseal centers one would expect them to close within the next 12 to 18 months.

The hand and wrist have a complicated series of joints since so many bony structures are involved. The radius, the ulna, the metacarpals, and the phalanges are basically tubular bone. The carpal bones tend to be rounded and peculiarly shaped in order to produce the flexibility and motion so necessary for that joint. Fractures of the carpal bones rarely occur in children. Since these bones are high in cartilage content, they tend to move or roll with trauma and therefore dislocate more frequently than fracture. After growth and molding of the carpal bones is completed, these bones are subject to the same traumatic effects as other bony structures.

However, because of their unique position, we rarely see fractures of the capitate, hamate, and lunate. We do, however, see dislocations of the lunate. The navicular is the most frequently fractured carpal bone, the lunate the most frequently dislocated. This does not imply that fractures and dislocations cannot occur in other carpal bones.

The hand is not only subject to trauma, but also mirrors many endocrine and metabolic changes. Case UX-20 was shown as an example of hyperparathyroidism. In fact, the hand is probably the most critical place to look for this process. We will not present another example of hyperparathyroidism in the Hand section, but we will bring out other systemic changes that are seen. As a general rule, the hand and wrist are the most sensitive areas to determine bone age. Many standards are available for comparison, and the multiple bony structures that are present in this relatively concentrated space give an excellent sampling of bone growth development and general metabolism.

Case UXH-5

Case UXH-5 is an elderly female who had fallen on her outstretched hand, and was admitted to the emergency room with a deformed wrist.

The fracture of the radius is quite apparent. There is impaction of fragments along the fracture line. Instead of a sharply defined fracture line, there is deformity, impaction, and fragmentation of bone. In the lateral view the long slender arrow is directed dorsally. The arrow is placed to show the angle of the articular surface of the radius, which is dorsally tilted nearly 30°. In the AP projection it will be noted that the articular margin of the radius sets proximal to the distal portion of the ulna.

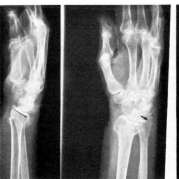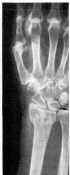

Case UXH-5

A solid dark arrow on the AP film parallels the distal portion of the ulna, and is directed toward a fracture of the ulnar styloid. The fracture of the ulnar styloid has little in the way of therapeutic or physiologic importance, but it is a classic component of the Colles' fracture.

There is moderate demineralization of bone, but no other significant changes are identified. Final diagnosis: Colles' fracture of the wrist. Colles' fracture must include a fracture through the distal radius with dorsal tilting of the articular margin, and a fracture of the ulnar styloid. As a general rule there is shortening of the radius, which is one of the most important aspects of this fracture. For good results from treatment, the length of the radius needs to be restored, and the articular angle tilted slightly forward.

Case UXH-6

Case UXH-6 is a 58-year-old woman injured in a fall.

On first surveying the radiograph one has the feeling that this is a comminuted Colles' fracture. There is a small questionable traumatic ossicle at the tip of the ulnar styloid. There is some loss of length of the radius. More importantly, however,

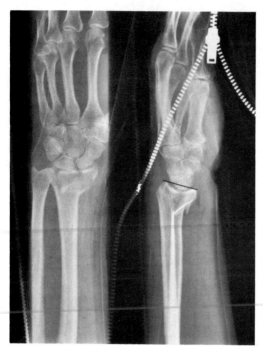

Case UXH-6

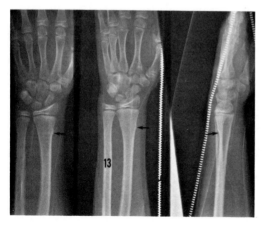

Case UXH-7

the lateral film indicates that the articular angle of the wrist, instead of being displaced upward as would be the case with a Colles' fracture, is tilted downward approximately 10 to 15 degrees. This is reverse displacement from that seen in Colles' fractures. This fracture is referred to as a reverse Colles' fracture, or for those who prefer eponyms it is a "Smith's fracture."

The reverse Colles' fracture does not occur as frequently as a Colles' fracture, its significance however, is much the same. These patients are not casted with the wrist in flexion, but depending on the patient's condition, are either casted with the wrist straight or modestly dorsiflexed.

Case UXH-7

Case UXH-7 is a 13-year-old boy who had fallen from a horse. He was admitted through the emergency room, and was wearing a plastic air splint. Radiographs were made through the splint.

The radiographs of the wrist and the forearm are AP, lateral, and oblique. The zipper that is clearly evident is part of the air splint. Linear folds over the hand and wrist are dressing for the comfort and safety of the patient. The splint and dressing are not altered. The solid dark arrow is directed toward the significant pathology. The margin of the radius at a point approximately 2 cm proximal to the epiphyseal line is altered. It is best visualized in the lateral view where there is clearly a wrinkle in the dorsal cortex. The ulna is uninvolved.

Other bony structures are consistent with the patient's age and show no evidence of injury.

The final diagnosis is a torus fracture of the distal radius. This is an incomplete fracture involving principally cortical buckling. It occurs only in persons with considerable elasticity in their bony structure. If this patient had been older, he would probably have a Colles' fracture rather than this simple fracture. It is one of the most frequently seen fractures of children. Therapy is supportive and protective. Good results are anticipated.

Cases UXH-8 and UXH-9

Cases UXH-8 and UXH-9 show the thumbs of two different patients. Case UXH-8 is an adult as evidenced by closure of all epiphyses and the presence of mature, well-formed bony structures. Case UXH-9 is a 15-year-old boy who had fallen. Both patients have sustained fractures at the base of the thumb metacarpal, however, the two cases are presented together since there are some very important differences.

The fracture in Case UXH-8 does extend into the articular surface and therefore, involves the joint space. As a result, there is loss of length of the thumb with the medial fragment lying high in position. Actually the medial fragment is occupying the normal position of the thumb, and the rest of the thumb has been displaced proximally. This is Bennett's fracture, which will require aggressive reduction in order to prevent degenerative disease in months and years to come.

Case UXH-9 shows a fracture at the base of the thumb metacarpal. This fracture does not enter the articular margin. The metacarpal shows very little displacement. The length of the thumb is reasonably well maintained. The joint surface remains smooth. The term "Bennett's fracture" has been used with virtually all fractures at the proximal end of the thumb metacarpal. More accurately it should be limited to those fractures that involve the

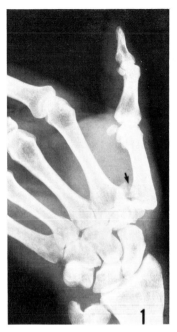

Case UXH-8

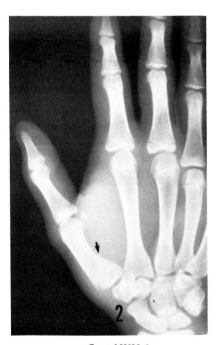

Case UXH-9

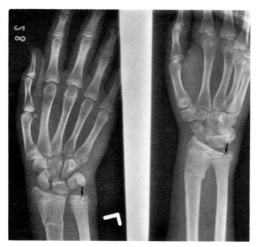

Case UXH-10

The study is primarily presented because of the unque type of injury shown in the distal ulnar epiphysis. The solid arrow is directed toward the fracture line that splits the epiphyseal plate. This is an excellent example of the Salter type III fracture (See chart 1, page 221).

Cases UXH-11 through UXH-13

These three cases are examples of fractures of the carpal navicular. This can be a diffiult diagnosis to make. Since the injury does carry a high nonunion rate, it is important to make the diagnosis as promptly as possible.

The navicular is the most frequently fractured carpal bone. The fractures usually occur through the mid portion of the navicular, but fractures can occur at either end. We routinely take an oblique film of the wrist to open the navicular to radiographic examination. Even so, there are times when special views of the navicular are needed. The specialized view most frequently used is an AP projection of the wrist with the wrist in ulnar deviation. Unfortunately, if the radiographer is too vigorous with ulnar deviation, the fragments can be separated. This makes the diagnosis easy, but probably is harmful to the patient.

joint space. Case UXH-9 has only an undisplaced fracture at the base of the thumb metacarpal, a much less serious fracture than that of case UXH-8.

Case UXH-10

Case UXH-10 is a 12-year-old girl injured by a fall. The radiograph shows an obvious transverse fracture of the radius with wrinkling of the cortex and dorsal tilting. Very little loss of length is present.

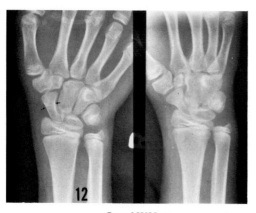

Case UXH-11

Case UXH-11 is a 12-year-old youngster with pain in the wrist following a fall.

The AP radiograph was made in slight ulnar deviation. A very faint fracture line is visible between the two small dark arrows in this view. The oblique film, which is usually very good at opening the navicular to our sudy, fails to show the fracture. Later, a more vigorous film in ulnar deviation separated the fragments and confirmed the diagnosis.

Case UXH-12 is a 28-year-old adult who had also fallen and had pain in the wrist.

The AP radiograph of the wrist shows an impacted-type fracture of the navicular with a line of increased density between the two small dark arrows. A radiolucent line is barely visible laterally. The oblique film does, in this instance, help us, and shows very clearly a radiolucent line at the articulation between the navicular and capitate. No additional views would be required.

Case UXH-13 is an 18-year-old youth who had injured his wrist several months previously. A fracture of the ulnar styloid is evidence of the old injury. In addition, there is an evident fracture in the carpal navicular, with some reabsorption of bone about the fracture line.

Tomograms are also shown here and are presented only to demonstrate the striking amount of bone absorption about the fracture line. The inferior insert, as evidenced by the small dark arrow, shows demineralization of the navicular extending along its lateral wall. A poorly defined fragment, which is somewhat increased in density, is seen in the fracture area.

As a general rule the term nonunion does not apply to fractures that are less than 6 months of age; and this fracture was slightly less than 6 months. However, it seems unlikely that this fracture will heal since the fragment of bone seen in the central portion of the navicular is dense, and there is associated local demineralization. Aseptic necrosis is a frequent complication of navicular fracture. Final diagnosis: Fracture of the carpal navicular with Case UXH-13 showing the effects of time and incomplete union.

Case UXH-14 through UXH-16

These three cases are typical examples of varying types of metacarpal fractures.

Case UXH-14 is that of a 24-year-old

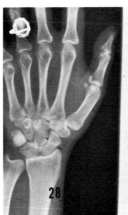
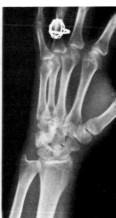

Case UXH-12

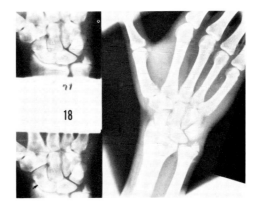

Case UXH-13

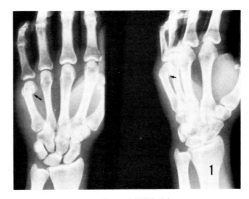

Case UXH-14

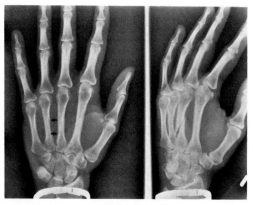

Case UXH-15

man who had been involved in a fight.

The fracture, as seen here, is a classic example of the type that results from a transmitted injury through the fist. This fracture has even been referred to as the "boxer's fracture" or the "fist-fight fracture." The fracture line is through the neck of the fifth metacarpal with the head tilted into the palm. This results in shortening of the fifth metacarpal and some distortion and angulation of the metacarpal. Restoration of the metacarpal length will be needed.

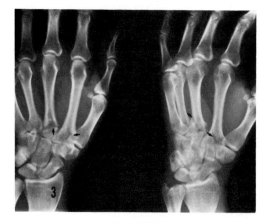

Case UXH-16

The second in our series of metacarpal fractures is a 20-year-old woman (Case UXH-15) injured in a car accident. This is the typical spiral fracture that occurs in the shaft of any long bone. In the AP projection arrows point to subtle changes that might be suspected of being fractures, but are certainly less than diagnostic. The oblique films clearly show the extensive fracture line. There is little or no displacement. Articular margins are not involved.

The third in our series of metacarpal fractures is a 38-year-old man (Case UXH-16) who had been involved in an auto accident. The fracture here is more subtle, but after it is identified by means of the solid arrows, it too is clearly evident. It is difficult to identify the fracture line in the AP view. The oblique projection helps considerably. Lateral views are of value, but because of space they are not included here.

As was the case in our first example, there is some loss of length of the involved metacarpal. There is some angulation toward the palm of the hand. Reduction and restoration of length will improve the subsequent function of the hand.

Cases UXH-17 through UXH-20

Our next series of four films represents unusual fractures in the carpal bones.

Here is a good clinical rule of thumb: "A sprained ankle is a sprained ankle, but a sprained wrist is a fractured wrist." Therefore, look hard and carefully at all wrist injuries. It is for this reason that we are presenting these relatively infrequent injuries. These infrequent manifestations relate to bones that do not ordinarily fracture. It is always well to know unusual manifestations of common disorders. In this instance we are presenting fractures, a common disorder, but in this instance in some unusual locations.

Case UXH-17 is a 15-year-old boy with a painful wrist following a fall.

Growth and development are consistent with the stated age. The solid arrow is directed toward a fracture line in the triquetrum. It is best visualized in the oblique projection; however, it is barely visible in both the AP and lateral view. Note the rather marked soft-tissue swelling over the dorsum of the wrist.

Case UXH-18 is a 40-year-old man with a painful wrist following injury.

Multiple radiographs were taken of this patient before the tangential view of the pisiform actually demonstrated the fracture line extending from the articular margin to the surface. The break in the cortex is barely visible in the AP projection. There is no displacement.

Case UXH-19 is a 21-year-old man with a painful wrist after an auto accident. Only the AP projection shows the fracture of the heavy, bony structure of the capitate. The oblique view does show the articulation of the capitate with the lunate and navicular, but the fracture line is lost with this slight rotation.

Case UXH-20 is a 23-year-old man who hit a solid object with his fist.

This is a variation of the "boxer's fracture" (UXH-14) described previously. However, in this instance the force was transmitted through the fifth metacarpal without breaking it, down to the hamate where a shearing force fractured the lateral articular surface of the hamate. The fifth metacarpal remains with the small shallow bone, and is displaced toward the palm and proximally. In the AP view there is obvious forward angulation of the fifth metacarpal, and shortening of this digit. In the oblique view we see a portion of

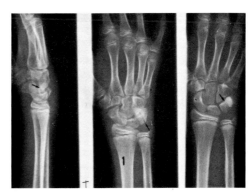

Case UXH-17

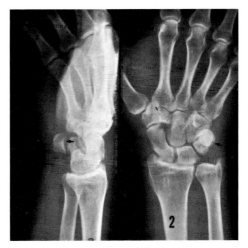

Case UXH-18

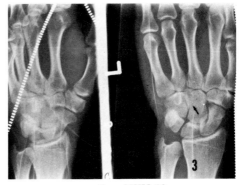

Case UXH-19

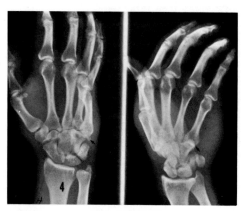

Case UXH-20

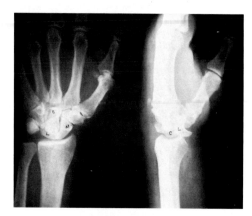

Case UXH-21

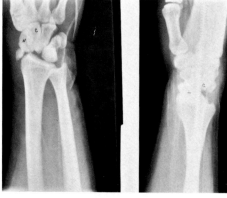

Case UXH-22

the hamate superimposed on the base of the fifth metacarpal.

Carpal bones may be dislocated as well as fractured. Dislocation, like fractures, can involve virtually any of the carpal bones. However, by far the most common dislocation in the wrist is one that involves the lunate.

Case UXH-21

Case UXH-21 is a 35-year-old man who had fallen from a scaffold. Marked swelling of the wrist is noted.

Radiographically, there is evident foreshortening of the wrist. The distance from the base of the metacarpals to the radius is relatively short. On more careful observation, it is noted that the capitate actually is seen superimposed on a portion of the lunate and the navicular. In the lateral view the lunate, instead of articulating with the radius has been dislocated toward the palm, and now is located in the periarticular tissues very much resembling a quarter moon. The capitate has fallen proximally and now articulates with the radius.

This is a classical semilunar dislocation.

Case UXH-22

Case UXH-22 is a 30-year-old man who fell on his extended wrist. The radiographs obtained are actually semioblique in each projection. However, the film that approximates an AP projection shows a fracture in the radial styloid, again with some modest foreshortening of the wrist. The lunate is lost from view, for it is superimposed on other bony structures. In the lateral view the lunate remains articulated with the distal radius and the dislocation is between the articulation of the capitate and lunate. The capitate now sets posterior to its normal position. It does not articulate with the radius for that position is still occupied by the lunate.

This is a classical perilunate dislocation with an associated fracture of the radial styloid.

Case UXH-23

Case UXH-23 is a 60-year-old man admitted to the hospital with a complaint of stiffening of the joints. Clinically the complaints seem referable to thickening and swelling of soft tissues rather than to actual joint disease.

The radiograph of the hand shows that the articular joint spaces have been well maintained, but that there is soft-tissue swelling and thickening about all joints. Some bony proliferation is noted at the proximal interphalangeal joint of the index finger; rather marked bony proliferation noted at the terminal tufts of all fingers. The bone trabecular pattern is rather coarse.

The final diagnosis was that of acromegaly. Changes in the hand as well as thickening of the heel pad (soft tissue) are quite characteristic of the disease. The hypertrophy of terminal tufts is seen in a high percentage of acromegalics.

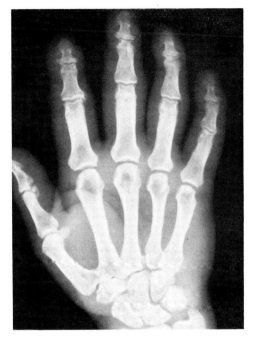

Case UXH-23

surface is quite tilted, rather than being relatively horizontal as would be expected in an adult.

Significant delay in bone age associated with the change in the articular angle at the wrist and general demineralization

Case UXH-24

Case UXH-24 is a 22-year-old woman. In the film, the fingers appear long and delicate. Bony structure is demineralized and since we have been given the age of 22 it is apparent that the bone age is quite retarded. The epiphyses of the distal radius and ulna are still open, and the epiphyses of the middle phalanges have barely closed. In addition, the articular angle of the radius with the carpal bones is more acute than is usually noted. The dark black lines along the articular alignment of the distal radius indicate that this

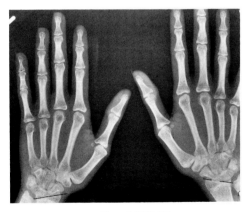

Case UXH-24

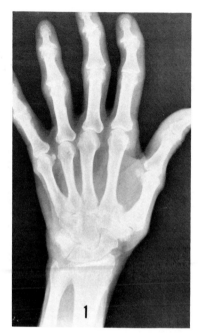

Case UXH-25

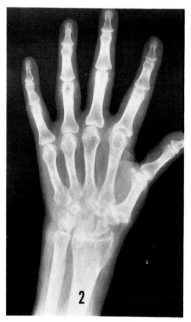

Case UXH-26

should mean Turner's syndrome (ovarian agenesis). This diagnosis was confirmed by the laboratory.

Cases UXH-25 and UXH-26

The radiographs of these two cases are presented together for their comparative value. Case UXH-25 is a 64-year-old man. Case UXH-26 is a 58-year-old woman. Both are patients on the rheumatology service complaining of "arthritis."

Case UXH-25 has osteoarthritis. Case UXH-26 has rheumatoid arthritis. Each patient shows some early and some late signs of their respective disease. A number of points are helpful in the differential diagnosis. In classical cases the two entities are easily separated. However, there are times when the two processes occur in the same patient, and the distinguishing features are much more difficult to ascertain. In general, osteoarthritis (degenerative arthritis) involves the distal interphalangeal joints and the articulation between the first or thumb metacarpal and the greater multangular. Unless the disease is extensive, it will generally spare the proximal interphalangeal joints, the metacarpal phalangeal joints, and the radial carpal articular joints.

Rheumatoid arthritis (atrophic arthritis) tends to initially and most severely involve the proximal interphalangeal joints, the carpal radial joints, and the metacarpal phalangeal joints. It tends to spare the distal interphalangeal joints. This distribution of the disease is a helpful place to start a differential diagnosis. Unfortunately, there are many individual exceptions.

In Case UXH-25 there are some classical osteoarthritic changes. The sclerosis of bone and the narrowing of the joint space with thickening of the adjacent bone seen at the articulation between the thumb metacarpal and the greater multangular is characteristic of this form of arthritis. The same can be said for the spur formation and lipping that has developed at the articular portion of the distal phalanx. The overall bone density in a patient with osteoarthritis is reasonably normal, with only slight periarticular demineralization.

Case UXH-26 demonstrates a number of classical features of rheumatoid arthritis. First, there is overall generalized demineralization of bone, with very intense demineralization of bone noted about the periarticular areas. This may be true even before there is joint space loss and bone erosion. Note, the proximal interphalangeal joint of the index finger, where the joint space is reasonably maintained, and no erosions are noted, but there is evidence of demineralization. The proximal interphalangeal joint of the third finger shows the same demineralization, but also shows a characteristic erosion of the articular margin of subchondral bone of the middle phalanx. The fourth proximal interphalangeal joint shows evidence of articular erosions on both the medial and lateral sides of the joint. Joint spaces here are only slightly narrowed.

At the level of the metacarpal phalangeal articulation of the index finger, the erosion is more striking and a large cystic-type area is noted in the head of the index metacarpal.

The carpal radial articulation is severely involved with a great deal of cartilage loss and erosion on the carpal bones to the point where the normal configuration is lost. The lunate is poorly defined, and the navicular appears triangular. There are also prominent cystic regions in the subchondral area of the distal radius. The ulna may show erosions on its distal aspect to the point where it has a "pencil" or "pointed-stick" contour. Soft-tissue shadows here are generally atrophic, except where there is an acute periarticular process, and there is some swelling. This is also noted at the index metacarpal-phalangeal joint.

The earliest radiographic sign of rheumatoid arthritis involves periarticular soft tissue swelling, and demineralization of bone. This is secondary to the inflammatory reaction in the synovium. The erosions of subchondral bone and the loss of cartilage are subsequent responses to this same synovial inflammatory process.

The films we are presenting do not show the end product of these arthritides. The subluxations and gross deformities of the hand and wrist that occur with rheumatoid arthritis are evident clinically as well as radiographically. If you have an understanding of the evolution of the process, these end stage deformities are not mysterious.

8

The Lower Extremity

PELVIS AND HIPS

Discussion of the lower extremity must begin with the pelvis and hips. Some discussion of the pelvis and hips was included with the films of the abdomen in the GI and Genitourinary sections. See also those sections.

CASE PRESENTATIONS

Case LX-1

Case LX 1, our model normal pelvis, is that of a 30-year-old woman. The contour and shape indicate that it is a female pelvis. The gynecoid contour of the true pelvis and the widely separated ischial spines are characteristically female.

The trabecular pattern of the bone varies with the stress that is transmitted through that bone. The femoral neck characteristically shows curvilinear stress-line patterns of a structure bearing considerable weight, while the iliac crest presents its trabecular pattern in a more punctate and disorganized fashion.

Arrows and numbers of varying types have been used to direct your attention to certain anatomical details. The open-faced large arrow is directed toward the intertrochanteric ridge on each side. The greater trochanter is seen at the top of this ridge. The lesser trochanter, which is

barely visible here, is an area of increased density at the inferior margin of the ridge. The femoral head is directed into the acetabulum, and the portion of the femur between the head and the intertrochanteric ridge is the femoral neck. The acetabulum is identified by short dark arrows. These arrows are directed from the soft tissues to the lateral edge of the acetabulum. The joint space width between the femoral head and the acetabulum is symmetrical and normal on each side. The gently curved arrows seen in the medial aspect of each pelvis point toward the ischial spines. These are important in the birth canal since they represent the critical level of the mid plane of the pelvis.

When the spines are seen in the lateral female pelvis radiograph, they identify the level of the cervix. In men, the spines are less important but are an anatomical landmark. The very short curved arrow used on the right (not on the left) is directed toward the pelvic wall and is the base of the ischial spine. The sharply curved arrows seen inferiorly are directed toward the descending ramus of the pubis as it approaches junction with the ischial tuberosity. The ovoid bone structure that extends laterally from the arrow and upward toward the medial femoral neck is the ischial tuberosity. Relatively long and delicate arrows point toward each sacro-

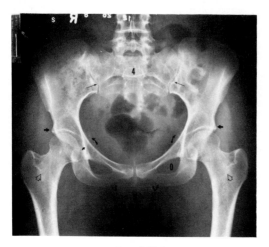

Case LX-1

iliac joint. The arrows point toward the lower portion of the sacroiliac joint. It is only the lower two thirds of the sacroiliac joint that contains a true synovial lining

The number 4 is placed on the promontory of the sacrum. The multiple grooves and margins of the sacrum are reasonably well outlined until the lower sacrum and coccyx are lost in the gas of the rectum. The study also shows the fifth lumbar body and a portion of the fourth. These

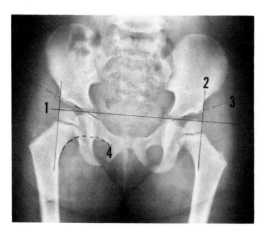

Case LX-2

have been reviewed in other sections.

The "0" seen on the left identifies the obturator foramen. One is present on each side; only the left side is labeled. A small isolated bone density is seen in the right proximal femur. This is in the proximal portion of the neck, just at the base of the femoral head. This is considered to be a sclerotic bone island and is of no great significance. The anterior and posterior margins of the acetabulum are seen superimposed on the medial portion of the femoral head and cast a faint line across the head, proximal to the bone island described.

Even though we are considering this a normal pelvis, we should comment that the hip joint is relatively shallow. The entire femoral head is not covered by the acetabular roof. Another way of describing this hip is to say that it represents half a lemon (cut across its long axis). A more desirable description of the acetabulum would be that of half an orange, with the acetabular roof completely covering the head of the femur.

Case LX-2

Case LX-2 is a three-year-old girl that we are presenting as having a normal pelvis. This film is presented not only to show the growth and development patterns of the pelvis, but to orient you to some basic lines that are used in pelvis evaluation. These lines are particularly helpful in pediatrics when trying to identify hip dislocation. They are also helpful in minor displacements in the adult pelvis secondary to trauma.

The femoral head epiphyses are well formed and symmetrical on each side. The epiphyseal line is running nearly at right angles to the weight-bearing axis of the body. The greater trochanter is seen only as a tiny epiphysis. The lesser trochanter is not yet formed. A defect in the descending ramus of the pubis just below the number 4 is simply an area of cartilage that has not been ossified. The line numbered 1 is the "Y" line of the pelvis. The line extends through the Y epiphyses of the acetabulum on each side. It should be at a right angle to the axis of the lumbar spine.

Line 2 is a line at 90 degrees from the Y line, placed in such a position that it drops through the lateral margin of the acetabulum. You will note that lines 1 and 2 cross and that the femoral head is in the inferior medial quadrant of the four quadrant intersect.

Line 3 is a line drawn through the slope of the acetabulum, and it measures or defines its slope. Line 4 is a curved line that extends from the inferior margin of the femoral neck through the roof of the obturator foramen to the inferior ramus of the pubis medially. This should be a smooth, unbroken line and is referred to as Shenton's line.

To evaluate the patient positioning on the pelvis film, the tip of the coccyx should be perfectly aligned or actually sitting in the superimposed symphysis pubis. If the coccyx is not seen this far down, it should be simply aligned with the pubis. We should also be seeing the femoral head epiphyses as sharp parallel lines for if the femur is flexed, this line will become distorted.

Case LX-3

Case LX-3 is a newborn girl. Clinically the infant was suspected of having a congenital dislocation of the left hip.

The lines drawn on the previous pediatric pelvis are not drawn for you here; however, they are easy to mentally con-

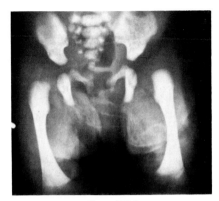

Case LX-3

struct. It is apparent that there is no ossification of the femoral head epiphysis; therefore, one can only surmise where it may be. However, by constructing the lines drawn previously, it is apparent that the left femoral shaft sits lateral in position, and that if there were a femoral head present it would not be in a medial quadrant of the intersect, but either in the lateral inferior or upper lateral quadrant. Shenton's line on the right, while separated by considerable cartilage, still can be drawn and appears smooth, while it is broken on the left.

A tentative diagnosis of congenital dislocation of the left hip is made. It should be stated that it is risky to make a diagnosis of congenital dislocation of the hip radiographically at this age. This is especially true if the infant was a breech delivery. With the stresses of breech delivery, the femurs may be lateral in position and will return to normal in a week to ten days. Apparently this child was not a breech delivery, so the diagnosis of congenital dislocation of the left hip is more firmly grounded. If there is doubt, the study should be repeated at a later date. No harm comes from a modest delay in treatment at this very early age.

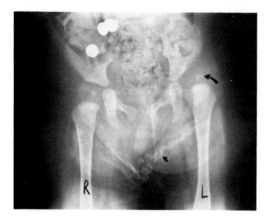

Case LX-4

Case LX-4

Case LX-4 is a 6-month-old boy, who, when seen by his pediatrician, was believed to have an abnormal left hip.

The AP radiograph of the pelvis is a classic demonstration of congenital dislocation of the left hip, sometimes referred to as a dysplastic hip. Our earlier example of a dislocated hip (Case LX-3) was a young infant, and the femoral head epi-

physes had not yet formed. These normally form at four to six months of age. The radiographic diagnosis of dislocation of the hip is easier and more reliable in this age group than in the infant.

The following signs establish the diagnosis.

One: The femoral head epiphysis is smaller on the side involved than on the normal side.

Two: The femoral head epiphysis is not in the medial lower quadrant of the intersect, as described with Case LX-2, but is in the upper lateral quadrant.

Three: The left femur is higher in position than the right.

Four: The acetabular shelf on the left is more sloping than the right.

Five: The entire left ilium is more hypoplastic or somewhat less developed than the ilium on the right.

Final diagnosis: Congenital dislocation of the left hip.

Case LX-5

Case LX-5 is a 40-year-old man who was involved in an auto accident. There are multiple fractures here. Each represents a relatively frequent type of bony injury. The pelvis is a series of bony ovals. Whenever an oval is fractured, the fracture usually occurs in two places. There are, of course, exceptions to this rule, such as single undisplaced fracture, but whenever one fracture is found, a second should be looked for. For example, the left pubic arch in this patient shows an apparent fracture at the junction of the descending ramus of the pubis and the ischial tuberosity. This is indicated by the heavy sloping arrow. This is a frequent site of injury in the pubic ring, and one that can be

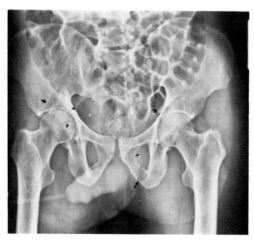

Case LX-5

quite subtle. In this instance, the second fracture is quite subtle and is at the inferior margin of the symphysis pubis, as indicated by a short dark arrow pointing toward the fracture line. The arrow lies in the obturator foramen.

The patient has bilateral acetabular fractures indicating that the force was probably transmitted upward through the femurs. Short heavy arrows indicate the fracture line on each side. On the right the fracture line is relatively wide, and shows only moderate distortion of the acetabular roof. Smaller arrows indicate multiple fracture lines through the acetabulum, indicating that this portion of the pelvis has been crumpled like an eggshell.

On the left a bony fragment projects into the pelvis. This is indicated by the heavy dark arrow. The acetabular margin appears intact. There is a questionable line seen through the mid portion of the acetabulum, superimposed on the femoral head. A point of interest on the left is the asymmetry of the lower portion of the sacroiliac joints. A dotted black line shows that the sciatic notch is continuous with the sacrum on the right, but on the left there is approximately 1 cm cephalad displacement of the ilium. Minimal asymmetry is noted at the crest of the ilium, and the lesser trochanter of each femur appears to be at the same vertical level. These somewhat contradictory findings suggest that additional studies will be needed before the probable diagnosis of separation of sacroiliac joint can be firmly established. The femurs appear intact. There is a catheter in the bladder. Moderate distention of the intestinal tract indicates a nonobstructive ileus.

Final diagnosis: Bilateral acetabular fractures. Fracture of the descending ramus of the pubis on the left (two places),

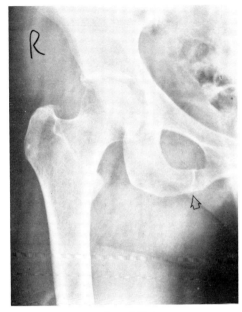

Case LX-6

probable left sacroiliac joint separation. Additional films, possibly even tomograms, will be needed to prove or disprove the sacroiliac injury.

Case LX-6

Case LX-6 is a 64-year-old woman admitted to the emergency room following a fall. She complained of pain in the hip.

Patients have trouble distinguishing the origin of bone pain. Most pain in the entire hemipelvis is referred to the patient's hip. Even clinicians examining patients may order films specifically designated for the hip, and find a fracture of the descending ramus of the pubis. The line of increased density in the descending ramus of the right pubis is identified by the open faced arrow. This is a classical location and fractures frequently appear in this area. It is probably the single most common fracture in the pelvis. While

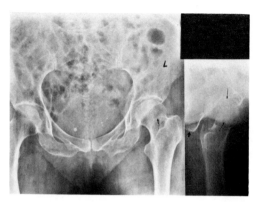

Case LX-7

painful, It carries a good prognosis. There may be a second fracture involving the obturator ring, but it is not identified here, nor was it seen on other films. Final diagnosis: Fracture of the descending ramus of the right pubis.

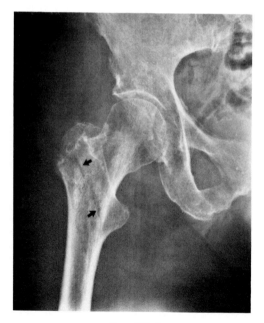

Case LX-8

Case LX-7

Case LX-7 is a 78-year-old woman who had fallen. The patient was admitted to the emergency room with pain in the left hip.

On the AP radiograph of the pelvis and hips, a small solid arrow points to a line of slightly increased density. Certainly this, in itself, is not enough to make a diagnosis of femoral neck fracture. However, there are other subtle signs seen on the film. The lesser trochanter on the left is much more evident than on the right, indicating external rotation of the leg. Shenton's line, which is perfectly smooth on the right, is broken on the left. The femoral neck also appears to be shorter on the left than on the right.

Of even more value is the lateral view. Note the two long solid black arrows. These arrows are not pointing toward a specific line or structure, but the arrow overlying the femoral neck identifies the alignment of the femoral neck, while the arrow pointing down the femoral head indicates general alignment and position of the head. There is evident angulation or posterior rotation of the femoral head.

All of the features mentioned above add up to make a diagnosis of an impacted femoral neck fracture on the left. These signs, once seen, are rather evident and the supportive signs (those signs other than the fracture line itself that indicates fracture) are extremely important in this case, and in all cases where the fracture is subtle.

Case LX-8

Case LX-8 is a 79-year-old woman that had fallen and was admitted to the emergency room with pain in the hip.

A single AP radiograph of the hip is presented here. It is sufficient for making the diagnosis. The arrows identify a fracture line running just posterior to the intertrochanteric ridge. The line extends down to the inferior margin of the femur. There is no appreciable displacement of fragments. The lesser trochanter is frequently split from the shaft with this type of injury, but in this case the lesser trochanter remains intact.

There is an important distinction between intertrochanteric fracture of the femur and femoral neck fractures. Most of the blood supply to the hip comes to the proximal femur through the capsule. The capsule inserts along the intertrochanteric ridge, so the blood supply to the intertrochanteric portion of the femur is very good. The blood supply to the femoral neck enters the head through the acetabulum, and the supply to the femoral neck is relatively poor when compared to either the head itself or to the intertrochanteric region.

Since the blood supply to the intertrochanteric fracture is quite good, it is possible for this fracture to heal without surgical pinning. However, most orthopedists find it more desirable to use an internal fixation device so that the patient can be up and about shortly, with reduced pulmonary and renal complications.

Femoral neck fractures, if in a very good position, may be pinned, but if the patient is elderly and there is any concern about repair, the femoral head will be removed and a prosthesis inserted. Final diagnosis: Undisplaced intertrochanteric fracture.

Case LX-9

Case LX-9 is an 86-year-old woman who was admitted to the emergency room following a fall. There was considerable pain in the left hip.

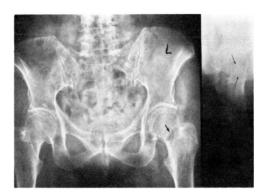

Case LX-9

This radiograph is presented not only for the left femoral neck fracture, of which it is a classic example, but for the general bone pattern as well. The dark arrow directs attention to the fracture line, as seen in the AP view. The long arrows again show the axis of angulation of the neck with respect to the head in the lateral view. There is generalized demineralization of bone. Very fine areas of punctate bone loss are noted in each intertrochanteric and subtrochanteric region. This is the type of demineralization that usually accompanies aging. Even along the lateral walls of the pelvis, as one approaches the superior ramus, there appears to be periosteal elevation. This is actually not periosteal elevation, but subperiosteal absorption of bone. This patient shows minimal atherosclerosis; however, such patients frequently show heavy vascular calcifications.

Final diagnosis: Generalized demineralization of bone. Fracture of the left femoral neck. This is not classed as a pathological fracture, although the generalized demineralization probably predisposed the patient to the fracture.

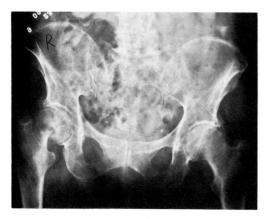

Case LX-10

Case LX-10

Case LX-10 is a 72-year-old woman complaining of severe pain in the right hip following a relatively minor injury.

The fracture of the right femoral neck shows most of the same basic signs described with earlier cases. In addition, it should be noted that the lesser trochanter rides considerably higher on the right than the left. Shenton's line is clearly broken on the right side, and the diag-nosis of an intracapsular fracture of the femoral neck is relatively easy.

The study is presented to show other features of bone pathology, as well as the fracture of the femoral neck. Multiple radiolucencies are noted throughout the bony areas. These are larger than were described with the demineralization of aging. In the area of the femoral neck fracture, there appears to be loss of a rather large portion of bone. Although there are evident degenerative changes in the lower lumbar spine, the pedicles are poorly defined, and one has the impression that there is destruction of bone along the lateral aspect of the fourth lumbar body.

Further investigation into the history indicated that the patient had a previous malignant tumor of the breast. Final diagnosis: Pathological fracture of the right femoral neck secondary to bony metastasis. The history indicates the primary tumor in the breast.

Case LX-11

Case LX-11 is a 69-year-old woman admitted to the hospital with generalized skeletal pain. There had been a history of relatively minor injury to the anterior portion of the pelvis three days earlier.

Bony structure is markedly demineralized, with generally decreased bone density. Close inspection shows multiple punctate areas of bone loss. These are somewhat larger than those seen with the osteoporosis of aging. They are smaller and more diffuse than was noted with metastatic disease. There is an apparent fracture involving the pubis on the left, with a small fragment of bone avulsed from the superior margin of the symphysis, and another small fragment of bone extending into the left obturator foramen.

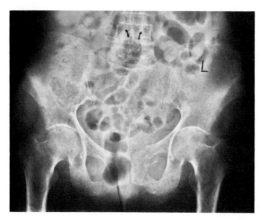

Case LX-11

Wrinkling of the cortex of the left descending ramus of the pubis indicates that there is further injury here.

The two curved arrows point to poorly defined pedicles of the fourth lumbar body. On the original film it is evident that the pedicles are still present on these bodies. The fifth lumbar body is compressed.

A differential diagnosis from a radiographic standpoint must include metastatic disease and multiple myeloma. Since the pedicles are intact, the bony structure is so diffusely involved, one's preference would be for a diagnosis of multiple myeloma. This diagnosis was confirmed by other laboratory studies.

The pelvis is one of the key areas to examine when suspecting multiple myeloma, for it represents a large volume of bone marrow. Multiple myeloma lesions tend to be intermedullary and extend out to involve the cortex. Failure to involve the pedicle is certainly not a pathognomonic sign of multiple myeloma, but we know that the marrow content of the pedicle is relatively small, and its peripheral blood supply is rich. Therefore, its involvement with metastatic disease is more likely than with multiple myeloma. Final diagnosis: Diffuse involvement of the pelvis with multiple myeloma, with a pathological fracture involving the left pubis.

Case LX-12

Case LX-12 is a 65-year-old woman injured in an automobile accident. When the patient was seen in the emergency room, there was marked flexion, internal rotation, and adduction of the femur. The image on the right was obtained.

There is apparent dislocation of the femoral head from the acetabulum. The

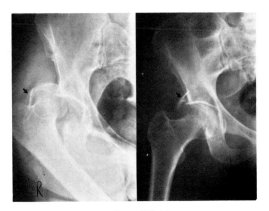

Case LX-12

dark solid arrow above the femoral head points to a wedge of bone that is more easily identified after reduction.

The image on the left is a post-reduction film. The head is now directed into the acetabulum. A wedge of bone is seen just above the acetabular shelf.

This is the classical presentation of posterior dislocation of the hip. As the hip dislocates posteriorly, it invariably fractures the posterior roof of the acetabulum. This type of injury occurs when the body suddenly decelerates in a sitting position (sitting in a car seat with forcible stop so that the weight of the body is directed through the femurs toward the dashboard or floorboard). Once dislocated, the strong adductors of the thigh produce the deformity seen clinically.

Even if the patient's dislocation is reduced prior to the radiographic study, and if the fragment of bone seen here in the post-reduction film can be identified, one can postulate with certainty that there was a posterior hip dislocation. Final diagnosis: Posterior dislocation of the femoral head, with fracture of the posterior margin of the acetabulum.

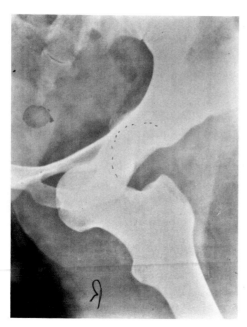

Case LX-13

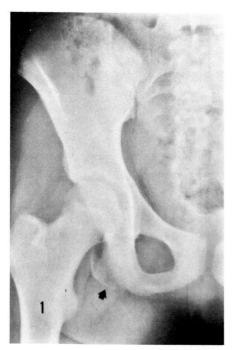

Case LX-14

Case LX-13

Case LX-13 is a 30-year-old woman involved in an auto accident.

The study is presented to show another dislocation of the hip, in which the dislocation is strikingly different from that seen in case LX-12. The acetabulum is marked with a dotted line. However, the head's location is inferior to this point, and the femur is sharply abducted. Note that the femoral head sets in, or is directly superimposed on the obturator foramen. Final diagnosis: Obturator foramen dislocation. This is a relatively rare form of hip dislocation, but one that is not unknown in areas where trauma makes up a considerable portion of the clinical experience. Since the head is directed toward the patient's blood supply, the chances of avascular necrosis are less with this injury than with posterior dislocation.

Cases LX-14 and LX-15

Two different cases are presented together here on a single film because the mechanism of injury is the same.

Case LX-14 (the side of the film with a "1" on the femur) is a 13-year-old girl who had been trying out for the cheerleading team and had been doing "splits." She complained of gluteal and groin pain.

Case LX-15 (the side of the film with a "2" on the femur) is a 14-year-old boy who had been trying out for track.

Heavy dark arrows point to portions of avulsed bone from the pelvis.

Case LX-14 is an avulsion of bone from the ischial tuberosity, secondary to a muscle pull from doing "splits." The fragment is separated slightly from the main portion of the tuberosity. This helps very much with the diagnosis. Had there been little or no displacement, the diagnosis would be extremely difficult.

The young man trying out for track has what is sometimes referred to as "hurdler's injury" where there is avulsion of the anterior-inferior iliac spine, again due to muscle pull of a vigorous type. Both patients were admitted with localized findings and symptoms. Radiographs identify the severity of the injury. The extent of the muscle tear is impossible to determine from radiographs. Final diagnosis: Avulsion or tearing-type fractures, involving the ischial tuberosity in Case LX-14 and the anterior iliac spine in Case LX-15.

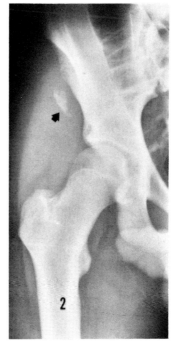

Case LX-15

Case LX-16

Case LX-16 is a 61-year-old woman admitted to the hospital for a general checkup. During the course of her hospitalization, it was found that she had an elevated alkaline phosphatase

The radiograph of the pelvis is generally normal for a patient of this age, with the exception of the margin of the right side of the pelvis. The two curved arrows indicate the pathology. There is some thickening of the cortical bone and even some expansion of the lateral margin of the superior ramus of the pubis. Compare this margin of the pelvis with the normal left margin; the expansion of bone and thickening of the cortex is evident. Paget's disease classically increases the size and density of bone involved.

Final diagnosis: Paget's disease with early changes in the pelvic brim, the so-called "brim sign." These patients do have an associated elevation of alkaline phosphatase. The lesion may be asymptomatic or quite painful. The pelvis and the skull are the best sites to examine when looking for early changes of this disease.

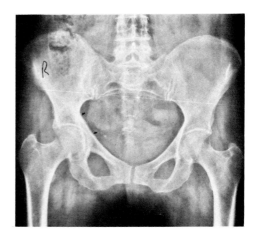

Case LX-16

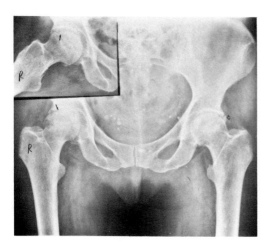

Case LX-17

Case LX-17

Case LX-17 is a 56-year-old female alcoholic who was admitted with right hip pain.

The radiographs of the hip are reminiscent of the shoulder radiographs in Case UX-17, a case of avascular necrosis of the humeral head. There is some fragmentation and a break in the cortex of the articular surface of the femoral head, as evidenced by the small arrow.

The left hip is normal; however, the open-faced arrow calls attention to an os acetabuli, which is a common normal variant. There are multiple phleboliths in the pelvis.

Avascular necrosis of the hip occurs in patients who have been on steroids or have collagen diseases or are alcoholics and a few are idiopathic. In a sense, it is an adult Perthes' disease. However, the prognosis is not as good, since the adult does not have the ability to reform and remodel to the same extent as the child. Final diagnosis: Avascular necrosis of the right femoral head.

Case LX-18

Case LX-18 is a 15-year-old girl complaining of right hip pain. The patient is moderately obese.

Marked asymmetry in the hips is noted. On the left the femoral head is located in a normal position with the epiphyseal line at its base, and a weight-bearing line, if one were to draw it, would fall through the head, epiphyseal line, and neck.

On the right considerable difference is noted. The head is rotated inferiorly, so that the weight-bearing line now extends through the acetabulum into the femoral neck traversing only a portion of the femoral head. This had resulted in the loss of considerable effective length of the femur on the right. The pelvic tilt that is noted to the right is an attempt to compensate for this loss of length.

Shenton's line on the right is distorted, with the line extending above the obturator foramen as it passes in this direction. The inferior margin of the femoral head, however, is transected by this imaginary line.

Slipped femoral epiphyses occur in teenagers, more frequently in boys than

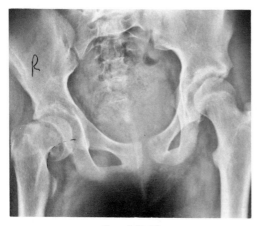

Case LX-18

in girls. These patients are usually obese. The cause is not known but maybe traumatic. Reduction and surgical fixation are generally required.

Case LX-19

Case LX-19 is a 4-year-old boy with a history of two days of pain in the left hip. The pain was quite severe.

Changes here are subtle, but important. The joint space width on the left is approximately 1 mm wider than that seen on the right. The soft-tissue planes about the capsule of the hip joint show moderate distention but are in other areas quite indistinct. The right side appears normal.

Even slight asymmetry in joint space width implies effusion. If the patient is in pain, this implies an effusion under pressure. The most important diagnosis under this circumstance is that of pus in the hip joint, or a septic joint, and the clinician should not wait for further radiographic changes.

In this instance, the needling of the hip revealed only clear fluid. The child's symptoms disappeared, and there were no sequelae demonstrated in follow-up studies over the next two months.

The final diagnosis here is synovitis of the hip. It is probably a reactive snyovitis. The child did have an upper respiratory infection. These are thought to be viral or reactive in their origin. It is most important that the joint space alteration be noted and that the diagnosis of septic hip be ruled out. If pus remains in the joint space, it destroys the cartilage, and the patient ends up with a disabled hip. The findings on this film are indistinguishable between the benign process, as this case turned out to be, and the much more important septic joint.

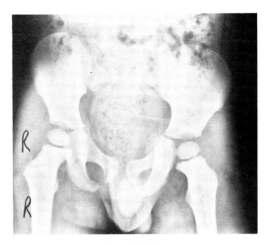

Case LX-19

Case LX-20

Case LX-20 is a 7-year-old boy. The patient complained of right hip pain of insidious onset.

The radiograph of the pelvis is presented so that the two sides of the pelvis and the two hips can be compared. On the left the femoral head appears somewhat mottled and is smaller than the corresponding epiphysis on the left. There is also slight irregularity on the lateral edge of the epiphysis, as seen in the AP projection. The lateral view shows rather

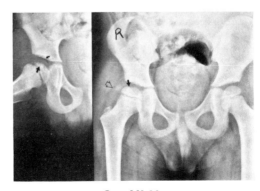

Case LX-20

marked irregularity and impaction of the posterior portion of the femoral head epiphysis. These areas are identified by short heavy dark arrows. The joint space is normally maintained. A short curved arrow is directed toward a crescent radiolucent shadow in the joint space. This represents the so-called "vacuum phenomenon," in which by some means or another, usually a traction-type injury, nitrogen is released in the joint space. It can be produced deliberately with a strong, sharp pull on the extremity. Aspirations of these small radiolucencies have confirmed the presence of nitrogen. They are nonspecific findings. This phenomenon may be seen in patients with painful hips and shoulders without traction injuries. The presence of this radiolucency does imply the absence of joint fluid. If fluid were present, this radiolucency would be displaced to the superior part of the hip and not be visualized radiographically.

The open arrow is directed toward the distention of the capsule on the right. Soft tissues are more prominent in the hip area on the right than the left. All of these features are findings in Perthes' disease, or avascular necrosis of the femoral capitate epiphysis. Of all of the avascular necroses that involve the epiphyses, this one is probably the most frequent in occurrence. It occurs three times as frequently in boys as girls, and the usual time of onset is between ages five and seven.

The outcome of the disease depends on the severity of the involvement. Some patients show minimal head deformity and heal with little or no residual change. Others show a great deal of fragmentation of the femoral head, so that when healing occurs the head becomes broad and flat.

This results in degenerative disease later in life.

The radiographic features of this disease are quite variable. This example is one of moderate involvement. Progressive fragmentation and destruction of the head will occur, and the remodeling process occurs subsequently.

Other texts will cover this entity in more detail. Except for the "vacuum phenomenon," we have presented the classic radiographic changes here. These changes will vary in degree from case to case.

THE KNEE

The knee is a major weight-supporting joint. It is a simple hinge joint with a complex soft-tissue supporting system. Fractures and other injuries occur in the knee. Consequently many radiographs are taken. However, of all of the joints in the body, the knee probably has the highest percentage of negative studies. This implies that there is a great deal of soft-tissue injury (we know this to be true) about the knee. Because the bones are strong and heavy, fracture is less likely.

CASE PRESENTATIONS

Case LXK-1

This patient is a 51-year-old man with history of recurrent knee pain. The basic anatomy of the knee is relatively simple. The distal femur articulates with the tibia. The fibula joins the lateral margin of the tibia with only soft-tissue support. No weight is supported here. The patella is a sesamoid bone in the heavy tendon of the quadriceps muscles. The small, bony density seen posterior to the femur is the fabella, which is in the lateral head of the gastrocnemius, another sesamoid bone (curved dark arrow in each projection).

The patella in the AP projection tends to ride higher than one would expect. In each view the patella is indicated by the open arrow. Small dark solid arrows are used to point to the area of fusion of the anterior tibial epiphysis, especially as it curves downward in the anterior portion of the tibia. Similar arrows are used to identify the site of closure of the distal femoral epiphysis. In this patient the epiphyses have long been closed since the patient is 51 years of age. Soft-tissue planes about the knee are of some diagnostic interest. Their absence implies an inflammatory process. Displacement of the suprapatellar fat line indicated by the straight solid arrow usually means a suprapatellar effusion.

As with most tubular bones, both the femur and the tibia show a relatively thin cortex in the metaphyseal and subarticular regions, but the cortex becomes quite dense as the bone constricts and the diaphysis is formed.

Special views of the knee can be obtained. The standard AP and the lateral view is shown here. The lateral view is taken with the knee slightly flexed. The leg is straight in the anterior-posterior-projection. Tunnel views are used to show the intercondylar portion of the femur. Special patellar views can be made with the incident beam directed longitudinally between the femur and the patella, with the knee moderately flexed. For cartilage and ligamentous injury, clinical examination and arthrography are required.

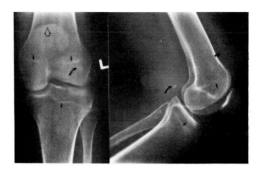

Case LXK-1

Case LXK-2

Case LXK-2 is a very active 12-year-old boy who was complaining of moderate pain over the upper anterior portion of the tibia.

A lateral view of each knee is presented. The left knee is normal. It is presented at this point to demonstrate the appearance of the normal epiphyses of the growing knee. The anterior tibial epiphysis actually curves downward and is the source of development of the anterior tibial prominence. This view also shows the epiphyseal line of the proximal fibula and distal femur.

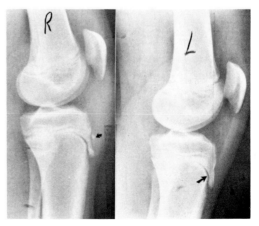

Case LXK-2

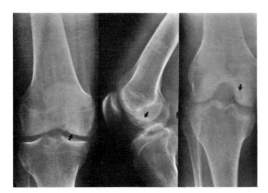

Case LXK-3

The right knee shows some fragmentation of the anterior tibial epiphysis as indicated by the short curved arrow and the soft-tissue swelling over this prominence.

Our final diagnosis here is a normal knee on the left with Osgood-Schlatter disease on the right. The process is considered active because of the soft-tissue swelling. Since we know that epiphyses can fragment normally, the diagnosis of Osgood-Schlatter disease cannot be made on the basis of fragmentation alone. It must be correlated with clinical symptoms and/or soft-tissue swelling.

Osgood-Schlatter disease is one of the more frequently occurring avascular necrosies of a growing epiphysis. It is usually considered traumatic in origin. It has an excellent prognosis.

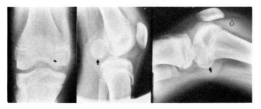

Case LXK-4

Case LXK-3

Case LXK-3 is a 21-year-old man who had fallen on his knee. The injury was not severe. The history indicated that he had had knee discomfort for some time.

The study is a classical demonstration of osteochondritis dissecans. This is also thought to be an avascular necrosis of the subchondral bone. This diagnosis may not be made until later in life. Symptoms may be locking of the knee or general discomfort or it may be asymptomatic.

The solid dark arrows point to saucer-ation of the medial condyle of the femur with a small, dense, bony fragment remaining in the saucer. When this fragment of bone shells loose from the condyle, it serves as a loose body that may produce locking of the joint. Spontaneous absorption of the fragment has been observed. In symptomatic patients, surgery is usually required.

Case LXK-4

Case LXK-4 is a 13-year-old boy who had suffered a clipping injury in football.

The three images presented show the advantage of even slightly different projections. The two lateral films both appear to be acceptable in their positioning. However, the lateral view in the center panel shows gross displacement of the medial portion of the distal femoral epiphysis, with the medial portion displaced posteriorly. The second lateral view, which was made cross-table (a valuable technique when it is difficult for the patient to move), shows not only the displaced epiphyseal fragment posteriorly as indicated by the heavy arrow, but also demonstrates a fat/fluid level beneath the patella as indicated by the open-faced arrow. This implies bleeding into the joint space, with fat floating at the top of the blood.

The AP view of the knee is surprising with its nearly normal appearance. The short curved arrow does point to the rather subtle vertical fracture line in the epiphysis. Our final diagnosis is a Salter type III * fracture of the distal femoral epiphysis.

Case LXK-5

Case LXK-5 is a 35-year-old woman who had fallen from a ladder.

An AP radiograph of the knee and a cross-table lateral film are presented. The lateral film shows the fat/fluid line as indicated by the open arrow. The solid dark arrow in the lateral view shows some superimposed bone, indicating that there is fragmentation and some impaction as the fracture line is increased in density. The AP projection reveals a faint fracture line extending through the midline of the articular margin, as indicated by the small dark arrow. The heavy dark arrow identifies the fracture line extending from the medial side of the metaphysis of the tibia upward to the vertical line and again laterally to the metaphysis producing an inverted "Y" fracture line. The tibial plateaus remain remarkably horizontal, and the joint space is considered normal.

Final diagnosis is an inverted "Y" fracture of the proximal tibia with fragments of the proximal tibia (each plateau) in reasonably good position. Every attempt will be made by the orthopedist to maintain the fragments in this position during healing. Since the plateau is quite level as viewed in the AP projection, pinning may not be necessary.

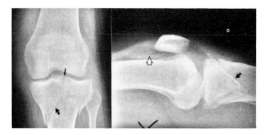

Case LXK-5

Case LXK-6

Case LXK-6 is a 78-year-old woman who tripped over her cane, falling on her knee.

The radiographs of the knee show generalized demineralization of bone. There is an obvious fracture through the distal femur (supracondylar area). Even more important, however, is a vertical split in the distal femur as indicated by the two solid arrows in the AP projection, which implies that both femoral condyles have been split. This is in addition to the trans-

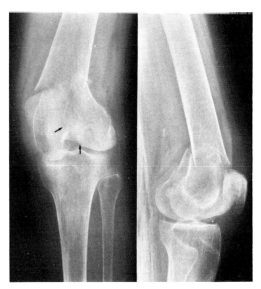

Case LXK-6

---

*See Chart #1, page 221.

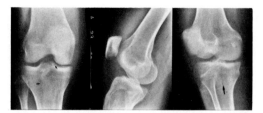

Case LXK-7

verse fracture in the supracondylar area. The tibia appears to be intact.

The final diagnosis is a supracondylar fracture with an associated split of the femoral condyles (T-type fracture). This is a very unstable distal femur. After reduction, it was treated with surgical fixation by means of an intracondylar pin and a lateral femoral plate.

Case LXK-7

Case LXK-7 is a 32-year-old woman with pain in her knee following a fall.

This study is presented to show the value of additional views, and to warn observers that minor changes in the AP and the lateral projections may be very important. The initial study was an AP and lateral radiograph as indicated here.

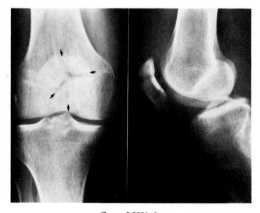

Case LXK-8

The small solid arrows suggest a fracture line, but there is no displacement and the line could merely be a prominent trabecular line. The lateral projection gave no clue as to the injury.

An oblique film was obtained. The solid dark arrow now points directly upward into the fracture line, which can be followed all the way to the articular surface.

This is a stable fracture. The condyles have not been displaced. Healing in this position should give a good result. However, whenever a fracture line enters a joint surface, the possibility of degenerative change in later years is increased.

Case LXK-8

Case LXK-8 is a 36-year-old man who had fallen forward on his knee. There was rather marked soft-tissue swelling and a great deal of pain.

Radiographs of the knee show a stellate-type of fracture in the region of the patella as seen in the AP projection. Four arrows point toward the suspected fracture lines. A lateral view also reveals some deformity along the inferior margin of the patella, with a slight offset at the level of the upper open-faced arrow.

Fractures of the patella sometimes are difficult to diagnose because of variations in the patellar development. Bipartite and tripartite patellae are not infrequent findings. (See Case LXK-10.) Films of the opposite knee may or may not help since the bipartite or tripartite patella may be a unilateral developmental variant. Clinical correlation is important.

Special views of the patella, such as the "sunrise view," may be difficult to obtain because of the patient's pain. Tomograms and oblique views usually will help distinguish between normal variations in the patella and fracture lines.

Case LXK-9

Case LXK-9 is a 55-year-old man who unfortunately was the pedestrian in a car-pedestrian accident.

The radiographs of the knee show marked changes that can be quite confusing. The solid dark arrows in the AP projection locate the patella. The medial joint space of the knee appears somewhat widened. In the lateral view the patella is superimposed on the distal femur. A small bone fragment is seen between the fabella and the femoral condyle.

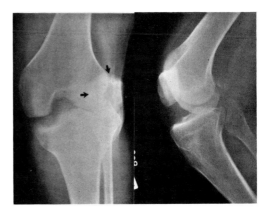

Case LXK-9

The patella usually rides in the intercondylar groove, but dislocations of the patella laterally are not uncommon. These may occur from muscular injury or direct force on the patella. In this case we assume that there has been a great deal of direct force on the knee joint, damaging the medial ligaments and forcing the patella laterally. Final diagnosis: Dislocated patella with associated soft-tissue injury to the knee.

Case LXK-10

Case LXK-10 is a 17-year-old boy radiographed because of an injury to the knee.

The images presented represent one of the confusing points in reference to patella injuries. The heavy dark arrow is directed toward a smooth line as it curves across the upper quadrant of the patella. In the lateral view there is a less well-defined line that is also identified by the heavy dark arrow.

This is a bipartite patella. It is a normal variant and should not be confused with a fracture. Comparison views of the other knee may be helpful, but usually are not. A similar line may involve the medial portion of the patella, giving three segments, a so-called tripartite patella. The bipartite patella is more frequent than the triple ossicle variety. Final diagnosis: Bipartite patella, a normal but sometimes confusing variation.

Case LXK-11

Case LXK-11 is a 13-year-old boy who had been actively involved in track ("sprints"), and now was complaining of pain in the upper leg.

The most significant radiographic change is indicated by the vertically directed small dark arrow. Note the increased band of radiodensity across the upper tibia. There is also some periosteal thickening posteriorly at the level of this increased

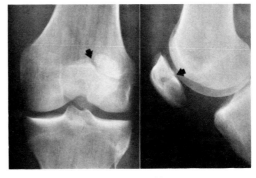

Case LXK-10

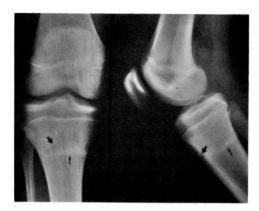

Case LXK-11

density. The epiphyseal lines are not remarkable.

The heavier dark arrow is directed to a shadow seen frequently on the AP film of the upper tibia. This is a curved radiolucent line and is of no significance, for it represents a portion of the anterior tibial epiphysis. The same type of dark arrow is

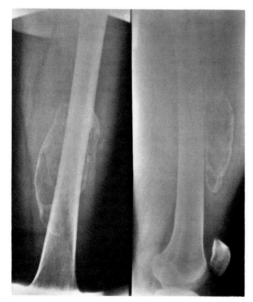

Case LXK-12

directed toward the base of the line as seen in the lateral view. Our normal case LXK-1 demonstrated a similar line.

Final diagnosis is that of a healing stress fracture of the proximal tibia. The evidence for the healing is the increased density. During the acute onset of a stress fracture, the radiographs are usually normal. It is only over a period of time, with increased osteoblastic activity, that the fracture becomes evident. Nuclear bone scanning will give a positive scan prior to x-ray changes.

Case LXK-12

Case LXK-12 is a 32-year-old man admitted because of a firm mass in the anterior thigh. The history indicated that there had been an injury four months earlier

The radiographic changes seen here are quite classical. In the AP projection, there is a large, partially calcified mass. Most of the calcification is noted in the periphery of the mass. In the AP projection one cannot be certain that the femur is involved. However, the cortex of the femur appears to be intact, as seen through the mass.

The lateral projection shows that the mass is lying anterior to the femur and that it does not have a periosteal component. Soft-tissue planes are displaced around the mass.

Final diagnosis: Myositis ossificans. The patient's injury had led to a hematoma, which is undergoing calcification. The important point here is that it not be diagnosed as a malignant bone tumor. When there is soft-tissue density seen between the bone in question and the mass, the diagnosis of myositis ossificans can be made with confidence.

Case LXK-13

Case LXK-13 is a 14-year-old boy who complained of pain and swelling in the knee. He attributed the discomfort to an injury one month earlier.

The radiograph of the upper tibia in the AP projection shows a large area of bone destruction involving the metaphyseal portion of the fibula. New periosteal bone is noted, and a great deal of bone destruction is identified. The new bone appears to be forming at right angles to the shaft. There is no margin limiting the lesion on the tibial side. A soft-tissue mass was noted clinically and is seen radiographically with the aid of bright light.

The final diagnosis is osteogenic sarcoma of the fibula. The lesion is malignant. It appears aggressive. There is bone destruction and bone production. The soft-tissue mass completes the classic triad of a malignant primary bone tumor.

Seventy-five percent of malignant primary bone tumors occur about the knee, with the peak-age incidence in adolescence. Primary bone tumors are rare in infants and very young children. In fact, although they are not totally unknown, if a bone lesion turns out to be a primary malignant tumor in a child under the age of four, the case is worthy of adding to the medical literature.

Case LXK-14

Case LXK-14 is a 13-year-old boy with a six-month history of knee pain and discomfort. In this case, the large destructive areas are in the metaphysis of the tibia. There is periosteal new bone formation along the medial side of the tibia. A soft-tissue mass is present. The lesion, while limited by the epiphyseal plate, has

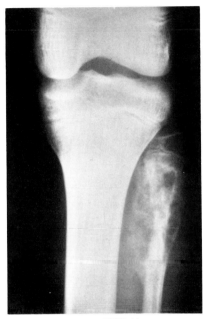

Case LXK-13

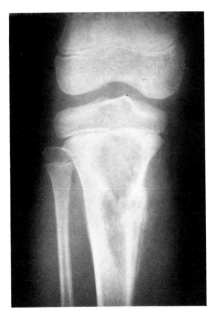

Case LXK-14

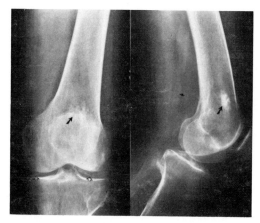

Case LXK-15

broken through the periosteum along the medial metaphyseal portion of the tibia.

The final diagnosis is osteogenic sarcoma of the tibia. The findings are much the same as that seen in Case LXK-13, except that the bone involved is different, and there is more bone destruction and less bone production than in the previous case.

The appearance of primary osteogenic sarcoma may vary from almost complete bone production to virtually complete

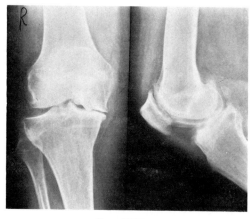

Case LXK-16

bone destruction. This is an extremely malignant tumor. The radiographic demonstration of any unexplained bone lesion in an adolescent deserves consultation and detailed evaluation.

Case LXK-15

Case LXK-15 is a 77-year-old man complaining of back and knee discomfort.

The radiographs of the knee in the AP and the lateral projections show generalized demineralization of bone. This is consistent with the patient's age. The most important finding on the radiograph is evidenced by the open-faced arrows, as they are directed to a fine lacy calcification in the knee joint. This represents calcification of the cartilage of the knee and is abnormal.

A second peculiar type of increase in bone density is seen in the distal femur. This is pointed out by sloping solid arrows toward a poorly defined area in the medullary canal of the distal femur. There is no bone destruction. Vascular changes and soft-tissue findings are not evident.

The third abnormal finding is identified by a small solid black arrow in the soft tissues posterior to the knee. It identifies a linear calcification.

Our final diagnoses are (1) arteriosclerosis of the popliteal artery (indicated by a small solid arrow on the lateral film). (2) enchondroma of the distal femur (indicated by sloping solid black arrows); and (3) chondral calcification (indicated by open arrows).

Calcifications of cartilage can have several causes. They may be degenerative in origin—in a man of this age this is the most likely cause. They can be produced by hyperparathyroidism and pseudogout. This latter diagnosis has some features of gout and may even respond to therapy like gout. The diagnosis can be established by finding pyrophosphate crystals in the joint fluid.

The enchondroma seen here is an incidental finding. At this age and in this location, it is of little or no significance.

Case LXK-16

Case LXK-16 is a 79-year-old obese female, with discomfort in both knees.

The patient has similar radiographic changes in both knees. However, only the right knee is being presented. The bony density is normal. There is narrowing of the medial side of the joint space, and a small amount of spurring is present on the articular margin of both the upper medial tibia and distal medial femur. The lateral portion of the knee joint space appears wide, indicating that the patient when standing is "bow-legged." The lateral view demonstrates spurring on the patella and on the anterior and posterior margin of the femur. The articular surface of both the tibia and the femur appears somewhat dense and sclerotic.

The final diagnosis is osteoarthritis of the knee. It is also called hypertrophic arthritis or degenerative arthritis. It is especially important to patients that are overweight, for the mechanical problems of the knee with time and trauma result in disability. Because of the bowing of the knee it may be necessary to do an osteotomy of the upper tibia, or even do a total knee replacement if the pain is severe.

This type of arthritis may result from the wear and tear of living, but of course it is markedly accelerated if there have been injuries or mechanical problems directed toward the joint. This disorder rarely occurs in people of normal weight, unless there has been an injury or some

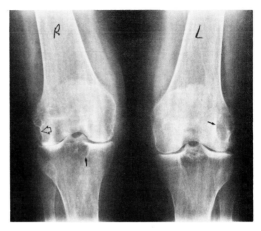

Case LXK-17

superimposed mechanical problem that adds special stress to the joint

Case LXK-17

Case LXK-17 is a 56-year-old female suffering from rheumatoid arthritis. Other joints were more severely involved than her knees.

AP radiographs of each knee are presented. The lateral views did not add to our findings. There is generalized demineralization of bone. Bony and soft-tissue structures appear relatively atrophic. There is joint space narrowing on both sides of the knee joint. The narrowing is more marked in the lateral portion of the knees than the medial. Despite the generalized demineralization of bone, the articular surfaces of both the femoral condyles and tibial plateaus are locally sclerotic. There are marginal erosions laterally, indicated by open arrows. Pseudocysts are seen on each side and are indicated by small solid arrows. The alignment of the femur to the tibia is relatively straight. However, these patients do develop flexion deformities.

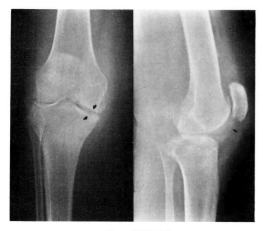

Case LXK-18

Comparison of this case with the one presented previously makes the differentiation of osteoarthritis and rheumatoid arthritis quite simple. Needless to say there are times when these entities are not so well defined, and there are times when the two processes occur together. Final diagnosis: Rheumatoid arthritis involving both knees.

Case LXK-18

Case LXK-18 is a 67-year-old woman who had been in the hospital for mitral valve surgery. She had recovered uneventfully from this and subsequently came to the hospital with "severe arthritis" of the knee.

There are features of both rheumatoid arthritis and osteoarthritis of the knee. However, there are some features that separate this from either of these two entities. The curved arrows in the AP projection point to areas where the well-defined articular surface has been destroyed. The small dark arrow on the lateral view directs attention to a locally demineralized area of the femoral con-

dyle. The lateral view also indicates that the femur is anterior in alignment, compared to the tibia. There is evident soft-tissue swelling about the knee.

The patient undoubtedly has degenerative disease of the knee, but now because of the cartilage destruction and marginal destruction of bone, the diagnosis of septic arthritis is in order. This, of course, is correlated clinically with fever and local pain. Subluxation of a joint from pus formation is not unusual. However, subluxation is more commonly seen in the shoulder and hip than in the knee.

Septic arthritis, as seen here, requires vigorous therapy if the cartilage is to be preserved and a functioning joint to result.

THE ANKLE

The radiographs of the normal adult ankle are routinely taken in the AP, lateral and oblique projections. The AP and the lateral views are self-explanatory. The oblique view is made with the foot and the knee rotated medially between 30 and 45 degrees. In this view it is important that the foot be held in slight dorsal flexion so that the os calcis does not obscure the tip of the fibula.

The ankle is a remarkably sturdy joint. The ankle joint itself only permits flexion and extension. Inversion and eversion of the foot are motions that occur in the subastragalar area and do not actually involve the normal ankle joint. The medial wall of the hinged joint that we have described is supported by the medial malleolus, which is an extension of the tibia. The lateral wall of this joint is supported by the fibula with the actual weight-supporting portion of the joint being across the tibia and talus.

Films made for ankle evaluation are made principally to identify the distal tibia, the fibula, and the talus. The lateral film, and occasionally the oblique view, will show portions of the os calcis and the tarsal bones and perhaps even the bases of the metatarsals, but ankle films are made distinctly different than foot films as will be described later.

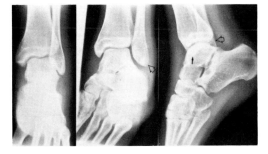

Case LXA-1

CASE PRESENTATIONS

Case LXA-1

Case LXA-1 has films of an adult man. The standard three views of the ankle. This patient shows no bone pathology. There is, however, some soft tissue swelling over the lateral malleolus indicating soft-tissue injury. In the AP projection the lateral portion of the tibia and the fibula are somewhat superimposed. In the lateral view it is always surprising how far forward the medial malleolus projects. This is indicated in the lateral view by the solid black arrow. By the same token, the fibula is relatively posterior when viewed in the lateral projection as indicated by the open faced arrow. The same open-faced arrow is directed toward the tip of the fibula in the oblique view. Note how well the fibula tip is seen in this projection.

The trabecular pattern of the bone is quite well outlined. The trabecular pattern tends to align itself along weight bearing directions. Stress lines in the talus tend to culminate in the superior portion of the talus, directly beneath its articulation with the tibia. The same stress lines can be seen extending both forward and backward and tend to be aligned with the supporting lines of the os clacis and tarsal navicular.

Case LXA-2

Case LXA-2 is a 10-year-old boy. The films are presented in an AP and a lateral projection only. They are presented principally to be consistent with the previously described anatomical areas where at least one pediatric case is presented to show growth and development. Two normal variants are identified here. The

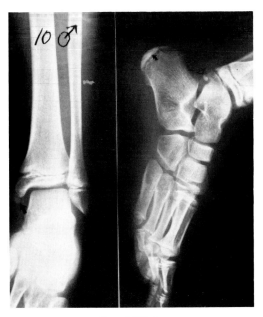

Case LXA-2

heavy dark arrow is directed toward an accessory epiphysis at the tip of the medial malleolus. This can be confusing if the patient has pain and injury at this site. However, the margins are always smooth and, while they may be somewhat smaller than the ones shown here, this is the characteristic appearance of this normal variant.

The second normal variant that is seen on the lateral view is identified by an open arrow. It represents the development of the os trigonum. This is one of the many supernumary ossicles that occur about the foot and ankle. This ossicle may occur in 20% of the population. It occurs so frequently that it should not be a source of confusion.

A short curved arrow is directed toward the epiphysis of the os calcis. This case is normal. The epiphysis is considerably more dense and somewhat amorphysis in its appearance compared to the rest of the os calcis. Just above the dark arrow is a line that suggests fragmentation. Certainly normal epiphyses may appear fragmented. A fragmented, dense epiphysis usually means avascular necrosis. The one exception to that statement is the epiphysis of the os calcis, which is invariably more dense and is frequently fragmented. What could be considered abnormal in other sites must be called normal in this important area.

Cases LXA-3 through LXA-5

Each of these three cases represents a slightly different type of fracture of the os calcis.

Case LXA-3 is the classical presentation of the fractured os calcis that occurs from a falling injury, with the patient landing on the feet. The usual story is of a patient falling from a ladder or from a roof, with the direction of force down through the ankle. The longitudinal arch of the foot is decreased, principally due to the impaction and the fracture through the os calcis. In the lateral view the fracture line is indicated by heavy dark arrows. A tangential view of the os calcis shows a long, diagonal fracture line, extending from posterior to anterior, with the os calcis being nearly split down the center. The value of the tangential view of the os calcis is evident. This is made with the patient lying on the back, the film under the heel, and the incident beam entering the sole of the foot at an angle of 45 to 60 degrees.

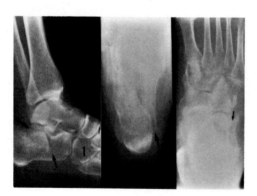

Case LXA-3

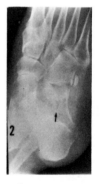

Case LXA-4

Case LXA-4 has a more subtle injury. The fracture of the os calcis, as identified by the smaller solid dark arrow, could not be seen in the lateral view of the os calcis or a tangential view. Fortunately, the patient had films of the foot; and the AP and the oblique foot images show the vertical fracture lines in the anterior portion of the os calcis. There is some impaction of fragments near the articulation with the cuboid. The double density seen over the lateral margin of the cuboid is ossification in the peroneus tendon. It is much more evident in the oblique projection.

Fractures of the os calcis can be very subtle. All are painful, and in the presence of a weight-bearing injury, multiple films may be needed to demonstrate the fracture.

Case LXA-5 demonstrates another subtle fracture of the os calcis. The open arrow is directed toward a faint fracture line in the anterior-superior beak of the os calcis. In some instances the fragment isolated by this type of fracture is larger than seen here and grossly displaced. The example we are presenting shows little or no displacement with a very faint fracture line beneath the tip of the arrow. This fracture will show only in the lateral projection.

This sequence of films has demonstrated the most frequently occurring fractures of the os calcis: (1) a longitudinal fracture through the body of the os calcis with resulting loss of the longitudinal arch of the foot, (2) a fracture of the anterior os calcis with a longitudinal fracture line that is incomplete but with anterior marginal impaction, and (3) a fracture of the anterior-superior portion of the os calcis (a "beak fracture").

Case LXA-6

Case LXA-6 is a 20-year-old man who had been involved in an auto accident. The images of the ankle presented here are AP and lateral views. The curved dark arrow directs attention toward a fracture line in the mid portion of the talus. There is no appreciable displacement of frag-

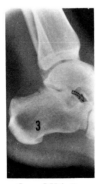

Case LXA-5

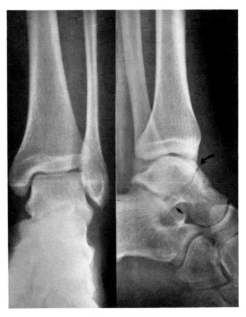

Case LXA-6

ments. The fracture line is not visible in the AP view. Most fractures of the talus tend to be slightly more forward in their position than in this example. Displacement, of course, varies with the severity of the injury. The anterior portion of the articular margin is involved in this instance.

The smaller dark arrow points to an incidental finding, which is a bony bridge between the os calcis and the talus. This is a relatively uncommon bony bridge, but one that should be recognized as a variant. Final diagnosis: Nondisplaced fracture of the talus. Bony bridge between the os calcis and the talus.

Case LXA-7

Case LXA-7 is a 57-year-old woman injured by a fall. The radiographs of the ankle are presented in the AP, the lateral, and the oblique projections. Clearly there are multiple bone injuries present. The curved, small, dark arrow is directed toward the fracture line involving the medial malleolus. In the AP projection the overlying zipper of the air splint is somewhat distracting, but the fracture is evident. In the oblique view it is more ob-

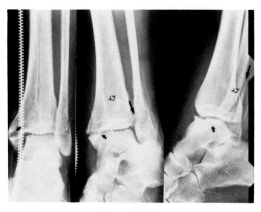

Case LXA-7

vious, the curved arrow isolates the distal fragment. The fracture line is approximately parallel with the ankle joint. In the lateral view the curved arrow again identifies the fracture in the medial malleolus. The fragment is separated by several millimeters from the remaining tibia, and the fragment itself is slightly greater than a cubic centimeter.

The open arrow is seen only on the oblique and lateral views. It is superimposed on the distal posterior tibia. In the lateral view it is very difficult to be certain that there is a separate fracture in the posterior tibia, for the fracture lines in the fibula are superimposed. However, by following the posterior margin of the tibia downward, a break in the cortex is seen just below the tip of the open-faced arrow. The faint fracture line on the oblique view, indicated by the open arrow, is helpful here. Fortunately, this fracture line does not extend down to alter the articular surface of the tibia.

The longer solid dark arrow is directed toward the fracture of the distal fibula. In the lateral view it can be seen that this is a long, diagonal fracture line, starting relatively high above the ankle, and extending down to the level of the ankle joint. The AP projection fails to visualize this fracture completely; and there is very little, if any, alteration of the ankle mortise.

The final diagnosis is that of a trimalleolar fracture of the ankle. Instead of presenting individual cases of malleolar fracture or even fracture through the medial and lateral malleolus (Pott's fracture), we felt that the diagnostic points of a trimalleolar fracture could cover the aspects of each of these injuries as they might be encountered individually. Certainly a diagonal fracture of the distal fibula, as an isolated injury, is the most frequent fracture about the ankle. Bimalleolar fractures are probably the next most frequent injury. Isolated medial malleolar fractures and trimalleolar fractures, occur at approximately the same incidence. None are rare. The degree of involvement of the posterior margin of the tibia is always the most difficult to determine radiologically. If the injury is severe and the fragments are grossly displaced, the problem is much greater in management than in diagnosis. In this case there is little displacement of fragments, and one might expect satisfactory results without surgical intervention. However, nonunion in the medial malleolus results in an unstable ankle; therefore, screw fixation of this fragment to the shaft of the tibia is a frequent form of therapy.

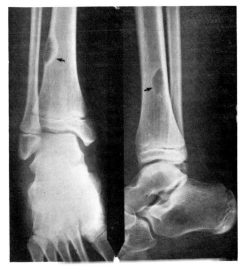

Case LXA-8

Case LXA-8

Case LXA-8 is a 12-year-old girl who had radiographs made of the ankle following an injury.

There is no evidence of bone injury. There is, however, some soft-tissue swelling over the lateral malleolus, consistent with a sprained ankle. The solid arrows are directed toward the incidental lesion of interest. Note that it is an expanding lesion within the cortex, and that it has some very fine septa within it (septa are not important in this diagnosis). There is no periosteal reaction and no evidence of unusual bone response to the lesion. Such lesions are frequently rimmed by sclerosis.

This is a simple, fibrous cortical defect. These lesions occur in 2% to 5% of children. They start just proximal to the epiphyseal line and move toward the diaphysis as the child grows. By the time growth is complete, these lesions usually disappear. They are asymptomatic and of no clinical significance, except that they should not be mistaken for more serious lesions. Their most frequent sites of occurrence are in the tibia and the distal femur, although they can occur in virtually any long bone. Once you know of the lesion and have seen one, its diagnosis should be no problem.

Case LXA-9

Case LXA-9 is a 15-year-old girl with a past history of multiple fractures. The patient's sister had a similar history.

The radiographic visualization of the leg from the ankle to the knee shows generalized demineralization of bone with a relatively thin cortex on all bony structures. The trabecular pattern of the bone is prominent, but still considerable space is seen between trabeculi. In this instance, there is bowing of the tibia and the fibula with what appears to be healing of an old fracture in the mid fibula. The ankle joint tilts to the medial side, while

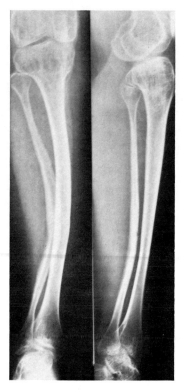

Case LXA-9

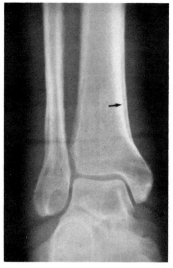

Case LXA-10

the knee compensates by tilting slightly in the opposite direction. The soft tissues appear somewhat atrophic.

The final diagnosis is osteogenesis imperfecta. Two forms of this genetically transmitted disease exist. One is so severe that the infant rarely survives the neonatal period. The other is osteogenesis imperfecta tarda, which implies that the infant survives and that the process is evident in childhood years. These patients generally show some improvement after puberty; but even with this improvement they are still subject to multiple fractures.

Case LXA-10

Case LXA-10 is a 60 year old man admitted to the rheumatology service because of multiple areas of bone pain and joint stiffness. A routine chest film showed what appeared to be a primary pulmonary neoplasm.

The radiographic changes of the distal tibia and fibula are quite striking. The solid black arrow points to the periosteal new bone formation along the medial margin of the tibia. This formation is also present along the lateral margin of the fibula, and to a lesser extent, along the lateral portion of the tibia near the upper portion of the film. The joint appears to be well preserved and normal. There is some soft-tissue thickening.

This is a classical example of pulmonary osteoarthrophy. The term implies that it is a joint problem. Usually complaints of the patient are related to joints. Radiographic changes are principally those of new subperiosteal bone formation, just as seen here. The periosteal bone formation is demonstrated with no evidence of bone destruction.

There are many interesting and unexplainable facets of this disease. We know that the skeletal changes do not represent metastatic lesions. In fact, the skeletal symptoms and findings will regress if the primary pulmonary problem is treated. Even in the absence of cure, a resection of the lung tumor results in improvement of bone symptoms. It has also been reported that vagotomy relieves some of the discomfort. No mechanism is offered to explain this feature.

The findings are predominantly in the peripheral extremities, with the lower extremity being more frequently involved. Ninety percent of the cases of pulmonary osteoarthrophathy are produced by malignant disease. Of these, metastatic disease rarely produces the problem. The other 10% of the cases are secondary to lung abscess, bronchiectasis, or, less likely, pulmonary emphysema. Tuberculosis rarely results in pulmonary osteoarthropathy.

Case LXA-11

Case LXA-11 is a 12-year-old boy who was admitted with swelling and some discomfort over the lateral aspect of the ankle.

The radiographic changes are striking and certainly indicate an expanding bone lesion. Despite the expansile nature of the lesion, the cortex remains intact except for a small area just above the epiphyseal line in the fibula laterally. Even here there is no significant alteration in the prominence of the mass outline. There appears to be well-defined new periosteal bone formation in the superior margin of the lesion. Even though the bone is expanded, no actual soft-tissue mass is identified.

This demonstrates most of the qualities of a nonagressive benign bone tumor. The diagnosis established here was that of an aneurysmal bone cyst. The patient was

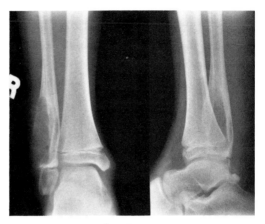

Case LXA-11

treated by curettment and packing with bone chips.

This lesion differs from the malignant bone tumors in that the new bone formed here is well organized and is tending to wall off the lesion. There is no break in the cortex altbough cortical thinning may be marked. There is no evidence of a soft-tissue mass.

THE FOOT

There is a tendency to compare the hand with the foot functionally. The foot does not have the fine motion and agility of the hand; it is designed principally for weight support and transport. It is a different and simpler structure. The opposable thumb of the hand has been replaced by the rigid

---

*NOTE: An area of increased density is seen through the talus in the AP view. This is the density produced by a rather prominent os trigonum. It is seen on the lateral view just above the superior margin of the os calcis. It was described in Case LXA-2.

supportive great toe. The tarsal bones are easy to remember, for the first, second, and third cuneiform articulate with the corresponding first, second, and third metatarsal. (See Case LXF-1, an example of a normal foot.) The relatively large block of bone that supports the foot between the base of the fourth and fifth metatarsals and the os calcis is the cuboid. The only remaining tarsal bone is the tarsal navicular. The talus and the os calcis, of course, have been mentioned in our views of the ankle. The talus, while actually a tarsal bone, is a major functioning component of the ankle.

CASE PRESENTATIONS

Case LXF-1

This case is our model of a normal foot. Multiple lines and angles can be drawn in the foot; however, there are two that are especially useful. On the lateral view we have constructed Bohler's angle. This is constructed by drawing a line through the anterior and posterior-superior facets of

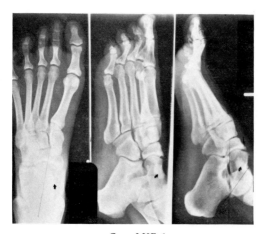

Case LXF-1

the os calcis and intersecting it with a line drawn from the anterior edge of the articular margin of the talus to the posterior-superior tip of the os calcis. This angle should be from 30 to 40 degrees. If the angle becomes less than this, it implies an impacted injury or a fracture of the os calcis.

A second line that is occasionally helpful is a line in the AP projection drawn through the central portion of the talus to indicate its central line of direction. This line should pass through the navicular and the first cuneiform and into the shaft of the first metatarsal; or it may actually fall, as in this case, slightly lateral to the first metatarsal. When the first metatarsal lies lateral to this line, it implies a pronated foot.

A straight solid arrow is directed toward the bony ossicle in the lateral view. This sits at the superior margin of the navicular and actually is an accessory navicular, another normal variant in the foot.

A second curved arrow is directed to an area of increased bone density in the talus. It is identifiable in each of the three projections. This is considered to be an internal cortical thickening and is of no clinical significance. It has been described as a healed fibrous cortical defect and its cortical position makes this a feasible suggestion.

Case LXF-2

Case LXF-2 is a 4-year-old girl. Films of the foot are presented only to show the pattern that exists in childhood. The growth and the development between this and the previous case are apparent. Note the rounded nature of the tarsal bone, the fragmentation of some of the epiphyses, and the cup-shaped metaphyseal end of the metatarsals. Note also that the epiphysis of the great toe is at the proximal end of the metatarsal instead of at the distal end as it appears on the second, third, or fourth metatarsal.

Some soft-tissue swelling is noted over the dorsum of the foot; however, this is probably less than it appears since most children tend to have prominence of the fat pad over the dorsum of the foot.

Case LXF-3

Case LXF-3 is a 5-year-old boy with obvious flat feet. Actually this child had been followed since infancy with bilateral flat feet and a reversal of the longitudinal arch of the foot, the so-called "rocker bottom foot." The radiographic findings are those that confirm the clinical observation that the arch is lost; however, it is important to note that the talus is essentially vertical. The dark line through the upper part of the talus is between 30 and 35 degrees from the horizontal, which is approximately the normal angle of the talus at this age.

Final diagnosis is a congenital variation, "vertical talus," resulting in a reversal of the longitudinal arch of the foot— "rocker bottom foot."

Case LXF-4

Case LXF-4 is a 35-year-old woman, radiographed because of trauma to the fifth metatarsal.

There is no evidence of bone injury here; however, the arrow is directed toward a normal variant. This variant has been confused many times with fresh or even old un-united fractures. It occurs in about 10% to 15% of children and adults. This is a true sesamoid bone, having its origin in the tendon of the posterior tibial muscle. As the bone matures, the sesa-

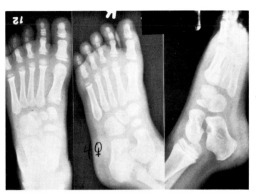

Case LXF-2

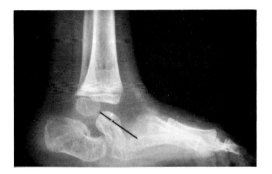

Case LXF-3

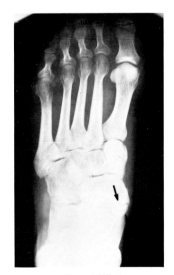

Case LXF-4

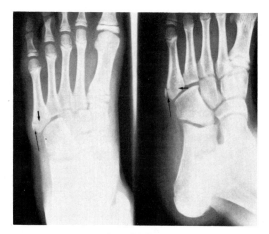

Case LXF-5

moid may escape from the tendonous site of origin, and become a true accessory navicular lying adjacent to the posterior tuberosity of the navicular.

This variation may become symptomatic, especially if the foot is pronated (loss of the longitudinal arch); and this portion of the navicular becomes unusually prominent. It may become irritated by footwear, or may even make shoes difficult to fit. From a radiographic standpoint, its

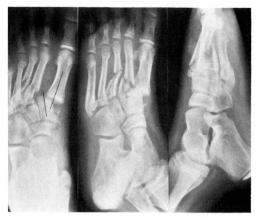

Case LXF-6

most important feature is not to mistake it for a fracture. Its size can vary from quite small to even larger than is demonstrated here.

Case LXF-5

Case LXF-5 is a 17-year-old boy with a twisting injury of the foot.

The radiographic finding here that is clinically significant is indicated by the short solid arrows. It is a line perpendicular to the long axis of the shaft of the fifth metatarsal. It represents a fracture.

The long slender arrow is directed toward an epiphysis at the base of the fifth metatarsal. This epiphysis is the only epiphysis in the body that runs parallel to the axis of a long bone. It is, therefore, frequently confused with a fracture.

The final diagnosis is an undisplaced fracture at the base of the fifth metatarsal. This is the most frequently occurring fracture of the foot, next to that resulting from a stubbed toe.

When it occurs in children, there are always problems with the epiphysis. A film of the opposite foot can be used, but should not be necessary. Remember that the longitudinal epiphysis is usual here, and that the lines that are significant in terms of trauma are like the one shown here, or similar to it.

Case LXF-6

Case LXF-6 is a 9-year-old boy who had been involved in a bicycle-automobile accident.

The radiographic changes here are striking. There are multiple fractures involving the proximal metatarsals. If all three views are carefully observed, it will be noted that the second, third, fourth, and fifth metatarsals all show fracture lines. The fourth metatarsal has a subtle fracture in the neck of the metatarsal, just proximal to the epiphyseal plate, seen best in the oblique film. The fifth metatarsal has a fracture line in the proximal shaft, also seen best in the oblique projection.

In addition to the obvious metatarsal fractures, the film is presented to demonstrate dislocation of the forefoot. In all views the first metatarsal is not directed toward the first cuneiform. The dark lines on the AP projection indicate the direction of the first metatarsal and the direction of the first cuneiform as visualized here. These lines obviously are not aligned. In the lateral view and in the oblique projection, the first metatarsal sets above the level of the first cuneiform. The fifth metatarsal is well directed toward the cuboid in each projection. Therefore, the dislocation does not involve this portion of the foot. There is so much comminution of the proximal ends of the second and third metatarsals it is difficult to be certain of the articulation; however, it appears that the stress line occurred across the fracture, and that the joints of the second and third metatarsals and their respective cuneiforms are intact despite the angulation and comminution of the fractures. A small fragment of bone is seen just medial to the first cuneiform. This presumably is an avulsion fracture of the cuneiform that occurred during the dislocation.

There is increased soft-tissue space between the first and the second cuneiform, and considerable generalized soft-tissue swelling, as would be expected. The final diagnosis is fractures of the second, third, fourth, and fifth metatarsals with dislocation of the first metatarsal, the first cuneiform joint with avulsion fracture from the first cuneiform.

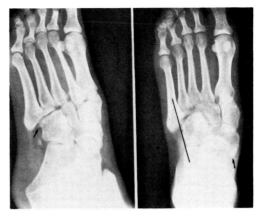

Case LXF-7

Case LXF-7

Case LXF-7 is a 29-year-old woman involved in an auto accident. She had jammed her foot vigorously against the brake. She has severe pain in her foot.

The radiographic findings are somewhat subtle. The anterior foot appears to be mildly pronated. The solid black line drawn through the lateral portion of the cuboid extends through the mid portion of the fifth metatarsal. Unfortunately, this black line passes directly over a tiny chip fracture, which is somewhat helpful in the diagnosis. The lateral line of the first cuneiform also is directed more toward the mid 1st metatarsal than is usually seen. The oblique film adds little to our findings, except to show the small avulsion fracture at the margin of the cuboid, as indicated by the short solid dark arrow. The second arrow in the AP view that is directed toward the medial side of the foot indicates an accessory navicular.

The diagnosis here is subluxation of the forefoot, the tarsal bones being deviated medially with respect to the metatarsals.

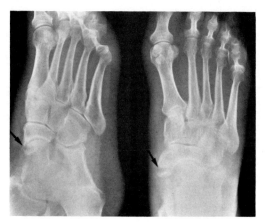

Case LXF-8

The patient's symptoms and complaints and physical findings were more striking than the radiographs. The lateral film did not aid us. This is another instance of being aware of normal anatomical relationships and correlating rather minor radiographic changes with the clinical findings. It is uncommon to see the fifth metatarsal as far lateral as we see it here.

Case LXF-8

Case LXF-8 is a 79-year-old woman with pain in her foot following a fall. The routine films of her ankle and the lateral film of her foot did not add to our findings.

There is considerable soft-tissue swelling. There are degenerative changes present about the foot and ankle. The dark arrows direct attention toward a transverse fracture line through a prominent medial navicular. The fragments are separated by 1 to 2 mm. It is seen quite clearly in the area of soft-tissue swelling in both the AP and oblique view. There is an incidental small accessory navicular present.

Fractures of the tarsal bones occur with surprising frequency. A fracture of the tarsal navicular does not have the same incidence of nonunion or avascular necrosis that is associated with carpal navicular fractures. Fractures of the navicular are less frequent than fractures of the cuboid. Fractures of the navicular tend to be more frequent in patients with a prominent medial navicular process. Final diagnosis: Fracture of the tarsal navicular.

Case LXF-9

Case LXF-9 is a 12-year-old boy who fell from a tree. He was experiencing considerable pain in the foot and could not walk.

The solid dark arrows in the AP view are to direct attention toward the fracture line in the cuboid. The oblique projection also shows poorly defined fracture lines running through the cuboid. Multiple lines are present, and there is some impaction of the bony fragments. The epiphysis at the base of the fifth metatarsal is noted. It apparently is uninvolved.

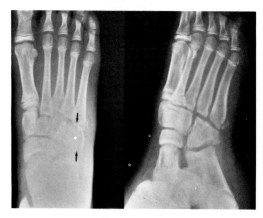

Case LXF-9

With support and immobilization the prognosis is good. Final diagnosis: Comminuted, mildly impacted fracture of the tarsal cuboid.

Case LXF-10

Case LXF-10 is a 20-year-old male athlete who was having considerable pain in the foot.

A film of the foot shows increased bone density involving the shaft of the second metatarsal at the junction of its middle and distal third. There is no appreciable malalignment. There does appear to be a break in the cortex medially. No joints are involved. Other views did not add to our findings.

The final diagnosis is a stress fracture of the second metatarsal. This has been referred to as a "march fracture." The pathology of a stress fracture is not well defined. However, the mechanism of its occurrence is related to persistent and unusual trauma. This is not trauma in the sense of a single blow, but trauma such as might be acquired by repeated incidences. It is a frequent finding in sprinters or other persons involved in athletic activities. It occurs more frequently in the untrained athlete than in the well-conditioned one.

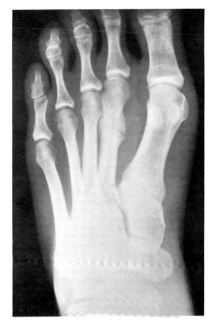

Case LXF-10

Cases LXF-11 and LXF-12

The AP studies of the foot are presented for two male patients. Case LXF-11 is a 12-year-old child that complained of discomfort in the foot when walking. The pain could be localized to the area of the second metatarsal. The long slender arrow points toward the epiphyseal center of the second metatarsal. It is flattened on the superior aspect and appears more dense than other metatarsal heads. The joint

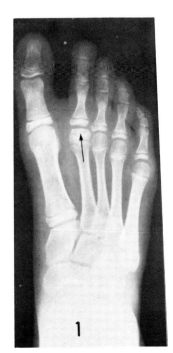

Case LXF-11

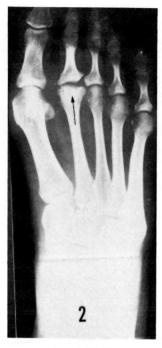

Case LXF-12

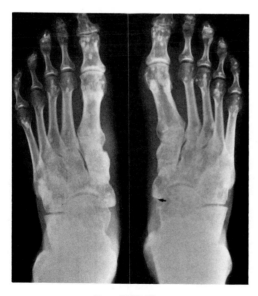

Case LXF-13

space is not involved. There are no fractures.

Case LXF-12 was a 38-year-old man who had fallen. The study of his foot was made because of the acute injury. The radiographic findings, indicated by the long slender arrow directed toward the head of the second metatarsal, are incidental. The patient was not symptomatic at this point. However, the patient did give a history of having had discomfort over the distal portion of the metatarsals in years past, but no therapy or radiographs had been done.

These two cases are examples of Freiberg's infraction, which is an avascular necrosis of the metatarsal head. It usually involves the second metatarsal, but has been seen on the third. It is probably related to the trauma of weight bearing, as the second metatarsal head shares most of the weight load with the first metatarsal. Except for the discomfort, the process usually is self-limited, and the only sequela is that of degenerative joint disease.

There is a great age difference between our patients. Case LXF-11, the boy, represents the acute process. Case LXF-12 represents the inactive process with residual deformity.

Case LXF-13

Case LXF-13 is an adult. The films were made as part of a skeletal survey.

The radiographic changes here are classical in appearance. Once seen they should not cause confusion in the future. Multiple small areas of increased density are seen scattered through the bones of the foot. They tend to be most frequent at the distal and proximal ends of the bone. The lesions tend to be ovoid in type, with the long axis of the oval being parallel to the long axis of the bone. They produce no reaction and no symptoms and do not convert to more complicated lesions with time. The arrow on one side is directed toward the coincidental finding of a small accessory navicular.

The final diagnosis is osteopoikilosis. It is an incidental radiographic finding.

Case LXF-14

Case LXF-14 is a 76-year-old woman who was admitted to the orthopedic clinic because of pain and discomfort in the area of the great toe. She was having difficulty in finding footwear to fit the foot.

The findings here are one of the most frequently seen abnormalities in elderly patients experiencing foot problems. The first metatarsal head is unusually prominent, and the proximal and distal phalanx of the great toe tends to be angulated away from the line of first metatarsal support. The patient also shows some prominent sesamoid bones with spur formation, a local degenerative change. Soft-tissue swelling is present over the metatarsal head. The first metatarsal, instead of pointing straight forward, is directed medially.

The generalized demineralization of bone is consistent with the patient's age. No evident vascular calcification is noted. The joint spaces between tarsal bones are quite well maintained. The final diagnosis is that of a bunion. This one is moderate in degree. Certainly there are times when the angle formed between the phalanges and the first metatarsal is more acute than is seen here.

Case LXF-15

Case LXF-15 is a 67-year-old male diabetic. He was admitted with pain and swelling of the fourth and fifth toes. There was no gangrene.

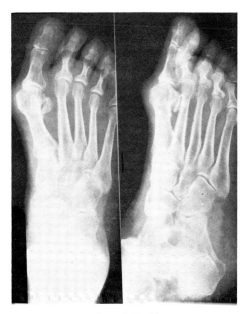

Case LXF-14

The radiographs of the foot show generalized demineralization. This is even greater than would be expected for the stated age. The patient's diabetes predisposes to peripheral vascular calcification. This is seen in the AP view between the

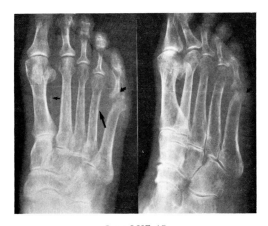

Case LXF-15

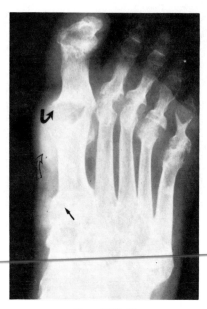

Case LXF-16

first and second toe, and indicated by a short, dark solid arrow.

The greatest changes are in the fourth and fifth toes. The proximal phalangeal metatarsal joint of the fifth toe has been destroyed. There is some subluxation here. Rather marked destruction of the head of the fifth metatarsal is noted. In addition, the large solid dark arrow points to an area of periosteal elevation in the mid portion of the fourth metatarsal. Final diagnosis: Osteomyelitis of the fourth and fifth metatarsals with septic involvement of the fifth metatarsal proximal phalangeal joint.

Diabetics are at high risk for foot infections. With the rapidly increasing number of diabetics, a corresponding increase in foot infections is likely. Despite prophylactic measures, these infections frequently lead to osteomyelitis or septic joint involvement. In nondiabetics the radiographic changes of osteomyelitis are rare.

Case LXF-16

Case LXF-16 is a 57-year-old man complaining of generalized joint pain and stiffness, as well as multiple soft-tissue nodules about joints.

The radiograph clearly shows involvement of the joint spaces, with the first metatarsal-phalangeal joint being most severely involved. The overall bone density of the foot is only slightly decreased. There are obvious areas of cartilage loss, particularly between the fourth and the fifth metatarsal and the articulating tarsal bones. Marked bone erosion is seen at the distal ends of the metatarsals, and there is some associated loss of cartilage. This film of the foot tends to show features of both rheumatoid disease (the erosions) and osteoarthritis (marginal bone spurring).

Virtually all erosive areas show overhanging edges. This is most evident at the base of the proximal phalanx of the great toe, as indicated by the curved dark arrow. The same type of process is seen at the first metatarsal-tarsal articulation as evidenced by the smaller black solid arrow.

The open-faced arrow is pointing toward a large soft-tissue prominence, which is reasonably circumscribed and shows some increased density compared to other soft tissues about it. The final disgnosis is gout. This is an advanced case. In other areas there were large tophi, similar to the ones identified here by the open arrow. In general, the end product of gout is osteoarthritis, for gout is a disease that undergoes remissions and recurrences. With this are problems of marginal bone injury and cartilage destruction that lead to degenerative joint disease.

Clinical and laboratory evaluation may give the diagnosis more rapidly than films, but the characteristic subchondral erosions with overhanging edges are quite characteristic.

Case LXF-17

Case LXF-17 is a 26-year-old man with a 13-year history of diabetes. He had burned his right great toe on a hot-water bottle two and a half years prior to this filming. An ulcer had been present on the toe since that time.

The radiographic findings here are striking. The normal left foot is shown for comparison. There are multiple areas of bone destruction involving the metatarsal head. Bone density is generally normal, with the exception of the fifth metatarsal, where there is some punctate bone loss as well as periosteal elevation on the shaft of the metatarsal. This is indicated by small dark arrows. There is lack of continuity of the periosteal elevation on the fifth metatarsal. Compare this with the periosteal elevation on the third metatarsal, as indicated by the long slender dark arrow. Here the bone has retained its density and there is no destruction, only new bone being produced. Even though the cartilage space of the joints is reasonably well maintained, the joint itself appears to be grossly abnormal and bone production is seen ringing the articular surface, particularly in the great toe.

The final diagnosis is that of neuro-

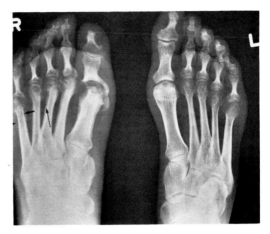

Case LXF-17

trophic joint disease of the foot. This diagnosis is made on the basis of bone destruction, bone production, and joint architecture distortion. This patient has a complicating feature—the fifth metatarsal demonstrates osteomyelitis. This toe subsequently was surgically removed.

Charcot's joint used to be considered pathognomonic of tertiary syphilis. However, with the vigorous therapy that syphilitic patients are now given, we rarely see Charcot's with that cause. Neurotrophic joints are now most likely of diabetic origin. Any joint from the spine to the distal interphalangeal joints may be involved. The lower extremity is generally involved with the disease more frequently than the upper extremity. The one exception is patients who have syringomyelia.

Glossary

Air Contrast A double contrast method to visualize the internal anatomy of a structure using air and a contrast media such as barium.

Air Fluid Level The interface between air and fluid which assumes a horizontal appearance, produced by the x-ray beam being parallel to the interface such as is seen in the upright or decubitus positions.

Anterior Refers to the front of the body or organ.

AP (anterior-posterior) Refers to the way an object is exposed to x-rays. The x-ray beam enters the anterior surface and exits posteriorly.

Arteriogram (angiogram) An x-ray technique using an intravascular catheter and contrast media injections to visualize the vessels and the organs of the body.

Artifact Changes on a radiograph that do not have an anatomic basis, but are technical errors produced by dirt, static electricity, or unwanted objects such as buttons or devices.

Barium Enema (BE) An x-ray technique to examine the colon, using barium introduced in a retrograde fashion through the anus.

Barium Swallow (esophogram) An x-ray technique using oral barium ingestion to outline the esophagus.

Blush Jargon for a radiograph made during the injection of contrast media (iodine) when the tissue of an organ or mass intensely opacifies.

Bronchogram An x-ray technique to outline the trachea and bronchi by instilling contrast material (iodine) into those structures.

Bucky A stationary or moving device used to eliminate scattered radiation. It is made of thin vertical lead strips and intervening spacers and is placed between the patient and film.

Comparison Film Radiographs that can be taken of the side opposite to the anatomical part in question so a comparison can be made and any deviation from normal variation can be seen.

Computed Tomography (CT, CAT) A specialized x-ray technique using a computer to produce cross-sectioned images of the body.

Cone-down View A radiograph produced by limiting the area exposed by collimating to a certain size so that better detail can be achieved.

Contrast Media A material of differing density used in radiology to outline organs or spaces.

Cystogram An x-ray technique to visualize the urinary bladder by instilling contrast material (iodine) through a catheter in the urethra.

Cystoscopy A method of directly viewing the lumen and mucosa of the urinary bladder.

Decubitus The position of the patient when lying on his/her side.

Density The degree of blackening on film. This may be more or less than surrounding structures, depending on objects studied.

Differential Diagnosis A list of diseases or abnormalities that produce similar appearances on a radiograph.

Double Contrast A technique to outline internal structures, using materials with different x-ray absorbing properties. Example: barium and air.

Endoscopy (colonoscopy, gastroscopy, esophagoscopy) A method to directly visualize the mucosa and the lumen of hollow organs such as the esophagus, the stomach, the duodenum, the colon, and the urinary bladder.

ERCP (Endoscopic Retrograde Cholangiopancreatography) A method used to visualize the pancreatic and the biliary duct systems using an endoscope and contrast material injection, which outlines their anatomy.

Excretory Urogram (IVP, intravenous Pyelogram) An x-ray technique using the injection of intravenous contrast material (iodine) to aid in visualizing the urinary system.

Exposure The act of exposing an object to radiation to produce a radiograph.

Filling Defect A space-occupying mass within a hollow organ.

Film A sheet of synthetic polyester covered with radiation-sensitive emulsion, upon which an image can be visualized after it is exposed to x-rays and the sheet developed.

Flatplate (KUB) Jargon for an abdominal radiograph that includes the kidneys (K), the ureters (U), and the bladder (B) areas.

Fluoroscopy The production of an x-ray image on a fluorescent screen that has been exposed by x-rays traveling through an object—a physician can study anatomic parts in motion using this method.

Gall Bladder Visualization (Cholecystogram, GB Vis., OCG) An x-ray technique to visualize the gall bladder utilizing oral contrast material (iodine) taken hours before its appearance in the gall bladder.

Hippuran Studies A special nuclear medicine study using radioactive iodine attached to ortho-iodohippurate to depict the anatomy and function of the kidney.

Hypotonic Duodenography A special x-ray technique to visualize only the duodenum with contrast media (barium and air) using a drug (usually glucagon) to inhibit duodenal motion.

Inferior Refers to the lower part of the body or organ.

Intravenous Cholangiogram (IVC) An x-ray technique using the infusion of intravenous contrast material (iodine) to visualize the biliary system.

Isotopes An element of different anatomic weight that emits electro-magnetic radiation. It may be used to image an organ or measure its function.

KV (Kilovoltage) The voltage or potential across an x-ray tube causing the acceleration of electrons.

Lateral Refers to the sides of the body or away from the midline.

Medial Refers to near the midline of the body.

Nuclear Medicine That subdivision of radiology that uses radioactive isotopes and their compounds to outline organs and structures in the body and their functions.

Oblique A position of the patient in which he/she is not straight but is turned so that the midline of the patient is angled more than 1 degree, but less than 90 degrees from the incident beam.

Old Films Radiographs made prior to the ones in question and used for comparison to detect the degree of change with time.

Osteoblastic A bone producing process—it increases the density of bone involved.

Osteolytic A bone destructive process—it decreases the density of bone involved. The increased lucency of bone results in a radiographic appearance blacker than normal.

PA (Posterior–Anterior) Refers to the way an object is exposed to x-rays. The x-ray beam enters the posterior surface and exists anteriorly.

Photon Bundles of energy (x-rays).

Posterior Refers to the back of the body or an organ.

Projection Description of the path the x-ray beam travels, beginning with the first anatomical location it passes through and ending where the beam exits. Example: PA, AP.

Prone The recumbent position of the patient when face down.

Pyelogram An x-ray technique to visualize the collecting system of the kidney and the ureter by instilling contrast material (iodine) in these structures.

Radiograph A developed piece of x-ray film on which an image has been produced by exposure to x-rays.

Radiologic Technologist (R.T.) A specially trained nonphysician working as an extension of the radiologist. The roles include patient routing and handling, and acquiring and processing films.

Radiologist A physician specializing in the use of x-rays and other forms of radiation in the diagnosis and treatment of disease.

Radiology That branch of medicine that deals with the diagnostic and therapeutic application of radiation energy.

Radiolucent (Lucent)—The black shadows on a radiograph produced as x-rays pass readily through less dense matter.

Radiopacity (Opacity)—The white shadows on a radiograph produced when x-rays are absorbed or impeded by a more dense matter.

Roentgenogram Another term for a radiograph.

Seldinger Technique A technique in diagnostic radiology to introduce a catheter into a vessel or organ so that the structure can be visualized.

Silhouette Sign A sign in radiology whereby the border of an organ or structure will disappear or become indistinct when an opacity with the same density is in contact with it.

Skull Series A routine set of radiographs of the skull, usually including PA, AP, and lateral views.

Small Bowel Series An x-ray technique using oral contrast material (barium) to outline the small bowel, especially the terminal ileum.

Superior Refers to the upper part of the body or organ.

Supine A recumbent position of the patient where he/she is face up.

Technique The technical factors (kilovoltage, time and amperage) involved in exposing an x-ray film to produce a satisfactory radiograph.

Tomography (laminography and planogram) A special x-ray technique that blurs out the shadows of superimposed structures in order to show more clearly the principal structures at a given level.

Towne's View A special AP view of the skull where the x-ray beam is angled approximately 35 degrees toward the feet to depict the posterior aspect of the skull.

TUR (transurethral resection) A surgical technique to excise tissue in or encroaching on the posterior urethra (prostate) through a urethral approach. It is done with cystoscopy.

Ultrasonography The use of sound waves to visualize internal structures and organs.

Upper GI series An x-ray technique using oral barium to outline the upper gastrointestinal tract.

Upright The position of the patient when sitting or standing upright.

Urethrogram An x-ray technique to visualize the urethra. It is accomplished by injection of contrast material into the urethra or visualizing the urethra during the voiding of contrast during a cystogram.

Venogram A special x-ray technique to visualize veins by injecting contrast material (iodine) into those structures through catheters or needles.

View Relates to the way the x-ray film images the patient and the position the patient has in relating to the film.

Voiding Cystourethrogram (VC) An x-ray technique using contrast material (iodine) instilled into the urinary bladder by catheter. Films are made as the patient voids after the catheter is removed.

Water's View A special PA view of the skull made with the chin on the film and the forehead elevated. It is used to show sinuses and facial bones.

X-Rays Electromagnetic radiation produced by bombarding an object with high speed electrons.

References

Birzle, H., Bergleiter, R., and Kuner, E. *Radiology of Trauma*. Philadelphia: W. B. Saunders Co., 1978.

Caffey, John. *Pediatric X-ray Diagnosis*. 7th ed. Chicago: Year Book Medical Publishers, 1978.

Edeiken, J., and Hodes, P. J. *Roentgen Diagnosis of Diseases of Bone*. 2 vols. Baltimore: Williams & Wilkins, 1973.

Felson, B. *Chest Roentgenology*. Philadelphia: W. B. Saunders Co., 1973.

—————. *Principles of Chest Roentgenology*. Philadelphia: W. B. Saunders Co., 1965.

Fraser, R. G., and Pare, J. A. *Diagnosis of Diseases of the Chest*. 4 vols. Philadelphia: W. B. Saunders Co., 1977–1979.

Heitzman, E. Robert. *The Lung*. St. Louis: C. V. Mosby Co., 1973.

—————. *The Mediastinum*. St. Louis: C. V. Mosby Co., 1977.

Keats, T. T. *An Atlas of Normal Roentgen Variants that May Simulate Disease*. Chicago: Year Book Medical Publishers, 1975.

Laufer, I. *Double Contrast Gastrointestinal Radiology with Endoscopic Correlation* Philadelphia: W. B. Saunders Co., 1979.

Margulis, A. R., and Burhenne, H. J. *Alimentary Tract Roentgenology*. St. Louis: C. V. Mosby Co., 1973.

Paul, L. W., and Juhl, J. H. *Essentials of Roentgen Interpretation*. New York: Harper & Row, 1972.

Peterson, H. O., and Kieffer, S. A. *Introduction to Neuroradiology*. New York: Harper & Row, 1972.

Schultz, R. J *Language of Fractures*. Baltimore: Williams & Wilkins, 1972.

Squire, L. F. *Exercises in Diagnostic Radiology*. 9 vols. Philadelphia: W. B. Saunders Co., 1970–1979.

—————. *Fundamentals of Radiology*. Cambridge, Mass.: Harvard Univ. Press, 1975.

Swischuk, L. *The Plain Film Interpretation in Congenital Heart Disease*. Philadelphia: Lea & Febiger, 1970.

Teplick, J. G., and Haskin, M. E. *Roentgenologic Diagnoses*. 2 vols. Philadelphia: W. B. Saunders Co., 1976.

Witten, D. M., Myers, G. H., and Utz, D. C. *Emmett's Clinical Urography*. 4th ed. 3 vols. Philadelphia: W. B. Saunders Co., 1977.

Index